PRAISE

The Healthy Bones Plant-Based Nutrition Plan and Cookbook

"*The Healthy Bones Plant-Based Nutrition Plan and Cookbook* is an important, groundbreaking book for everyone—no matter their eating style. Drawing on the latest emerging nutritional science, Dr. Laura Kelly assures us that we can live a vibrant, healthy life and protect and build healthy bones simply by knowing what combinations of whole foods nourish our cells, microbiome, organs, and especially our precious bones. It's the only book you need, not just for the empowering information but also for the enlightened recipes designed by Jummee Park, who guides and inspires us to prepare food with love, light, and lusciousness."

—**PAT CROCKER**, author of *The Juicing Bible* and *The Herbalist's Kitchen*

"*The Healthy Bones Plant-Based Nutrition Plan and Cookbook* is a fantastic practical guide to preventing osteoporosis and promoting long-term bone health. The authors simplify complex bone-health science and offer a wealth of delicious, nutrient-packed, plant-based recipes. Each recipe is easy to prepare, making healthy eating a delight. With clear, actionable advice and comprehensive meal plans, this book is an essential read for anyone committed to maintaining strong, healthy bones naturally. Highly recommended for its informative content and culinary creativity!"

—**KIA MILLER**, founder, Radiant Body Yoga

"*The Healthy Bones Plant-Based Nutrition Plan and Cookbook* is a must-read for conscious eaters. Laura Kelly and Helen Kelly provide a fascinating grounding in the science, and the book is made craveable by chef Jummee Park's beautiful recipes for the everyday cook. This is food as medicine in a deliciously digestible form."

—**ERIK OBERHOLTZER**, chef; cofounder of Tender Greens; author of *Ten Year Plan*

PRAISE FOR

The Healthy Bones Nutrition Plan and Cookbook

by Dr. Laura Kelly and Helen Bryman Kelly

"Dr. Laura Kelly and Helen Bryman Kelly thoroughly explain why osteoporosis is most often due to deficiency, not disease, and how and why to prepare traditional foods for bone health as well as overall gut health. Writing from firsthand experience, these authors have dotted every 'I' and crossed every 'T' when it comes to eating for bone health. This is a must-read for those looking to treat osteoporosis and for anyone looking to understand nutrition, eat traditionally, and thrive."

—**HILARY BOYNTON**, coauthor of *The Heal Your Gut Cookbook*

"*The Healthy Bones Nutrition Plan and Cookbook* is part of a sweeping change in the way scientists, practitioners, and writers are thinking about health care and how people can shift their state of being from chronic illness to good health. Readers who follow the guidance provided by Dr. Laura Kelly and Helen Kelly to create a personal nutrition plan will be empowered to interact with medical professionals in a new, more rational, safer, and less costly way. And they will enjoy much better health outcomes, relying on truths that are highly likely to endure."

—from the Foreword by
SIDNEY MACDONALD BAKER, MD

The HEALTHY BONES PLANT-BASED Nutrition Plan and Cookbook

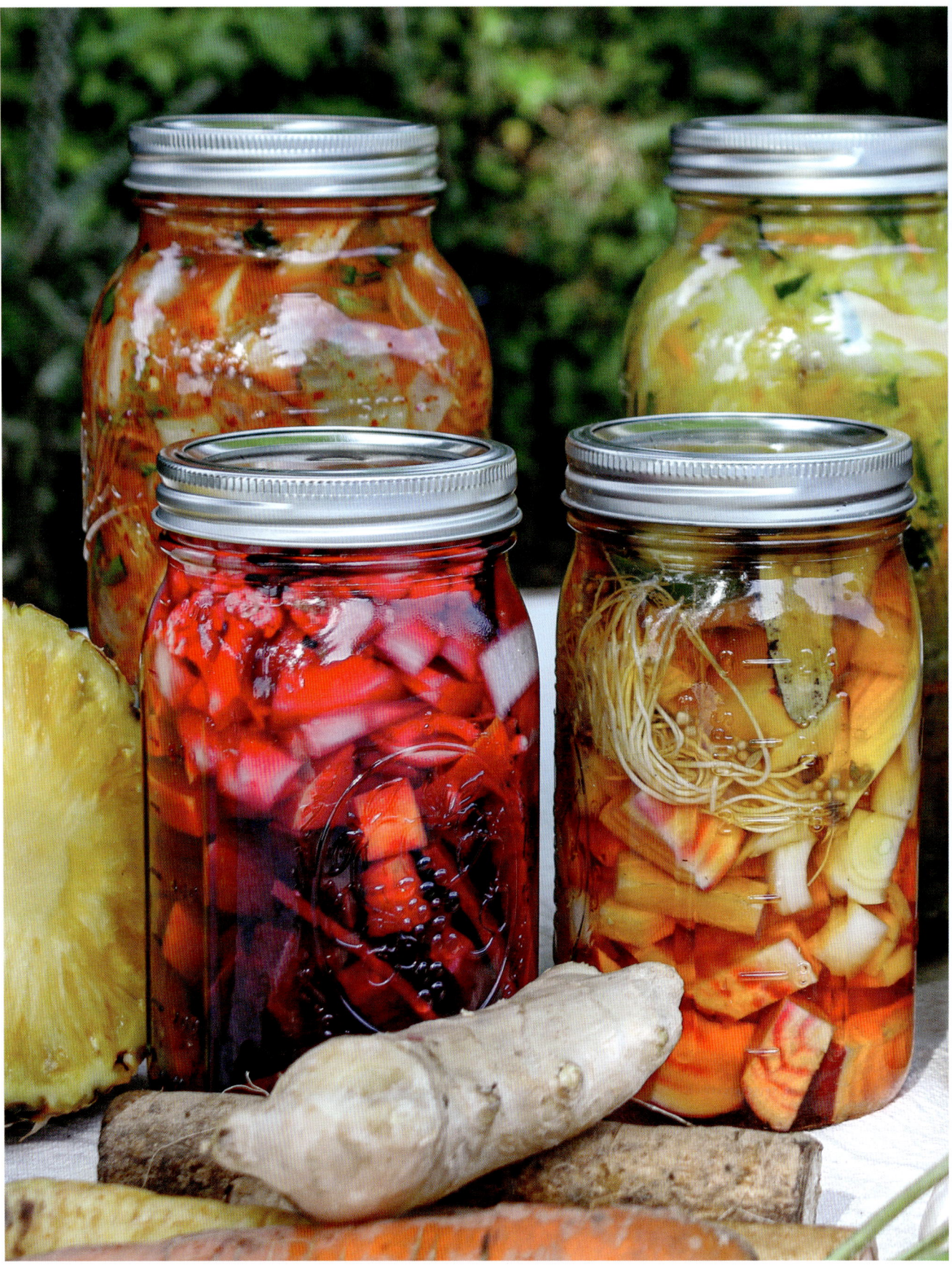

The HEALTHY BONES PLANT-BASED Nutrition Plan and Cookbook

How to Prepare and Combine Plant Foods to Maintain Optimal Bone Density and Prevent Osteoporosis

**Dr. Laura Kelly
Helen Bryman Kelly
Jummee Park**

Chelsea Green Publishing
White River Junction, Vermont
London, UK

Copyright © 2024 by Laura Kelly, Helen Bryman Kelly, and Jummee Park.
All rights reserved.

Unless otherwise noted, all photographs copyright © 2024 by Jummee Park.
Unless otherwise noted, all illustrations copyright © 2024 by Laura Kelly and Helen Bryman Kelly.

No part of this book may be transmitted or reproduced in any form by any means without permission in writing from the publisher.

Project Manager: Rebecca Springer
Editor: Fern Marshall Bradley
Editorial Assistance: Amalia Herren-Lage
Copy Editor: Deborah Heimann
Proofreader: Rachel Markowitz
Indexer: Elizabeth Parson
Designer: Melissa Jacobson

Printed in the United States of America.
First printing September 2024.
10 9 8 7 6 5 4 3 2 1   24 25 26 27 28

Our Commitment to Green Publishing
Chelsea Green sees publishing as a tool for cultural change and ecological stewardship. We strive to align our book manufacturing practices with our editorial mission and to reduce the impact of our business enterprise in the environment. We print our books using vegetable-based inks whenever possible. This book may cost slightly more because it was printed on paper from responsibly managed forests, and we hope you'll agree that it's worth it. *The Healthy Bones Plant-Based Nutrition Plan and Cookbook* was printed on paper supplied by Versa that is certified by the Forest Stewardship Council.®

Library of Congress Cataloging-in-Publication Data
Names: Kelly, Laura, 1967– author. | Kelly, Helen Bryman, 1942– author. | Park, Jumme, 1969– author.
Title: The healthy bones plant-based : nutrition plan and cookbook : how to prepare and combine plant foods to maintain optimal bone density and prevent osteoporosis / Dr. Laura Kelly, Helen Bryman Kelly, Jumme Park.
Description: White River Junction, Vermont ; London, UK : Chelsea Green Publishing, [2024] | Includes bibliographical references and index.
Identifiers: LCCN 2024019733 | ISBN 9781645022268 (paperback) | ISBN 9781645022275 (ebook)
Subjects: LCSH: Bones—Diseases—Prevention. | Osteoporosis—Prevention. | Vegan cooking. | Cooking (Natural foods) | LCGFT: Cookbooks.
Classification: LCC RC931.O73 K455 2024 | DDC 641.5/6362—dc23/eng/20240605
LC record available at https://lccn.loc.gov/2024019733

Chelsea Green Publishing
White River Junction, Vermont, USA
London, UK
www.chelseagreen.com

For my mother, the very definition of healthy aging and a continuous inspiration, and for my patients and other healthy-bones seekers who have pushed me to find ever better methods and helped me to have a hand in the healing of the world.
—Laura

For my daughter Laura, whose exceptional diagnostic skill and insight into nutrition and the mechanisms of aging are a privilege to behold, and whose guidance in these later years has helped me see that age really is just a number.
—Helen

For members of the online Healthy Bones Group—especially our first members Sylvia, Cynthia, Eva, Robin, and Anne—whose courage and questions continue to inspire us every day.
—Helen and Laura

To my mother, who expressed her love through food, and bore my existence from the seed of light in the womb to eternity.
—Jummee

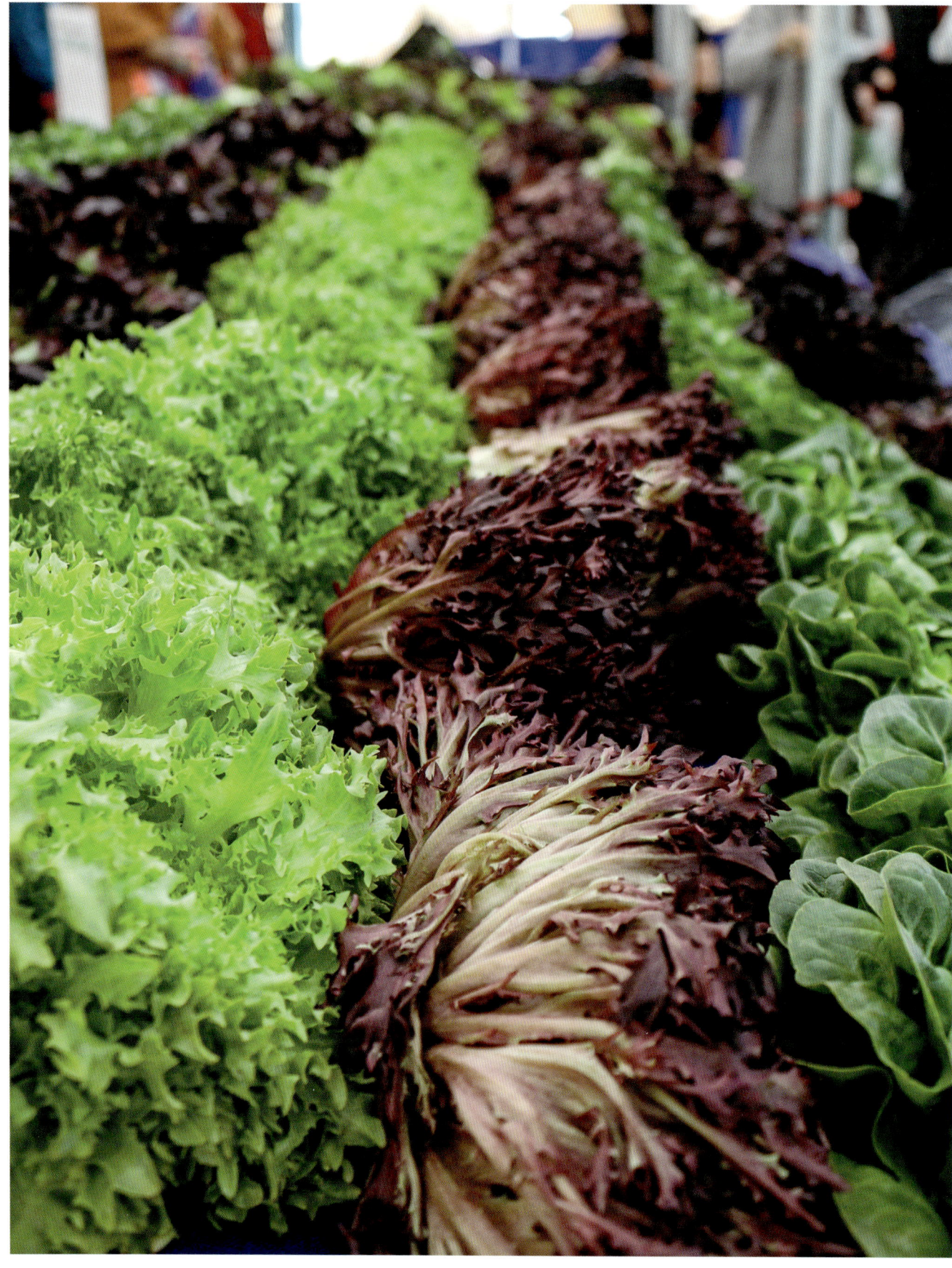

CONTENTS

INTRODUCTION
Plants and Bones: A Dynamic Relationship   1

PART I
How Plants Nourish Bones

1. Bones Are a Family of Cells   11
2. Feeding Your Bones   19
3. Managing Antinutrients and Acrylamide   41
4. Healthy Body, Healthy Bones   49
5. Healthy Bones on a Vegan Diet   69
6. Creating a Bone-Health Nutrition Plan   81
7. Ancient Medicine for Bone Health   91

PART II
Creative Cooking for Healthy Bones

8. Jump-Start Your Kitchen   101
9. Juices, Lattes, Milks, and Smoothies   107
10. Dressings and Pestos   119
11. Fermented Slow-Aged Pickles and Bone Vinegar   127
12. Dips and Breads   139
13. Small Meals   155
14. Broths, Porridge, and Soups   173

15.	Salad Meals	195
16.	Main Meals	215
17.	Super Side Dishes	243
18.	Good Sweets	263
19.	Meal Plans	283

Acknowledgments	289
APPENDIX	
Recipes for Paleo and Ketogenic Diets	290
Notes	293
Index	299

INTRODUCTION

Plants and Bones
A Dynamic Relationship

Plants and bones are the perfect pair. Plant foods are a rich source of the very vitamins, minerals, enzymes, and protein-building amino acids that help bones grow strong and stay dense. Despite that, there is evidence that bone density is lower and fracture risk is higher among people who rely mostly or solely on plant foods.[1] This perplexes physicians and patients alike and raises the question: Can people who wish to eat more, mostly, or entirely plant foods have healthy bones?

Our answer is yes, it's entirely possible to maintain bone health on a plant-forward diet, and this book explains the why (the science) and the how (what to eat and how to prepare it) and provides more than 100 recipes to support you on your journey.

Most of the nutrients humans need to absorb from food do exist in plant foods and edible fungi, including greens and grains, legumes, beans, fruits, edible flowers, nuts, seeds, and mushrooms. However, while the nutrients in animal foods exist in forms we humans can readily absorb, in concentrations we need, and include all the nutrients key to bone health, the same is not true for plant foods. The body does not readily absorb many key nutrients in the forms found in plant foods. Many of those precious plant nutrients end up being excreted. Plus, some of the natural chemicals in plant foods lock up nutrients and can be damaging to our health.

People on plant-forward diets also need to be aware that different types of plant foods vary widely in the amounts and kinds of nutrients they contain. This is especially important when it comes to amino acids, which are the building blocks of proteins. And only a very few plant foods supply any of the three key bone-health nutrients—vitamin B12, vitamin A, or iron—in a form that the human body can absorb.

Are these obstacles to bone health? Again, most certainly not. Preparing plants in a way that releases their nutrients and eliminates their interfering chemicals is quick and easy; combining plants to supply the full complement of nutrients is as simple as the click of an online nutrient calculator; and finding vitamin B12 along with vitamin A and iron the body readily absorbs is a matter of planning and a bit of knowledge, nothing more.

We wrote this book about food and healthy bones because we wanted you to know what scientists know and what Laura's clinical experience has demonstrated treating dozens of patients with low bone density and high fracture risk: No matter how far you are from peak bone density when starting this journey, and whether you are aiming to top up your bones' reserves against later decline, arrest bone density decline, or treat osteoporosis naturally, you *can* protect and treat bone health while eating some, mostly, or only plant foods. And, we are delighted to report, learning to cook with plant foods can have a very high return in overall health.

The Science and Art of Being Well

The Constitution of the World Health Organization states that "health is basic to the happiness of all peoples." If we, as providers and consumers, push this most basic right through access to nutritional medicine, the paradigm can shift and medicine can focus on the art of being well.

In the past twenty years, the United States government has taken big steps forward in changing the paradigm of the nutritional benefit programs they support. Medicaid-supported Food as Medicine pilot programs in Arkansas, California, Massachusetts, and Oregon specify and pay for prepared meals and groceries, including produce.

This is a welcome first step, because proper nutrition is the foundation for good health, and emphasizing that good food is prevention as well as medicine is exactly the shift we need. That said, the implementation is flawed. Policymakers have not yet established guidelines for premade meals that rule out highly processed ingredients and certain food additives and require whole foods that are properly prepared for nutrient absorption. Thus, not only is the situation ripe for quick-fix financial opportunism, but the meals are not yet being designed as true food as medicine.

Some medical schools are also starting to acknowledge the importance of nutrition in human health by offering their students nutrition courses and, in a few cases, cooking classes. However, conventional medicine's focus on pharmaceuticals is long-standing, and it will likely take a new generation of thinkers who have mastered the complexity of natural medicine to move a new paradigm forward.

Research is showing us how to use plants to prevent and treat disease and chronic illness. The science explains why natural biochemicals present in plant foods can protect bones, and we share this exciting science with you in this book. The chapters that follow make clear why nutrition is the foundation for healthy bones and provide a basis for understanding how to prepare and combine plant foods to prevent and treat osteoporosis.

Genetics, Nutrition, and Health

Here's a powerful truth: The nutrients in your food directly influence the action of genes, which in turn directly shape your health, your incidence of disease, and your longevity. This interaction is how food and nutrition influence health outcomes, and it happens via a mechanism termed *gene expression*. Simply put, we will not have healthy gene expression unless we eat foods that provide certain critical compounds that act as signals to activate or silence individual genes. This interaction is an exquisite chemical dance that happens in your body every day, and what it means is that you have a responsibility. Genes carry potential—potential for supporting health but also potential for favoring disease. And that potential must be regulated by you, through the choices you make about what to eat. We delve more deeply into this critical topic in chapter 2, including a specific discussion of how two common plant foods—beets and lentils—can be powerful superfoods that support DNA function.

The idea that all nutrients are, in fact, regulators of genetic expression is dramatic and exciting. After the first sequencing of the human genome in 1990, many scientists were drawn to the new field of *nutrigenomics*—scientific investigation that sheds light on the way components of food affect genes that influence health and disease. *Nutrigenetics*, the companion science to nutrigenomics, identifies genetic differences in an individual that influence the response to nutrients.

The use of nutrigenomics and nutrigenetics as a tool kit for health is set to become widely adopted within the next ten years. Such a tool kit would allow each of us, on our own or with a health care professional, to create detailed nutrient and food prescriptions to either prevent or treat chronic disease in an elegant and efficient way. We will have the ability to design nutrition to positively modify metabolism, creating a new and welcome medicine that is relatively low cost, environmentally positive, and accessible to all.

Laura's Story

I have learned a lot since 2016, when my mother and I put together our first book, *The Healthy Bones Nutrition Plan and Cookbook*. As the esteemed Dr. Sidney MacDonald Baker wrote in the foreword to that book, precision medicine—treating the individual, not the disease—has shown itself to be the most effective way to achieve health.

In applying precision medicine to bone health, I have been able to understand how an individual's genetic profile contributes to their bone density, and in this context know more precisely how to improve their recovery, as well as whether lifelong attention to their bone health is needed.

Using precision medicine in my practice has entirely changed how I practice, to great result. DEXA scan results show impressive gains for many of my patients—18 percent, 28 percent, 29 percent, 44 percent density increases. Some clients have achieved gains solely through attention to nutrition, while others have combined nutrition and estrogen (at very low dose) or in concert with pharmaceuticals. Even people with genetics working against them for bone health have increased their bone density.

These gains are far more impressive than the average increase that results from taking a bisphosphonate drug such as Fosamax, so you can confidently read this book knowing that anyone who tells you nutrition doesn't work for maintaining healthy bones is wrong. The most efficient way to bone health is to know how you are built (what your genes are) and what nutritional assistance you need, which can be determined by nutrition testing.

As it turns out, plant sources of calcium appear to trigger more helpful genetic expression, and build better bones, than rock calcium does, and plant protein can in many cases provide more health benefit than animal protein—so we know we can faithfully rely on plants to help us thrive.

I hope this book is a contribution to the knowledge of how to prepare and cook plant foods in ways that maximize their nutrient value, so that people of all ages may know how to protect body and bones and improve their health while enjoying more plant-based meals.

Helen's Story

Despite consuming greens, grains, mountains of calcium pills, and a wide array of dairy products, I was diagnosed with osteoporosis at age 48. For more than twenty years, every DEXA scan showed more bone loss. As Laura and I discussed this health dilemma, she had an insight that turned out to be powerfully consequential for my health: If we consume the nutrients our bodies use when making bone, and the nutrients are in a bioavailable (readily absorbable) form, we can prevent osteoporosis, arrest bone loss, and—depending upon age, lifestyle, nutrition status, and genetics—possibly grow new bone. We figured out what I should eat to supply my body richly with nutrients for building bone, and I followed that nutrient route for eighteen months. My next DEXA scan showed no bone loss in any region of my body. My doctor, incredulous, insisted I retest. With only nutrition as medicine, I had arrested osteoporotic bone loss—something my doctor had thought improbable if not impossible. As Laura began to work with patients using this approach and they succeeded, too, we decided to write our first book. Over time, we learned that there was one thorny issue that had to be addressed with greater attention: making sure that the nutrients in *plant foods* are bioavailable. This issue was the impetus for this second book on plants for healthy bones.

My doctor continues to be surprised; since that time I have experienced minimum bone loss in one site and grown some bone in another site. He has, reluctantly, agreed to read both books!

Working on our first bone-health book was the most interesting writing assignment I'd ever had. Laura looks, evaluates what she sees, and asks why, and then she digs. In true lean-management fashion, she digs for root causes. Armed with why, she illuminates the mechanisms and then, if a remedy isn't at hand, creates one. In that way, Laura discovered that in the simple act of eating the nutrients that nourish bone, one may rectify nutrient deficiencies and arrest the relentless march of bone loss.

I was looking forward to writing this new book, too, but I wasn't prepared to be surprised and delighted with new information. Yet I was surprised and delighted—not only by information about how nutrients influence genes and the important ways one may tailor plant choices when managing a chronic condition, but by the simple elegance of cells telling their stories about making and breaking down bone. I was fascinated to learn how directly we can intervene to influence those cycles in our favor, as long as we provide the nutrients that bones need and we are gentle and respectful of their inbuilt and beautifully executed steps. Throughout I was captivated by the science, at once complex and transparent, that demonstrates not only that plants nourish bones, and by the elegant mechanisms of the interplay between our genes and the nutrients we absorb from food. I invite you to share the excitement of discovery, of finding the wellspring of health in your own kitchen. I am 81 years old, and the enlivening experience of continuing to learn has left me knowing with absolute certainty that age is just a number, and health is just around the corner if you know where to look.

Jummee's Story

On Memorial Day in 1998, I boarded an airplane in Korea, and eighteen hours later I landed at John F. Kennedy International Airport in New York City. All I had with me was two suitcases and $2,000 in my pocket. My heart was filled with terrified enthusiasm and unwavering faith. I was on a mission to become a filmmaker and pollinate the seeds of hope in the hearts of people. I called it my version of the American Dream.

Like most immigrants, I worked diligently and found myself climbing the corporate ladder, eventually becoming a corporate executive. I achieved everything I'd set out to attain, following my mother's wish. She was a housewife who never had the chance to pursue a career but dreamed of freedom, financial independence, and power. But in the process of achieving her dream, I had become a workaholic who struggled with an eating disorder, and I found myself trapped in an endless loop of anxiety.

I came to realize that my unfulfilling job was separating me from my true purpose, and I plunged into a deep depression. What saved me was rediscovering my love for cooking. I enrolled in culinary school in the evenings, and cooking became my sanctuary, my escape from the monotony of life. Cooking was therapeutic and showed me a path to self-love.

I grew up in a somewhat chaotic family, but we always came together to eat. My body yearned for those peaceful moments, and cooking brought back memories that became my emotional security blanket. As I continued to cook, my body transformed, and I felt happier and healthier. I overcame my challenges, left my corporate job, and had the courage to follow my passion, becoming a food shaman who helps people overcome their obstacles through food and mindfulness.

My deep love for plants, my practice of Zen Buddhism, and my love for the Earth are my inspiration to create and share plant-based dishes. These passions led me to take on many clients who follow plant-based diets. One client had been a vegan for over two decades and struggled with complex allergies for which conventional doctors couldn't identify root causes. Working closely with this client to prepare medicinal meals from limited food choices, I gained the wisdom to transform the everyday guilty-pleasure dishes he had eaten for years into a diverse array of fresh, locally sourced

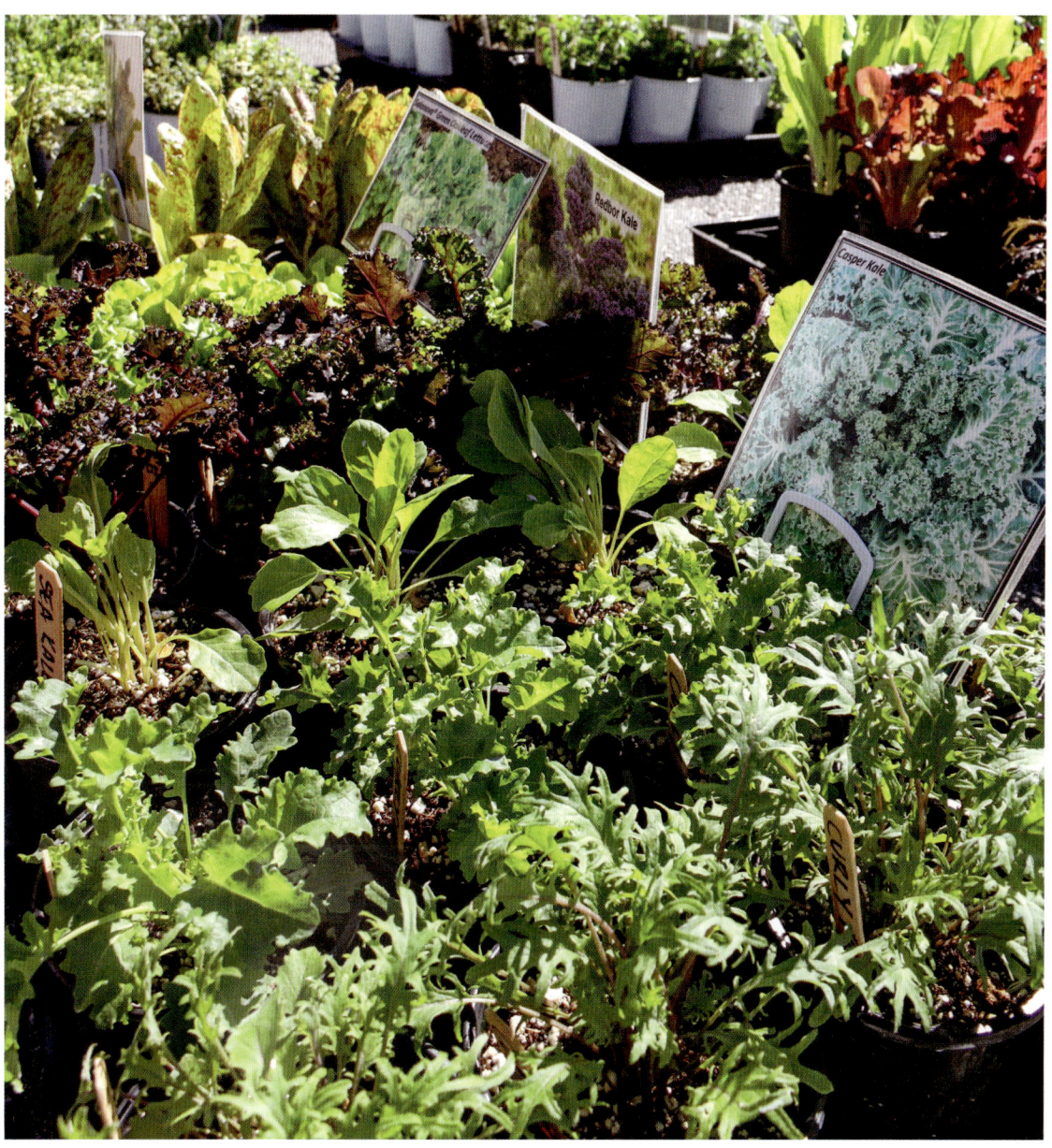

living foods. I cracked the code under almost impossible circumstances. Within six months, my client was free from all the allergies and medications he had been dealing with for years. Through this experience, I discovered that food could hold the major key to our emotions, body, and mind.

I also discovered, through signals from my own body, that sometimes our best efforts to eat well can be complicated by the hidden toxins within so many commercial food products in the United States. Around fifteen years ago, in the course of a perplexing mysterious illness, I discovered that I had a leaky gut. I began reading the ingredients label of every product in my kitchen, and I was astounded to find so many processed, harmful additives in them! This drove me to embrace local, seasonal, organic, farm-to-table whole foods. As a result, my leaky gut symptoms vanished entirely.

People often ask me about the secrets to staying young and maintaining ageless and radiant skin. One of my secrets is decades of following a macrobiotic diet while living in harmony with nature. Along with simple, local, seasonal, organic whole foods, I also include sprouted, fermented, and slow-aged foods to balance my body and mind. I believe this increases vitality and can lead to disease-free, ageless living.

When Laura and Helen approached me about working with them on a book, I was intrigued by Helen's concept of spreading knowledge on the importance of bone health through a plant-forward or plant-based diet. It allowed me to learn more about bone health with a beginner's mind. The journey of creating this book with them has been an eye-opening experience, highlighting how crucial bone health is as the foundation of a healthy body overall. Developing recipes, cooking tips, and meal plans based on this knowledge has deepened my appreciation of the fascinating relationship between food and bone health.

The main ingredients in my recipes are simple, easy, affordable, and accessible. I garnish with a "wow" factor well blended from decades of wisdom embodied in the Five Elements of Traditional Chinese Medicine, macrobiotic principles, biodynamic philosophy, and, of course, the Buddhist temple cuisine deeply ingrained in my bones and flesh, the culture in which I grew up.

Through the recipes in this book, I hope you will discover the pivotal role that cooking can play in unlocking your full potential. Cooking is not just a creative process; it empowers you and nourishes you as a whole. Whether you are seeking meaning and your heart's passion or are simply curious about how to unleash your inner superhuman, come back home to the kitchen. Peel the vegetables, clean them with gratitude, chop and cook foods you adore. Plate your dish with such beauty that it inspires you to eat it. Cherish that moment when you realize how much the food loves you, extending an invitation to a journey of self-discovery and perhaps even the doorway to enlightenment.

About This Book

You may be someone who enjoys eating meat and dairy but wants to add more plant foods to your diet. Or you may be someone who already includes plant foods in most of your meals. Or you may be a vegetarian or a vegan. This book is for all of you. The road to healthy bones is not limited to a strictly defined diet; rather, it is a journey that can include any of the whole foods you love, as long as they are properly prepared to release their nutrient stores and are combined strategically so that your meals provide the optimal nutrient levels that feed your body, your microbiome, and your bones. The three are inextricably linked together, and they help to ensure you will keep your skeleton healthy.

There is one exception to the choose-any-wholesome-food principle, and that applies to people who are strictly vegan. Too often vegans have low bone density and are surprised to find the cause is nutrient deficiency. With that in mind, in this book we provide detailed guidance on tailoring plant-food choices and strategies for mitigating nutrient deficiencies.

Part 1 of the book explains the mechanisms of bone-health nutrition and the roles that flourishing beneficial gut bacterial colonies and an overall healthy body play in skeletal health.

Nutrition Planning

Chapter 6, on nutrition planning, includes practical instructions for using an online nutrition calculator to keep track of the food combinations that supply the recommended dietary allowances for bone health. There are guidelines for vegans on how to plan meals to provide sufficient protein, iron, choline, and vitamin B12. Along with information on how to obtain tests for assessing bone density and your genetic propensities for bone loss, there is a worksheet for assessing bone loss. We explain how you can monitor nutrient consumption and modify as needed. Sometimes people will want to consider mineral supplements along with food-based nutrients. The test results will suggest your best course of action.

Learning to feed your bones is a journey of many steps yet one you may take at your own pace. So where best to start? How best to proceed? We provide a natural medicine plan that suggests steps to take each month for twelve months. Some people may take these steps over a course of twenty-four months; some, whose bones need more immediate attention, may move more quickly.

Part 2 is a cookbook bursting with plant-food recipes that supply the nutrients bones need in a form the body can absorb. It begins with guidance on preparing whole fruits and vegetables for cooking and lists of ingredients to assemble to support the recipes, from basics like Dr. Laura's Bone Vinegar (page 137) and homemade plant-based milks to a full range of small plates, soups, salads, main dishes, desserts, and more.

You Can Cook!

Cooking is a skill that is accessible and enjoyable to anyone. With each new technique you learn, you improve and empower yourself. The beginner's mind is the master's mind.

Your first step on your cooking journey is building a well-stocked pantry. In chapter 8 you'll find an essential pantry list that Jummee developed through years of trial and error. Follow her guidance and you'll be well on your way to making your favorite dishes in no time, turning your cooking into more joy.

We hope that preparing recipes from this book will become a creative and enjoyable weekend ritual and routine. Try setting aside a three- to four-hour block of time to spend in your kitchen. Consider it your self-love time. Cooking is akin to painting—there is so much opportunity for creative experimentation. Preparing extra portions during your weekend cooking will save you time during busy weeks, because you'll have meals ready to reheat and eat in less than twenty minutes. And as you do, it's easy to add something extra and give your dish a new twist.

These recipes are designed for versatility and are principally vegetarian; some are vegan, and one or two include an egg. The recipes are crafted from a vast array of plant foods—many of the ingredients will be familiar, a few may be new to you, but all are readily available at most grocery stores. You will be spoiled for choice.

We are delighted to say that you needn't have any experience creating recipes or tweaking them because each of our recipes is designed to provide a generous helping of the nutrients healthy bones require. We hope our recipes will inspire you to create some of your own.

The final chapter of the book provides four meal plans—one for each season—so you can get cooking and step into a world of plant-based dishes that will provide energy and culinary delight for you and whoever joins you at your table. Crafting a weekly meal plan that incorporates seasonal ingredients not only saves you time, it makes cooking easier and more enjoyable. This variety is pivotal for your overall well-being, rejuvenation, and longevity.

Cooking as a Radical Act

The natural world, in flow, contains everything your body needs to achieve long life in good health, starting at any age and at almost any health status. And food is the first, most important, and most effective tool of medicine.

But why bone health? Why health? Certainly, we want to feel well, to live without pain. But there is more. When ill, we must focus internally. But when we are healthy, we are able to reach outward, to others, to the world, to embrace and to connect. Our spirit is free to wander, and we can open ourselves to magic. Many things can be learned to achieve this sort of bliss through the connection with nature and food.

First, start with the basics. Eat a lot of different plants. Find sources of plant foods grown in soil and with water that are healthy and free of toxic chemicals. Eat plants that are in season, and prepare them so they are most nourishing and delicious. Use these plant foods, with guidance from your medical professionals, as part of managing chronic or intermittent health issues. Know your own health status and challenges, and eat for prevention.

In chapter 7 you will find some basics of food as medicine from the teachings of Traditional Chinese Medicine (TCM), which you can explore on your own or with a TCM practitioner, nutritionist, or health care provider familiar with the principles of food as medicine. This can add a layer to your understanding of which plant foods are most beneficial for you.

There is a bounty of information that can inform your food and cooking choices, and we encourage you to explore and identify your preferences and body's needs. Luckily our bodies are often aware of what we need, and if we are listening, we intuitively reach for the food that will meet the need.

Once you understand your constitution (from your own monitoring or from working with a professional nutritionist or physician), the season, and the nature of food, you can open up to another level of eating in harmony with your body, the foods, and nature itself. It is there that cooking becomes true alchemy.

So, as Laura advises all of her patients, listen to your body.

Second, appreciate the value of the food in your fridge or pantry, not only as sustenance but for the energy and effort that was required to grow it. Consider that the sprouts you are about to eat grew from nuts, beans, lentils, or seeds that were nourished, watered, protected, and harvested, probably by hand. Then they were dried and cleaned, packaged and shipped, stocked and sold, all by people you may never meet but who care about the plants that are going to help your body stay healthy.

Third, recognize that your feelings affect those around you and influence what you create. Infuse what you cook to nourish yourself and those you care for with what you wish to communicate. Your food can communicate love, generosity, and compassion. Should you doubt these subtle arts, please remember that we do not yet understand the physics underpinning our universe, and err on the side of love.

Cooking is a radical act. In the face of Big Ag, Big Chem, and Big Pharma, the choice to engage with your food—to spend your money on clean, well-grown, real food, to create bonds with your cooking companions, to nourish yourself and loved ones properly so you remain healthy—becomes a revolutionary act.

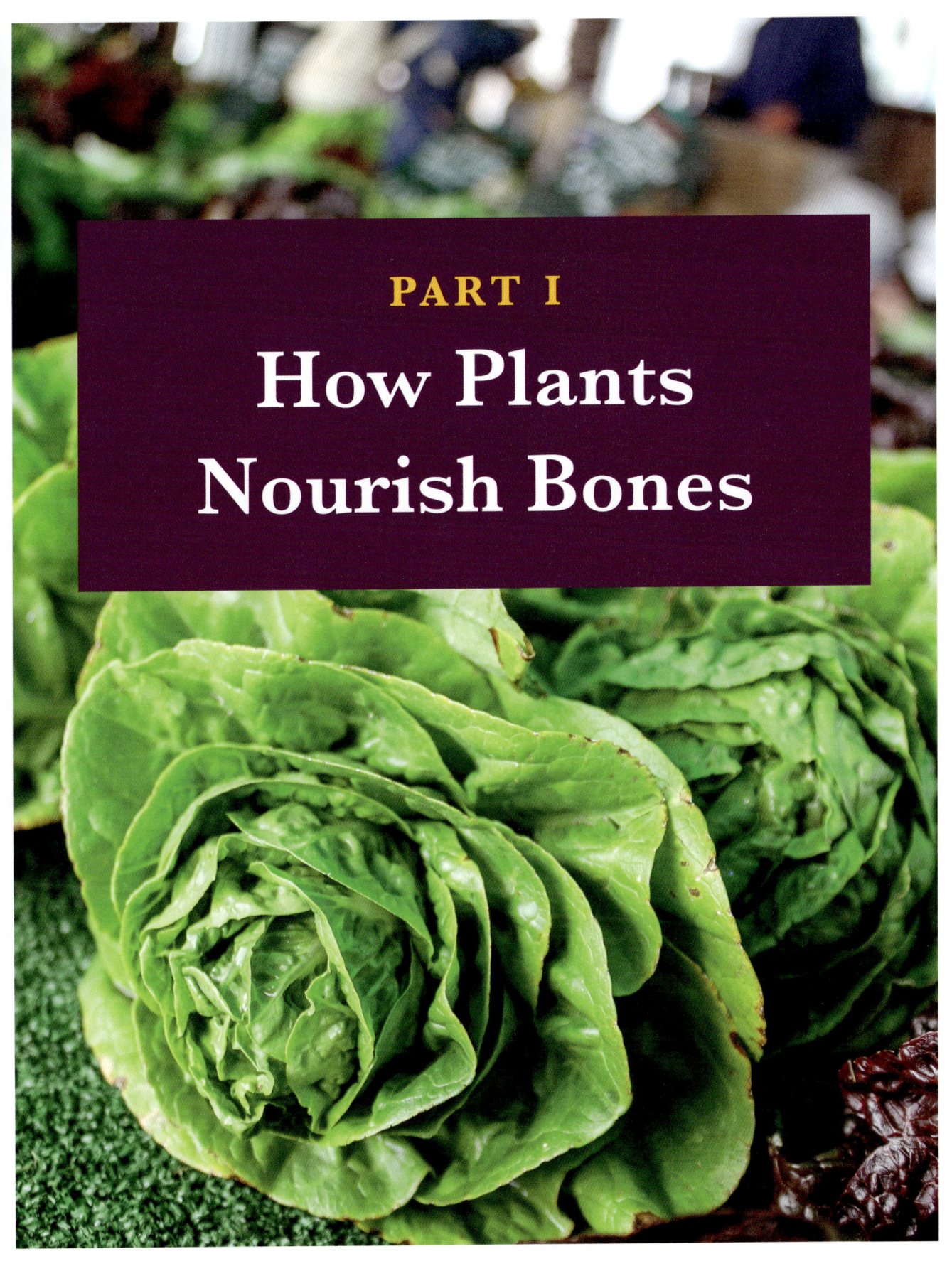

PART I
How Plants Nourish Bones

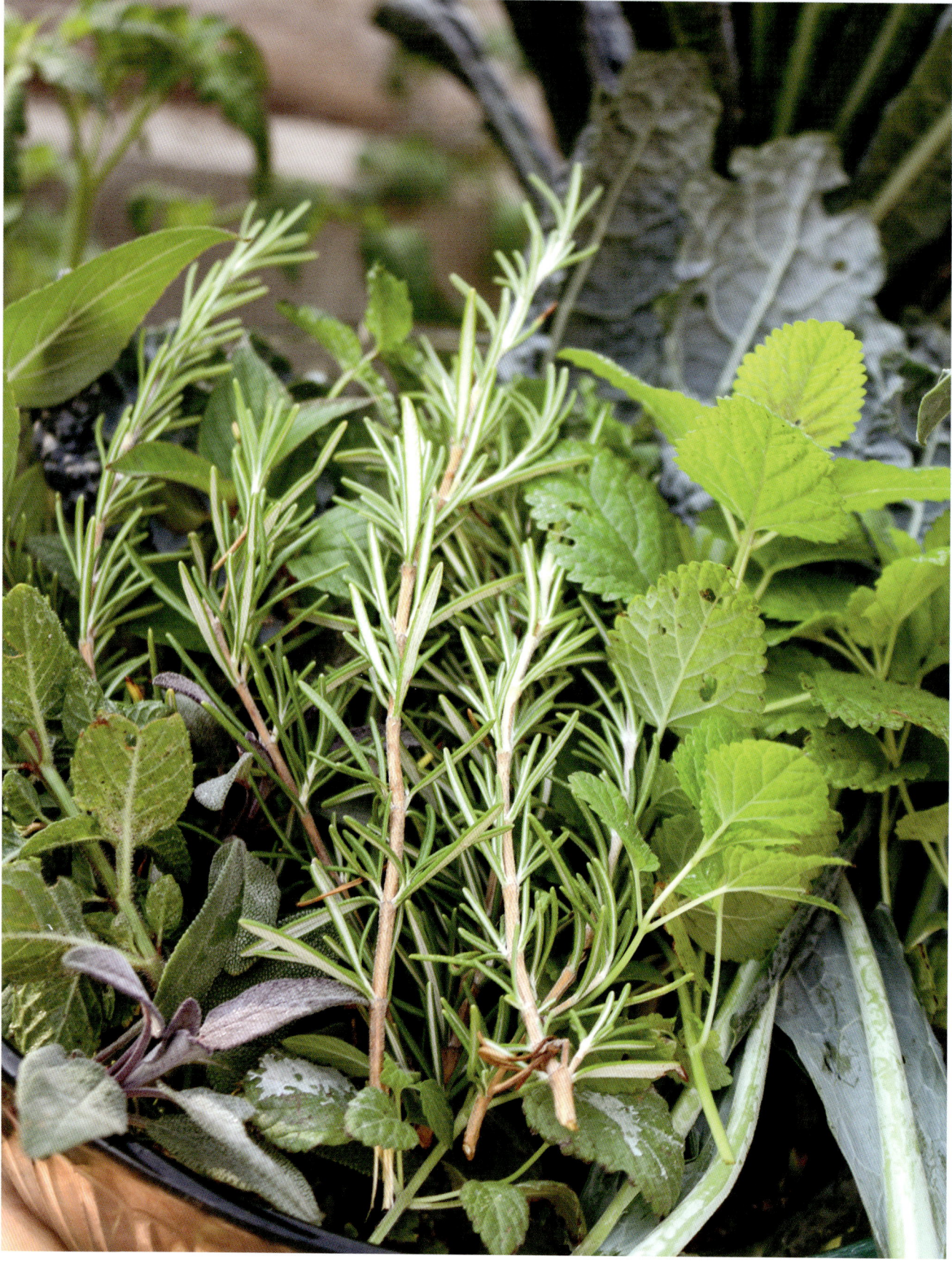

CHAPTER 1

Bones Are a Family of Cells

The body is a sturdy yet vastly complex engine relying on a precision mix of many and varied nutrients to keep its systems running. Because the bones function in the larger body system, complete nutrition is always required for the best overall health and the best bone health. As science and medicine find ever more evidence that maintaining ideal nutrient balances can keep the body in top form at any age, nutrition professionals are working to identify precisely which nutrients are protective and therapeutic for individuals and conditions, and the best whole-food sources of each.

Understanding your own personal nutrition requirements is important, as each of us has different requirements. When it comes to bone health, we are especially fortunate. We know which nutrients and roughly the measures and ratios that can help keep bones healthy.[1] A full mix of these nutrients can help to prevent and even arrest mineral loss. Thus, folks who wish to prevent and treat bone mineral loss have a reliable list of nutrients and foods to combine and consume.

Bone Density Is Gender Neutral

Bone density decline is tied to hormone levels in both men and women. What have researchers discovered about sex-based patterns of bone loss? Men reach peak bone mass by age 20, and their bone-density decline begins immediately afterward. Over time a man's hip bones lose mass faster than a woman's do. If a man breaks his hip, he is likely to die sooner after the break than an average woman would. And although from age 40 a man's bone loss patterns differ from those of a woman, by age 70 men and women lose bone at the same rate: rapidly.

Women reach peak bone mass around age 34. Density then declines steadily until menopause, when hormones begin to wane. After that, density may stabilize until age 65, when bone loss steps up, sometimes dramatically, leading to osteoporosis.

Fortunately, starting at age 30 and at any time after that, no matter your bone health status, you can interrupt natural patterns of bone-density decline by:

- consuming the nutrients that nourish bone
- promoting maximum absorption of those nutrients
- keeping your body healthy and as free as possible of chronic inflammation, so that it can make full use of nutrients

Patterns of bone-density decline can worsen if a person's gut health, immune system, or nourishment are compromised. For both men and women who routinely eat sugary and ultraprocessed foods, have diabetes, drink a lot of alcohol, use proton pump inhibitors, take steroid or NSAID medications, or take prescription medications for a variety of

> ## Men Get Osteoporosis, Too
>
> Both bone size and hormone levels influence bone density. Although men typically have larger bones and maintain hormone levels longer than women do, the risk of osteoporosis looms large for men who have, among other conditions, rheumatoid arthritis, chronic liver or kidney disease, overactive thyroid or parathyroid glands, celiac disease or other threats to gut health, or diabetes. Osteoporosis is also a risk for men who are clinically obese or who take glucocorticoids, anticonvulsant medications, hormone deprivation therapy for prostate cancer, or certain antidepressant medications. Men who smoke, are alcoholic, don't exercise, don't spend any time in the sun, or are clinically underweight are also at risk. A man who has osteoporosis may become shorter or hunched; severe cases may cause undiagnosed pain.

chronic conditions, bone thinning can begin in middle age. And since DEXA scans aren't among their routine screenings, men usually won't know they have osteoporosis until they break a bone.

Over the years, Laura has fielded many questions from her patients who are concerned about bone health. These are some of the questions that come up time and time again, along with Laura's replies.

Does eating for bone health require following a diet of specific foods?

Not at all. You can prepare and cook foods you love. Bone-health success depends upon consuming the nutrients that nourish bone, and regardless of your dietary style, you have a wide range of food choices available to you.

Can I strengthen my bones and improve bone density if I consume mostly or only plant foods and fungi?

Most certainly. You'll need to prepare certain types of plant foods in a specific way before eating them so they will release their nutrients properly in your gut. The preparation techniques are not hard to learn and in time will become second nature. You'll also need to combine ingredients thoughtfully to ensure that meals provide complete protein. Though many animal foods are good sources of readily absorbable iron and vitamin B12, few plant sources are. You will need to learn which foods supply these nutrients and incorporate them into your diet.

If I take pharmaceuticals that affect bone density, do I have to stop taking these medications in order to sustain bone density and maintain healthy bones?

Only your health care professional can advise about your medications, but I know from experience that adding the right nutrition to your treatment plan can help medication work even better.[2] For those who have chronic diseases that affect bone health, it is especially important to establish and maintain a healthy microbiome, make healthy lifestyle choices, and, if possible, test for and address nutrient deficiency.

If I want to reduce the amount of animal foods in my diet, but not eliminate them completely, which are the best ones to continue eating to support bone health?

Mozzarella and Gouda cheeses are good sources of vitamin K2. We also recommend pastured eggs, organically raised poultry, wild-caught salmon, trout, oysters, wild-caught shrimp, and pastured lamb. Other meats to consider are bison, venison, and ostrich.

Bones Are a Family of Cells

It is easy to take bones for granted. Without fanfare or fuss they support our bodies; they carry calcium reserves that nerves and cells use to communicate and stay healthy; they give birth to components of the immune system; and they generate blood cells. We may forget that bones themselves are living tissue comprising many types of cells among a rigid framework composed primarily of calcium and other minerals. Each bone cell is a microscopic engine that processes nutrients and oxygen that enter the bloodstream, from which our organs and other body systems may take them up.

Bones are stiff thanks largely to the minerals they contain, yet bone is a multilayered body tissue, as shown in figure 1.1. Each layer, and each cell type within it, requires a distinct nutrient profile to sustain health. The principal nutrients are calcium, collagen, and water, but a large cast of additional nutrients is required to grow bone tissue.

The innermost layer of a bone is the marrow, which produces stem cells, blood cells, and immune cells. The outer layers of bone contain blood vessels, nerves, other tissue components, and calcium. The periosteum is the dense, fibrous outer layer of bone. Though less than a tenth of a millimeter thick, it contains collagen, blood vessels, and neural pathways. The blood vessels carry nutrients and oxygen, and the nerves transmit signals when tissue needs growth or repair. The periosteum is protective and readily bonds with connective tissue such as tendons.

By structure, all bone is a scaffold made of collagen. A mineral compound called hydroxyapatite, which is composed of calcium and phosphorus, sits on the scaffold. The scaffold comes together inside bone as collagen filaments called fibrils that assemble randomly and then weave together in a process called crosslinking. The random, irregular pattern ensures that the structure will remain flexible despite impact from any angle or direction; crosslinking makes the structure strong. The density of this scaffold and its minerals are what a DEXA scan measures.

Types of Bone Cells

Bone has four types of living cells—osteoclasts, osteoblasts, osteocytes, and bone-lining cells.[3] Bone cells are born as stem cells. Most stem cells arise near or adjacent to blood vessels.[4]

> **Osteoblasts** are the cells that make bone.
> **Osteoclasts** are the cells that reduce bone.
> **Osteocytes** are mature osteoblasts. These cells live within the scaffold and help to maintain bone strength.
> **Bone-lining cells** are flat, inactive osteoblasts that sit on the surface of bone.

All these cells dance in a cycle of growth and retirement called turnover—a coordinated set of steps that break down old bone (a process called

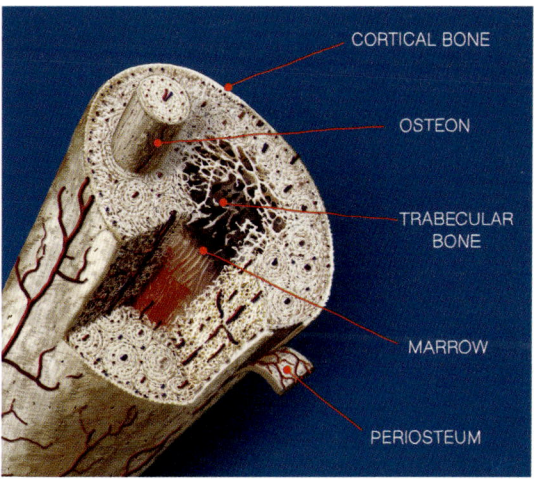

Figure 1.1. If you could see into the outer layer (periosteum) of a bone, you would observe the dense network of collagen and hydroxyapatite that gives a bone strength, along with the marrow at the center. *Illustration by Daniel Auber*

Bones Are a Family of Cells • 13

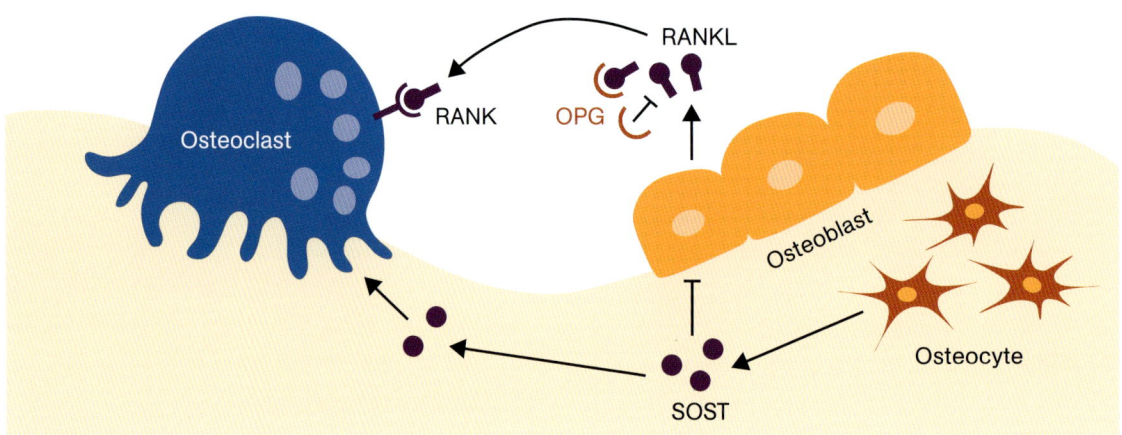

Figure 1.2. Bone cells communicate among one another and the body to regulate bone turnover.

resorption) and grow new bone, a daily process of keeping bones healthy and strong (see figure 1.2). Bone turnover is also referred to as bone remodeling. Osteoprogenitor cells, which arise from stem cells, are central to bone growth, remodeling, and repair, and to maintaining the strength and integrity of the skeleton. Osteoblasts and osteoclasts each pass through several different developmental stages before they mature and are ready to take up their functions in bone. Specific nutrients are required at each stage for successful transition to the next.

OSTEOBLASTS

Osteoblasts arise from stem cells, primarily, though not only, in bone marrow.[5] These stem cells arise from progenitor stem cells, which are cells that move through several stages of development. The first stage is known by two names, osteoblast precursor cell and osteoprogenitor cell. These early-stage osteoblasts have potential to migrate to bone's outer layer and become fully functioning specialized cells, but they remain precursors until cell signaling such as is needed for bone growth or repair triggers them to complete the developmental cycle. A wide range of nutrients catalyze preosteoblast transition to mature osteoblasts, which move to the bone surface, where they secrete and deposit new bone.

Osteoblasts live for up to 200 days. The genes that instruct bone marrow to make osteoblasts depend upon a sufficient supply of iron, which is why iron deficiency is associated with reduced bone density.[6]

Sclerostin (SOST) impedes osteoblast formation. Estrogen suppresses sclerostin, which is one of the mechanisms by which estrogen helps keep healthy bone mass.

OSTEOCLASTS

Osteoclasts arise principally in bone marrow, but osteoclasts do not arise directly from stem cells. Instead, they form from the fusion of two precursor stem cells. Some of these migrate to the surface of bone and differentiate to preosteoclasts before becoming active osteoclasts dedicated to bone resorption. This process is called osteoclastogenesis.[7]

Preosteoclasts respond to signaling and proteins, including the powerful RANKL system, as described in "Why Bone Density Declines," page 16. Osteoclasts live for up to twenty-five days.

OSTEOCYTES

Osteocytes are elder osteoblasts that embed within bone tissue and help to maintain bone strength. They may live for fifty years or for one year only, depending upon the extent to which they and the other bone cells are properly nourished. Osteocytes depend upon a healthy fluid flow for delivering nutrients to and removing waste products from bone and on a variety of other growth and signaling factors that are not nutritional.

BONE-LINING CELLS

Bone-lining cells populate the surface of the periosteum. They cover any areas not actively undergoing new growth or removal of old bone. These cells participate in bone growth as old cells retire.

Healthy Bone Turnover

Thinking about bone health, our first concern is usually about the bones that presently form our skeleton. But in terms of nourishing the skeletal system, it's also important to understand these other aspects of bone health:

- nourishing bone marrow—the birthplace of bone cells
- nourishing the cells that make new bone
- nurturing the cells that help worn-out bone to break down and be resorbed
- sustaining the cells that settle in bone for the long term to keep it healthy and strong
- nourishing the other tissues that make up our bones
- nourishing the proteins and enzymes that aid the body in absorbing nutrients and in the deposition of bone
- replenishing the matrix of bone mineral that can thin and lead to osteoporosis

Every cell has a life cycle: grow, maintain and repair tissue, retire. *Scientific American* reports that 1 percent of the cells in the human body—about 330 billion cells—are replaced daily.[8] In the course of three months, 30 trillion cells are replaced, which means that significant parts of your body are renewed four times a year. For all this turnover to continue across a lifetime, the fuel is nutrients, without which the cells would languish or die. (Nutrients play a pivotal role in all metabolic processes that include production of hormones and enzymes.)

The mineral framework of bone also undergoes turnover, about every three months. Gut and skin cells renew every few months; the liver, every few years; much of the skeleton, about every decade; osteocytes, every fifty years; the brain, very slowly over a lifetime.[9] Oxidative stress, inflammation, and poor nutrition, among other stressors, can affect turnover rates.

Telomeres

The nucleus of a cell contains DNA, formed into long strands called chromosomes, encoded with instructions for making the proteins that build or regenerate the body. The cell turnover process is managed by the telomeres, which are located at the end of each chromosome strand. Thus, the telomeres largely control the health of newborn cells.[10] These telomere caps also guard genome stability. Telomere length determines the integrity of cell copies during turnover replication.

As the body grows older (or sicker), and cells continue replicating, the telomeres themselves may shorten, and the reproduction instructions they send become less faithful. In this way, mistakes—mutations—arise. When human cells mutate, the results are usually not beneficial and are often detrimental to healthy cell function.

Telomeres rely entirely on nutrients for their own health, and thus adequate nutrition can help to mitigate the risk of mutations occurring. Astragalus and *Centella asiatica* have both been shown to increase telomerase, the enzyme that replenishes telomeres.

The entire cellular bonanza—including cell communication, cell turnover, and cell death—operates in a network of biochemical pathways including but not limited to hormones and enzymes. Chemical signals synchronize the whole. Consider that red bone marrow produces about 8 million new stem cells every second, and you begin to understand the scope and complexity of human metabolism. These stem cells differentiate to as many as twenty different types of cells.

Proper nutrition is vital to cellular health. Eating foods that contain protein provides the body with amino acids that are necessary for building cellular structures such as collagen and cell membranes. Carbohydrates from food provide energy cells need to function, and lipids provide material for cell membrane structure and function. Thus, proper nutrition keeps the basic engines of our health functioning at a cellular level. Without healthy cellular function, our bodies struggle to maintain critical processes such as ridding the body of toxins or fighting infection, and the malfunction of these processes can lead to a slow decline in health as we age. The good news is, genetic predispositions aside, the right nutrition can fortify healthy cell regeneration and keep our mechanisms in good working order as we age.

Why Bone Density Declines

Until roughly middle age, bone turnover seems to stay in the right balance naturally. With age, the balance can shift toward bone loss. Why does it shift? What is happening when normal bone loses density and becomes porous and weaker, sometimes at risk of fracture?

THE ROLE OF RANKL

Bone turnover is a subtle chemical choreography influenced by proteins, hormones, lifestyle, and nutrient sufficiency. The turnover controller responsible for keeping formation of new bone equal to or greater than bone breakdown is a protein with a very complicated name: *receptor activator of nuclear factor kappa-B ligand*. Scientists just call it RANK ligand (a ligand is a molecule that binds with other elements or compounds) or RANKL. RANKL has complicated and surprising functions in bone health. To understand what RANKL does, it's helpful to know that a receptor is a protein that sits on the surface of a cell and is available to bind with other, specific molecules or viruses. Binding triggers a signal that in turn triggers a reaction. For example, RANKL binds with a receptor on the surface of osteoclasts. That binding triggers a signal to start breaking down bone.

Osteoblasts (the cells that make bone) manufacture RANKL, but counterintuitively, RANKL stimulates the differentiation of progenitor cells to osteoclasts—the cells that break down bone. It also activates the osteoclasts.

Osteoblasts also secrete osteoprotegerin (OPG), a receptor that intercepts and binds with RANKL. When OPG attaches to RANKL, it changes the shape of the RANKL molecule. As a result, RANKL then does not fit into the receptor on the surface of an osteoclast, and thus the osteoclast will *not* receive the signal to start breaking down bone. In other words, the OPG decoy mechanism tricks bone breakdown into taking a break, and bone turnover stays roughly in balance. That is, until estrogen begins to wane, because estrogen is the main source of stimulation for OPG production. As estrogen declines, OPG production declines, clearing the way for more RANKL/ostcoclast binding and more bone resorption. Without intervention, there is a shift in balance from stable growth/resorption to more bone loss than growth. Among women, estrogen wanes during middle age. Thus bone density declines with age.

Magnesium also plays a part in this story, because it helps to regulate both RANKL and OPG. Magnesium is vital to body and bone, and magnesium deficiency—common in the United States—is correlated with increase in osteoclast number and lowered bone density.[11] A rough guess is that 50 percent of Americans are deficient in magnesium. For more information on magnesium, see page 32.

ENTER PHYTOESTROGENS

There is another player that can affect bone turnover balance: phytoestrogens. Phytoestrogens are secondary compounds produced by plants, and phytoestrogens have similarities to human estrogen. Phytoestrogens can stimulate OPG production, as shown in figure 1.3, and this is one of the critical ways nutrition impacts bone health. Phytoestrogens present in plant foods and mushrooms can regulate RANKL secretion as well as vitamin D3 production.

This relationship of OPG and RANKL is the foundational mechanism of osteoblast/osteoclast balance and, in the course of aging, the most potent influence on bone health and density. Hormones wane later in life for men than for women, which helps to explain why men who develop osteoporosis do so relatively late in life. (Onset can occur at younger ages if during prostate cancer treatment a man must take androgen deprivation therapy, which typically carries a high risk of osteoporosis.)

Along with helping to sustain bone health, phytoestrogens enhance bone response to exercise. Phytoestrogens have now been thoroughly researched, and high-quality research shows that phytoestrogen intake decreases breast cancer risk.[12]

ACTIVITY STIMULATES TURNOVER

Nearly all osteogenic precursor cells have the potential to become active osteoblasts, but whether they do so depends on demand. Walking and other forms of exercise signal osteoblasts to build more bone cells, thus helping to balance bone turnover. The less engaged bones are in activity, the fewer precursor cells differentiate to bone cells.

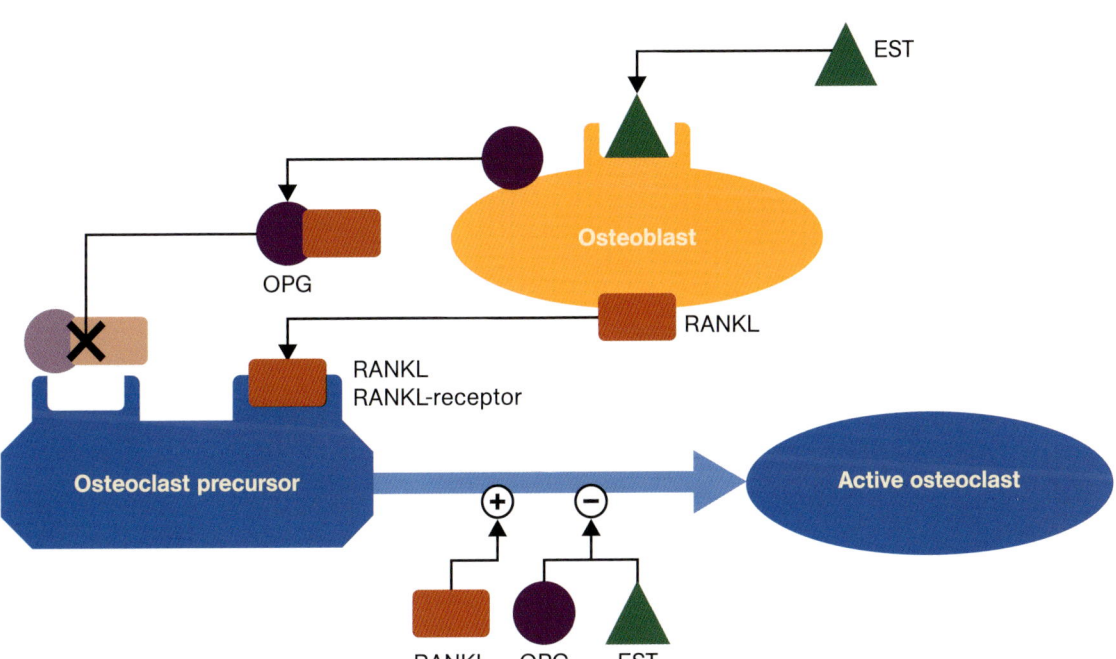

Figure 1.3. Bone turnover is regulated by phytoestrogens via a decoy system in which osteoprotegerin (OPG) attaches to the RANKL molecule, changing the shape of RANKL and preventing it from docking on the RANKL receptor. Loss of OPG allows RANKL to dock, thereby triggering osteoclasts that break down bone.

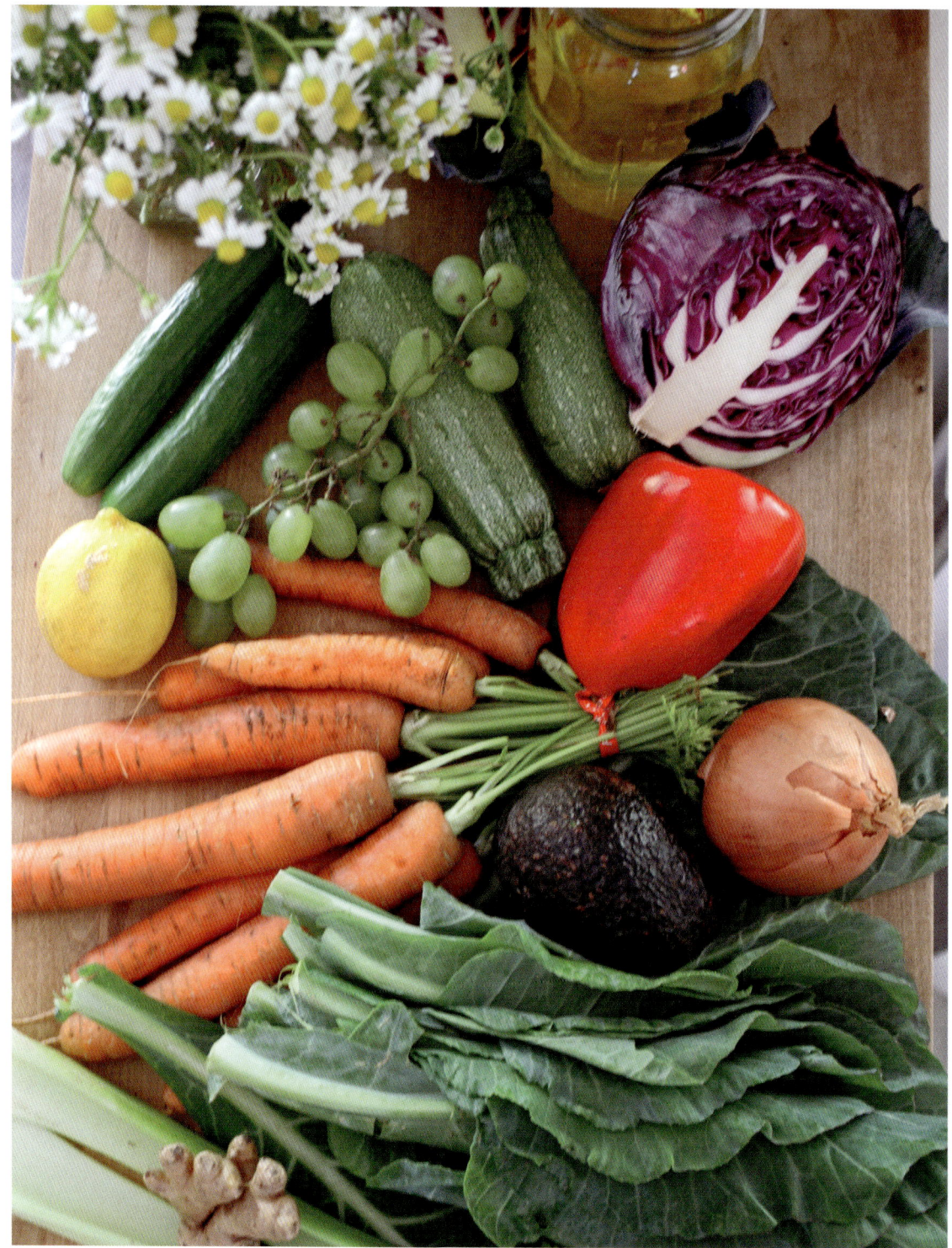
Figure 2.1. Shopping at a farmers market allows you to choose food that is in season where you live.

CHAPTER 2

Feeding Your Bones

At each stage of the life cycle of bone cells, as they grow and differentiate, their nutritional needs change. For the best bone-health outcomes, you must supply the nutrients the growing cells need as well as the nutrients that feed the environment within which they grow and mature. In this chapter, we dive into the details of specific nutrients that help to protect bone strength and redress bone loss, as well as the plant foods that supply them. Before the nutrition overview, though, let's look more deeply at how nutrition relates to the critical phenomenon of gene expression.

Gene Expression

As you probably learned in science class, DNA, the coded instructions for your body, carries thousands of individual sets of instructions for regulating every life function. Genes are segments of DNA specific to physical characteristics or functions. A gene's code is a set of instructions to make proteins that modify an aspect of the body's physiology, biochemistry, or behavior, such as eye color, enzyme, or immune system function. But the code can remain inactive until a signal prompts action. When the gene has received a signal and issued instructions, this is called gene expression. The gene itself does not change form, but its action varies depending upon the signal it receives and also the form of the gene's code itself, which can vary from individual to individual.

Two types of organic compounds act as signals—methyl groups and acetyl groups. Methyl groups most often work to silence genes, stopping their expression. This is called DNA methylation.

Acetyl groups work in the opposite direction, allowing access to the DNA, leading to activation of the gene. Both compounds are vital to healthy function, and both are formed from what we eat. You will not have healthy gene expression unless you eat the foods that provide methyl and acetyl groups.

If you are not supplying your body enough methyl groups, you will have impaired gene expression. If you are not supplying enough glucose or fatty acids, then you will not produce enough acetyl groups for healthy gene expression.

This is just the tip of the iceberg in how the food we eat is vital to our gene expression that decides our health. And what this means is that we have a responsibility. Genes carry potential—potential for supporting health but also for favoring disease. And that potential must be regulated by us.

Here's an example of how nutrition affects health in the most basic way. Beets and lentils contain high levels of methyl donors; they are in fact superfoods for the methylation process. Beets contain betaine, the most potent methyl donor of them all, and lentils contain folate, another powerful methyl donor.

If you do not consume enough methyl donors in your diet (or if your methylation is genetically impaired and untreated), you can experience a wide range of symptoms: lack of focus, inability to concentrate, poor short-term memory and organizational ability, lack of emotional stability, poor sleep hygiene, and impaired hormone regulation.

If the low methyl group state goes on for a long time, impaired DNA function can lead to chronic disease and damage.

Food Regulates Gene Expression

In 2016, French scientists researching one of the most lethal cancers, glioma, found that when some components of protein were intermittently limited, an important cluster of genes directed the death of the cancerous glioma cells, leaving normal cells alone.[1]

Two years later, an Italian research team made a similarly exciting finding: Epigallocatechin gallate (EGCG), a natural anti-inflammatory compound found in green tea, triggered genes that stopped cancer stem cells from activating.[2]

Research in nutrigenomics is exploding because nutrients, such as EGCG, easily and effectively target master genes that regulate many important body processes. And because such nutrients are available in common foods, people can enjoy their health-giving benefits naturally, safely, and relatively inexpensively.

In fact, scientists have been able to link specific nutrients to health outcomes at the most basic level. Healthy DNA is a basic requirement for all health, and in order for DNA replication to occur, cells need folate, vitamin B12, magnesium, zinc, and iron. Vitamin C, vitamin E, zinc, manganese, and selenium protect DNA against damage by free radicals (see "Oxidative Stress and Antioxidants" on page 63). Niacin, zinc, iron, and magnesium step in to help repair damaged DNA, helping to protect against mutations that can lead to cancer. Deficiency in these micronutrients increases DNA replication stress and instability of the genome, increases susceptibility to DNA damage caused by toxins, and disables normal control of healthy gene expression.[3]

The results of research about nutrient contributions to health are no longer the sole province of academic journals. Writing in a 2022 popular press article about how plants talk to genes, Monica Dus, professor of biology at the University of Michigan, used the example of honeybee development to illustrate the basis for confidence in nutrients to influence health at the genetic level. Worker bees, those that work nonstop, she wrote, are sterile and live only a few weeks. The queen bee lives for years inside a hive and is so fertile she gives birth to an entire colony. Yet workers and queen bees are genetically identical; the only difference between them is what they eat. Worker bees eat nectar and pollen; the queen eats royal jelly, a special substance containing nutrients that trigger genetic instructions to create the queen's unique anatomy and physiology.

> Like the switches that control the intensity of the light in your house, genetic switches determine how much of a certain gene product is produced. Royal jelly, for instance, contains compounds that activate genetic controllers to form the queen's organs and sustain her reproductive ability.[4]

Professor Dus also noted that a human baby's genes are responsive to nutrients in breast milk, and furthermore, that all foods—including plants—have genes that respond to and are shaped by the nutrients in their environment.

More about Nutrigenetics

As explained in the introduction to this book, nutrigenetics identifies genetic differences in an individual that influence the response to nutrients. For example, genetic variation explains why some people need only a small amount of vitamin D while others—including me (Laura)—require much larger amounts daily.

It also explains why my mother, Helen, needs to take a form of folate called methylfolate. A gene, the

MTHFR, directs a process that transforms folate from food to methylfolate, the form the body uses during the production of red blood cells, among other metabolic processes. In some types of MTHFR gene polymorphism, the transformation from folate to methylfolate is incomplete. This is Helen's situation. A concentrated form of methylfolate supplement allows her body to skip the transformational step. As is true when considering any supplementation, you must be guided by a health care professional, as too much methylfolate can also be deleterious to health. The highest levels of naturally occurring methylfolate are in sprouted legumes.

For vegans and vegetarians, this idea comes into full play with vitamin A. Vitamin A in animals is called retinol, which is the chemical form of vitamin A the human body uses. Our body cannot use the form of vitamin A found in plants, called carotene; our body, *via our genes*, must convert carotenes to retinol. In some of us, the genes responsible for this conversion do not work so well. This is why it is important, if you are going to rely on plants for vitamin A, that you know whether your genes for making this conversion are functioning optimally. In some of us they will be working well; in others the genes will be impaired, which suggests the need for a lot more carotene intake, or even supplementation, to reach recommended daily levels.

Macronutrients and Micronutrients

To sustain life, your body needs a range of macronutrients and micronutrients. The macronutrients are protein, glucose, fat, fiber, and water. The micronutrients essential for good health include vitamins, minerals, and plant compounds called polyphenols; these are needed by the body in relatively small amounts. These small amounts do not reflect their importance, as deficiency in any micronutrient can cause health issues either acute or chronic.

Protein is made up of amino acids and builds the collagen matrix that holds the calcium-rich hydroxyapatite that is most of a bone's density. Protein also maintains the production of hormones and growth factors, such as IGF1, that modulate bone growth.[5] Protein is also needed for repair of muscles and bones. It is now known that higher levels of protein intake positively impact bone health among people of all ages, including those who are elderly.[6]

Carbohydrates (and in some cases fats) become glucose, which powers the metabolic processes of all cells.

Fiber keeps the digestive system healthy by feeding the gut bugs; fiber also helps to balance cholesterol and blood pressure levels and helps prevent spikes in blood sugar levels. Fiber is fermented in the intestines, producing short-chain fatty acids (SCFAs). SCFAs positively regulate local and systemic immune function as well as inhibit osteoclast differentiation, thereby increasing bone mass. Research shows that a high-fiber diet and high levels of SCFA activity significantly increases bone mass and prevents postmenopausal and inflammation-induced bone loss.[7]

Clean water is also important for bone health, as it is for the health of all body systems. Water conducts electricity throughout the body, and this electrical activity is required for the nervous system to send signals to body and brain. Water also is the conduit for waste elimination through urine, perspiration, and bowel movements. Water containing electrolytes, such as mineral water and natural spring water, keeps tissues, joints, and the spine cushioned and lubricated. Laura advises her patients to drink water that is rich with a natural balance of minerals and filtered for removal of toxins. (See "Let's Start with Water," page 101.)

Fat supplies energy, protects organs, is a component of hormones, aids nutrient absorption, and appears to be closely related to bone mass density. Your body fat also helps to keep you warm. Eating

The Protein Debate

Research scientists and clinicians are studying and debating the effects of protein on health in general and bone health in particular, as well as the ideal amount of protein to consume as one ages. There is a fair bit of speculation about a correlation between protein intake and bone density.

This discussion stems from previous observations of a correlation between protein intake and calcium excretion. At the time, scientists ascribed the cause to meat and assumed that consuming meat had caused calcium to leach from bones. That was a brave leap, but the argument fell flat. In fact, there is a relationship between calcium excretion and eating more of some protein foods—such as animal protein, oatmeal, and walnuts—than the body can use at one time. These forms of protein create an acid residue, called ash, which is left after the body digests the food. Too much acid ash creates a pH imbalance (see "pH Balance and Bone Health," page 61) if not corrected by alkaline foods or a draw on calcium from the body. But the calcium does not come from the bones; it is calcium circulating in the bloodstream. Further, studies show that protein is correlated to slight calcium excretion if calcium intake falls short of recommended daily allowances, especially among postmenopausal women, men who smoke, and others at risk of bone density loss. However, when protein and calcium are both present in sufficient levels, protein improves recovery after fracture, may reduce age-related bone loss, and may increase bone density.

The most common recommendation for daily protein consumption is 0.8 grams per kilogram of body weight, which translates into about 1.2 ounces or 46 grams of protein (about the size of a deck of cards) for the average premenopausal woman who is sedentary, double

---

monounsaturated fats lowers blood levels of low-density lipoprotein (LDL) without lowering levels of high-density lipoprotein (HDL), which is the type of lipid that absorbs extra cholesterol from the blood. Triglycerides, a type of fat found in fatty foods, butter, and both animal fats and plant oils, is stored in fat cells and released when the body needs energy. Excess triglycerides promotes production of LDL, may reduce HDL levels, and disrupts blood vessel function, among other mischievous acts. Fatty acids, on the other hand, such as those found in salmon, flaxseed, nuts, and seaweed, can reduce triglycerides, inhibit deposition of plaque, and generally reduce the risk of cardiovascular disease. In practice Laura has seen fat malabsorption (too much fat passing too quickly through the gut and not being absorbed) linked to bone density loss, and this can be a hidden cause when everything else seems to be in line. Investigation into this effect of fat malabsorption is ongoing, as there is not much research yet available. Note that in Traditional Chinese Medicine one of the prime herbs for fixing bones is named "Tonify Bone Fat."

Favorite Foods for Bones

Thanks to systematic, rigorous research, scientists have identified dozens of nutrients fundamental to bone health, and nutritionists know which foods, salts, and oils are rich stores of each. Most plant

that for women who are active. Considering protein requirements for building muscle, that means 20 to 25 percent of your daily calorie intake should be protein if you are an athlete or trying to build muscle—about 2 grams per kilogram. As a comparison, Laura's estimated daily protein intake averages 80 to 120 grams per day (depending on exercise), equivalent to 0.8 to 1.0 grams per pound of body weight.

Protein and Your Bones

Even though there is no universal recommended daily allowance of protein, scientists know quite a lot about the role of protein in bone health.

Collagen requires a ready source of protein for ongoing scaffold renewal. Thus, consuming some protein daily supports healthy bone regeneration. However, if protein intake is too low, the whole process of bone building will slow down, as the body senses missing resources and gives priority to other critical metabolic functions. The body's precision in managing is quite elegant and exciting.

Average daily consumption of protein in the United States is generally regarded as more than a human body needs, possibly much more than needed, and that can be detrimental. The body converts excess protein to sugar and fat. A buildup of unused protein stimulates a metabolic pathway that plays a role in cancers and in shortened life span. This pathway is not activated when protein consumption is moderate, and reducing this overload seems to reset the body and defuse the pathway. Consuming excess protein also produces excess nitrogenous waste, which must be cleared from the bloodstream. The nitrogenous waste goes out with water, so if you eat a lot of protein, it's a good idea to drink lots of water to ward off the risk of dehydration.

Note that if you are very active, pregnant, or breastfeeding, your body will use more protein than the average sedentary person does.

---

foods that are grown in rich soil, without the use of artificial chemical fertilizers and pesticides, will supply your body with a wide variety of nutrients. But when whole foods are subject to industrial-scale processing, many nutrients can be lost. Reducing your intake of processed foods is one of the best first steps you can take toward protecting your bones.

Depend on Diversity

Most of us have favorite foods. Preparing and enjoying them are among life's pleasures. And most of us have heard about the longevity benefits of certain foods such as nuts, seeds, berries, and cacao. But can you be properly nourished on a steady diet of a few favorite foods? Almost certainly not. Here are the three key reasons why.

1. Consuming a diverse diet of clean whole food and water enhances the diversity of beneficial gut microbiota. The benefits of this include a healthy gut lining and maximum potential to digest and absorb available nutrients.
2. When adopting a plant-forward diet, consuming a broad range of plant types and colors increases the likelihood of consuming sufficient nutrients to promote healthy cell function overall and the specific nutrients required for bone health.
3. If you eat mostly or only plant foods, the broader the range of foods you choose, the

more likely you are to include the amino acids required for complete protein.

Better Together: Companion Eating

Certain food pairings improve nutrient absorption, and you can make that work to your advantage. Some of the best pairings nutritionally are a wonderful combination of flavors, too!

VITAMIN C AND IRON

Cells that carry oxygen depend on iron for growth. Animal foods supply heme iron, and plant foods contain non-heme iron. Though heme is the more readily absorbed form, you can render them essentially equal by consuming iron-rich plant foods with any vitamin C–rich food. So mix and match! Some recipes to try: Green Pea and Roasted Red Pepper Mash (page 248), Golden Triangle Indian Mash (page 162), and Black Bean and Tofu Scramble Wraps (page 220).

Sources of Non-Heme Iron	Foods High in Vitamin C
chickpeas	bell peppers
dark chocolate	broccoli
dried beans	Brussels sprouts
lentils	cauliflower
molasses	citrus fruits
pine nuts	guava
pistachios	kale
spinach	kiwifruit
tofu	mango
	papaya
	peaches
	pineapple
	strawberries

Try spinach and pine nuts or tofu and bell peppers. Fancy a dark chocolate fondue with strawberries?

VITAMIN D AND CALCIUM

Calcium shies away from absorption but smiles when vitamin D shows up. Some perfect pairings of vitamin D and calcium include salmon or fresh mackerel with broccoli, bok choy, or arugula. Try scrambled eggs with maitake mushrooms and broccolini for brunch, or sunned mushrooms and tofu for an appetizing starter.

TOMATOES AND OLIVE OIL

Tomatoes and olive oil feature in so many recipes and no wonder: Olive oil, unlike other oils, fosters the absorption of lycopene in cooked tomatoes. Lycopene acts powerfully against inflammation. Together with oleocanthal, a chemical in extra-virgin olive oil, these two substances act against debilitating diseases such as some neurodegenerative diseases and some cancers. Tomato seeds and skin are also rich in digestive enzymes and lycopene.

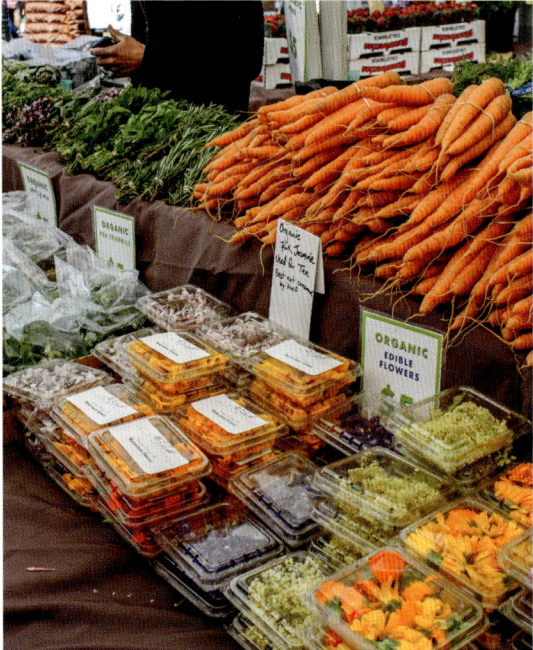

Figure 2.2. Floriphagia is a fancy term for eating flower petals. Edible flowers are gaining popularity at farmers markets because they offer not only beauty but nutrition, too.

24 ▪ *How Plants Nourish Bones*

BEANS AND RICE

The classic pairing of beans and rice provides the amino acid content for complete protein, and the beans supply fat with the fat-soluble vitamins A, D, E, and K. Peanut butter offers similar benefits to beans and rice and is self-contained, supplying in addition a healthy fat, peanut oil, and a luxurious level of vitamin E.

TURMERIC AND BLACK PEPPER

Turmeric is touted as a superfood, and indeed there are indications it has anti-inflammatory as well as other beneficial health and well-being effects. The assumed beneficial ingredient in turmeric, curcumin, is not easily absorbed, but an ingredient in black peppercorns, piperine, increases curcumin absorption by 2,000 percent. Fat is needed for full absorption as well. So add a piece of turmeric to tea; grate some into curries, rice, beans, juices, and smoothies; but don't forget to add a light shower of cracked black pepper and consume with or near a meal. Your bones will thank you.

Nutrients for Bone Health

Minerals such as calcium and metals such as iron are essential for building body structures such as bones and teeth. Calcium, magnesium, and phosphorus are key players here. They facilitate processes essential to life because of their roles in regulating cellular fluid balances and making hormones. And equally crucial, they help to boost the immune system.

We designate minerals as macrominerals and trace minerals. Macrominerals are those needed in larger amounts; they include calcium, chloride, magnesium, phosphorus, potassium, sodium, and sulfur.[8] The body stores smaller amounts of trace minerals, though they are equally essential to life. There are approximately seventy different minerals that the body needs in trace amounts for cellular function.

The popular press may lead one to believe that calcium and vitamin D are all that's required for healthy bones. However, although these two nutrients are key requirements—and bones would grow weaker without them—proper nutrient absorption relies on a much larger group of nutrients, including but not limited to vitamin D3, vitamin K2, magnesium, phosphorus, and trace minerals.

Bone RDA

Because genes play a role in how your body uses nutrients, as do your gut health and lifestyle, there isn't a one-size-fits-all recommendation for nutrient intake to ensure bone health. The RDA (recommended dietary allowance from the National Academies of Science, Engineering, and Medicine) and research-supported bone RDAs listed in table 2.1 are a general guideline. Laura strongly advises her patients to test nutrient levels in order to tailor their diets to their unique situation. A nutrition test will tell you what nutrients your body is absorbing and whether there are any nutrient deficiencies. Deficiencies may be due to lifestyle or genetics. A genetic test can rule out a genetic cause for a nutrient deficiency. (See "Summing Up Testing Needs" on page 85.)

The bone RDA (table 2.1, page 26) is for women ages 19 and up. The Office of Dietary Supplements at the National Institutes of Health lists RDA for women outside that range and for men of any age.[9]

Nutrient by Nutrient

Most bone-health nutrients are active at each stage of bone cell development, but some are prominent or unique to a particular stage and process. In this section, we present a summary of the nutrients that keep bone cells healthy from birth to sturdy skeleton. We focus on the roles each nutrient plays in bone health and offer a brief list of foods that are a particularly good source for each nutrient.

As you decide which foods to include when planning meals to support bone health, it's important to keep in mind that among the vitamins, some are water-soluble and some are fat-soluble. That is, to

Table 2.1. Bone-Health RDA Values for Protein, Minerals, and Vitamins

Nutrient	Recommended Daily Allowance
Boron	4 mg
Calcium	700–1,000 mg
Choline	445 mg
Chromium	50 mcg
Copper	2.5 mg
Fluoride	3–4 mg
Folate	400 mcg
Iodine	150 mcg
Iron	8 mg***
Magnesium	500–800 mg
Manganese	4 mg
Molybdenum	100 mcg
Phosphorus	700 mg
Potassium	4,300 mg
Protein	56 mg*
Selenium	100 mcg
Silica	180 mg
Strontium	20–50 mg
Sulfur	1,000 mg
Vitamin A (mixed carotenoids)	30,000–45,000 IU
Vitamin B1	1.1 mg
Vitamin B2	1.1 mg
Vitamin B3	14 mg
Vitamin B5	5 mg
Vitamin B6	1.3 mg
Vitamin B7	30 mcg
Vitamin B9	400 mcg
Vitamin B12	2.4 mcg
Vitamin C	900 mg
Vitamin D	5,000 IU**
Vitamin E	200 IU
Vitamin K2	350 mcg
Zinc	11 mg

* Minimum daily value for an average woman.
** Blood level 50–80 ng/ml.
*** Increase if menstrual periods are heavy.

be absorbed, the vitamin needs to be taken either with water or with fat. The water-soluble vitamins are the B vitamins and vitamin C. The fat-soluble vitamins are vitamins A, E, D, and K. For example, when enjoying spinach, carrots, or sweet potato (rich in vitamins A and E), you'll want to add a bit of coconut oil, butter, or ghee, because the fat in the coconut oil will facilitate absorption of the vitamins. The body can store fat-soluble vitamins; it generally does not store water-soluble vitamins. Without fat, vitamins A, E, D, and K are excreted.

For an overview of bone-health nutrients that includes more complete lists of foods, see table 2.2.

CALCIUM, OSTEOCALCIN, AND VITAMIN K2

The best way to obtain calcium and other key minerals is from food, but calcium alone cannot travel from your digestive system to your bones unless other nutrients are also present, including vitamins D and K2, magnesium, phosphorus, silicon, and trace minerals. For example, once you eat food that contains calcium, vitamin D3 fosters calcium absorption in the gut. In bones, calcium joins phosphorus and trace minerals to create hydroxyapatite. Amino acids, vitamin C, and trace minerals help collagen fibers crosslink and form the scaffold on which the bone mineral sits.

Vitamin K2 is rare in the diet though crucial for bones. Very few foods contain vitamin K2, and none that Westerners consume routinely. Laura recommends vitamin K supplements made from natto, one of the few foods that naturally contain K2, or supplements from bacteria that produce some vitamin K2 in the gut.

In the presence of vitamin K2, calcium binds with osteocalcin and remains in the bone. Osteocalcin is central to the binding of calcium to bone—a process called bone mineralization. The formation of osteocalcin happens through multiple metamorphoses. It is first pro-osteocalcin, which is not biologically active. Vitamin K is one of several nutrients required for the transformation of pro-osteocalcin to active

A Spinach Leaf

Spinach is recognized for its antimicrobial, anticarcinogenic, and antioxidant activity and is considered a highly bone-healthy leafy green vegetable. To help you understand exactly how nutrition nourishes bone, let's look at the nutrient content of the spinach leaf. Spinach is highly nutritious for bone health, but spinach also contains what is called an antinutrient, oxalate, a substance that binds to minerals and blocks or hinders our ability to absorb them. For this reason, we'll eat a wilted spinach leaf, because heat weakens oxalates and allows for better nutrient absorption. (Chapter 3 provides a detailed discussion of antinutrients and how to manage them.)

- The nutrient bounty in a spinach leaf includes protein and a good dose of fiber.
- Spinach contains high levels of micronutrients: 1 cup of cooked spinach contains 244 milligrams of calcium, 156 milligrams of magnesium, and 6 milligrams of iron (almost your daily need!) as well as vitamin K, zinc, copper, and manganese.
- Spinach also contains modest amounts of vitamins E, A, and C, as well as silicon, fluoride, boron, sulfur, folate, and vitamins B1, B6, and B2. That list covers the bases for all major nutrients required for healthy bones except vitamin D and omega fatty acids.
- If you eat spinach while sitting in the sun, you'll manufacture vitamin D, so critical for bone health. Eating spinach with chickpeas and sunflower seeds while sitting in the sun will provide complete protein and also a solid boost for your bone health.
- If you are flexitarian, eat spinach with pastured eggs or sustainable tuna, as they top the list for sources of vitamin B12.
- Spinach also contains phytoestrogens, wonderful molecules for bone health, as well as flavonoid polyphenols, necessary for bone and overall body health.

We find this bounty of nutrients in a spinach leaf wondrous. It offers a rich picture of the way a plant's nutrients act to nourish cells and life-sustaining processes such as cell metabolism and bone turnover, and it was our inspiration to gather together the discussion of bone-health nutrients that we present in this chapter.

---

osteocalcin. Vitamin D3 is also necessary for production of osteocalcin.[10] Vitamin K2 keeps osteocalcin in the bone, where osteocalcin binds to hydroxyapatite, the calcium and phosphorus compound that populates the collagen scaffold to create dense bones. If vitamin K2 is deficient, osteocalcin detaches from the bone and enters the bloodstream, where it can bind calcium. This compound circulates and may deposit in joints or blood vessel walls.

Keep in mind as well that calcium alone, such as one may consume in calcium pills, can settle in joints or blood vessels. If more than 500 milligrams of calcium is taken at one sitting, the excess is excreted. Calcium supplementation of 1,200 milligrams or more has consistently shown in research to correlate with increased cardiovascular events. If your health care professional advises that you take a calcium

(continued on page 32)

Table 2.2. Nutrition for Bones by Nutrient

Nutrient	Notes	Plant-food sources*		Bone RDA
B vitamins	Water soluble. Adequate B12 sustains bone density. Deficiency may imperil bone density and overall bone health. B12, B6, and folate break down homocysteine. High homocysteine may indicate vitamin B deficiency and lead to serious cardiovascular events.	nori nuts peas shiitake mushrooms		B1 1.1 mg B2 1.1 mg B3 14 mg B5 5 mg B6 1.3 mg B7 30 mcg B9 400 mcg B12 2.4 mcg
Boron	Vital for bone development. Helps to reduce calcium and magnesium excretion. Triggers vitamin D production. Enhances the body's use of estrogen, testosterone, and vitamin D. Boosts magnesium absorption. Raises levels of antioxidant enzymes. Protects against pesticide-induced oxidative stress and heavy-metal toxicity.	apples **avocado** bananas peaches peanuts	pears prunes, prune juice raisins sprouted beans walnuts	4 mg
Calcium	Principal mineral component (about 65%) of bone. Vitamin D must be present for proper absorption.	**arugula** bok choi broccoli dandelion greens dill fresh and dried figs nettle tea	sprouted almonds sprouted soybeans sprouted soy products (e.g., edamame, tofu, tempeh, miso, soy milk)	700–1,000 mg
Choline	For brain and nervous system, liver health, and cell membranes.	cruciferous vegetables shiitake mushrooms	soy products wheat germ	445 mg
Chromium	Enhances insulin's ability to promote glucose absorption. Enhances breakdown and absorption of carbohydrates, protein, and fats.	Brazil nuts brewer's yeast broccoli	grape juice, grapes whole grains	50 mcg
Copper	Aids in zinc absorption.	avocado basil blackberries chocolate cilantro **fennel bulb** mace nuts	pomegranates poppy seeds seeds spearmint turmeric wheat bran whole grains	2.5 mg

* Foods listed in bold are the richest sources of each nutrient.

28 ▪ *How Plants Nourish Bones*

Nutrient	Notes	Plant-food sources*	Bone RDA
Fluoride	Necessary for bones and teeth. Stimulates new bone formation and improves bone density in osteoporosis patients. Obtain fluoride from food.	**black tea** oatmeal potatoes raisins	20 mg
Iodine	Essential to healthy thyroid function. Thyroid or Hashimoto's disease patients should consult a health care provider before consuming seaweed regularly.	**kombu** nori wakame	150 mcg
Iron (non-heme)	Crucial for DNA replication, DNA repair, and health of oxygen-carrying cells. Found in plant foods. Absorption is improved with vitamin C. Vegetarians and vegans should consume many plants rich in non-heme iron (see page 75 for discussion of iron and vegan diets).	asparagus, beans, bok choy, chickpeas, **dark chocolate (minimum 70% cocoa)**, fennel bulb, kimchi, lemongrass, lentil sprouts, lentils, lima beans, molasses, morel mushrooms, mustard greens, onions, palm hearts, pea sprouts, peas, pine nuts, pistachios, pumpkin, red bell peppers, seeds and nuts, sweet potatoes, Swiss chard, tofu, tomatoes, wilted spinach	8 mg; increase if heavy periods
Magnesium	Prepares osteoprogenitor cells for mature roles in bone cell mineralization. Essential for bone health.	black beans, cashews, chia seeds, dark chocolate (minimum 70% cocoa), sprouted almonds, sprouted pumpkin seeds, tamarind, tiger nuts	500–800 mg
Manganese	Helps build connective tissue.	beans, black pepper, brown rice, **hazelnuts**, oatmeal, pecans, spinach	4 mg
Molybdenum	Unless otherwise advised by a health care provider, obtain only from food. Higher quantities than required can inhibit bone growth and lower bone mineral density.	beans, lentils, soy products (e.g., tofu, soy milk), soybeans, whole grains	100 mcg

* Foods listed in bold are the richest sources of each nutrient.

Feeding Your Bones

Table 2.2. (*continued*)

Nutrient	Notes	Plant-food sources*		Bone RDA
Omega-3 fatty acids	Anti-inflammatory. Important for reducing bone loss and reducing fracture risk.	algal oil Brussels sprouts chia seeds flaxseed	perilla oil soybeans walnuts	1.3 g
Phosphorus	Prepares osteoprogenitor cells for mature roles in bone cell mineralization. Joins with calcium to form the bone mineral scaffold.	Brazil nuts chickpeas sprouted beans sprouted lentils	**sprouted pumpkin seeds** sprouted sunflower seeds white beans	700 mg
Potassium	Prepares osteoprogenitor cells for mature roles in bone cell mineralization.	avocado **bananas** blackstrap molasses cantaloupe honeydew lima beans	nectarines parsnips potatoes spinach sweet potatoes Swiss chard tomatoes	4,700 mg
Protein	Human body is at least 20% protein. Collagen is a form of protein that builds bones.	amaranth buckwheat **hemp seeds** legumes Mankai duckweed mushrooms (shiitake, maitake, oyster, portobello, porcini)	nuts and seeds quinoa soy products spirulina sprouts whole grains	46 mg**
Selenium	Helps make DNA and protect against infection and cell damage. Essential to thyroid function. Limit consumption (see page 34).	asparagus **Brazil nuts** mushrooms	peas sesame seeds spinach	100 mcg
Silica	Promotes synthesis of collagen and hydroxyapatite (bone mineral) matrix mineralization.	bananas beer flour **green beans** mango	oat bran pineapple rice runner beans spinach	180 mg
Strontium	Absorbed and incorporated into bone. Found mainly in seawater. On a DEXA scan may impersonate calcium. May help balance bone turnover.	Brazil nuts carrots lettuce parsnip peas	root vegetable peels spinach wheat bran	20 mg
Sulfur	Helps the body make collagen and glucosamine for bone and joint health. Promotes absorption of heavy metals. For bone health, obtain only from food.	beans cruciferous vegetables nuts	onions seeds shallots whole grains	1,000 mg

* Foods listed in bold are the richest sources of each nutrient.
** Minimum quantity for an average woman.

Nutrient	Notes	Plant-food sources*		Bone RDA
Vitamin A	Fat soluble. Consume with olive, coconut, sesame, or avocado oil or other high-fat foods.	amaranth butternut squash carrots dandelion greens kale mango	orange squash red bell peppers spinach sweet potato Swiss chard turnip greens	30,000–45,000 IU mixed carotenoids
Vitamin C	Water soluble. Supports absorption of non-heme iron. Promotes collagen synthesis. Potent antioxidant.	acerola cherries bell peppers broccoli Brussels sprouts cabbage cauliflower citrus fruits guava kakadu plums kale	kiwifruit mango oranges papaya peaches **pine needle tea** pineapple strawberries	900 mg
Vitamin D	Fat soluble. Consume with oil or high-fat food such as avocado. Stimulates uptake of calcium from intestines. Important part in cell division. Supplement only if serum levels show deficiency.	**maitake mushrooms** other mushrooms, sunned		4 mg
Vitamin E	Fat soluble. Consume with olive, sesame, coconut, or avocado oil. Alpha-tocopherol (the form of vitamin E used by the human body) is a powerful antioxidant. Best to obtain from foods.	asparagus beet greens collard greens hemp seeds mangoes **peanut butter** pumpkin red bell peppers	spinach sprouted almonds sunflower seeds sunflower, safflower, and soybean oil wheat germ oil	200 IU
Vitamin K2	Fat soluble. Activates osteocalcin and keeps calcium in the bones. Increases collagen production and accumulation.	lacto-fermented foods	mk7 from natto **natto**	350 mcg
Zinc	Important to healthy DNA expression. Protects against free radicals. Helps repair damaged DNA.	avocado broccoli chickpeas hemp seeds kale lentils	nuts oats pumpkin sesame seeds spinach	11 mg

* Foods listed in bold are the richest sources of each nutrient.

> ### Make Your Own Calcium Supplement
>
> Eggshell calcium (calcium carbonate) is well-absorbed by the body. A homemade supplement is inexpensive to make if you or someone in your life eats eggs. We recommend eggs from pasture-raised hens because the nutrient value of both the egg and the shell will be higher. Here's how to make the calcium supplement.
>
> 1. Boil 12 eggshells for 15 minutes to sterilize.
> 2. Spread on a baking sheet and bake at 225°F (110°C) to dry completely, 15 minutes (or longer if you live at high altitude). Do not allow the shells to burn.
> 3. When shells have cooled, grind them to a fine powder in a coffee or spice grinder. Store in a glass jar.
>
> Half a teaspoon of this supplement provides approximately 400 milligrams of calcium.

(continued from page 27)

supplement, you may consider trying to increase your intake of calcium through foods, or by making your own eggshell-based calcium supplement (see above).

Although calcium is the main mineral component of bone, Laura has noted in practice that calcium deficiency is rarely the causal factor when a patient's bones have thinned; more often, deficiency of other nutrients is.

Favorite foods for calcium:
sprouted almonds, kale and other cabbage-family veggies, dandelion greens

MAGNESIUM

Magnesium is vital to more than 300 cellular processes. Magnesium affects osteocalcin levels and directly affects osteoblast/osteoclast differentiation and function, with a low concentration of magnesium inhibiting osteoblast activity, leading to increased bone breakdown.[11] Magnesium is also important for formation of enzymes that foster many processes involved in making bone. Protein, copper, and zinc are also needed for enzyme formation. In the presence of healthy levels of zinc, magnesium will be better absorbed. Pyridoxal-5-phosphate (the active form of vitamin B6) levels are also important, determining how much magnesium will be absorbed into cells.[12]

Favorite foods for magnesium:
dark chocolate, tiger nuts, leafy greens, edamame, pumpkin seeds

PHOSPHORUS

As noted earlier, phosphorus combines with calcium to create hydroxyapatite, the mineral that sits on a bone's collagen scaffold. Nonetheless, too much phosphorus and too little calcium from food raises parathyroid hormone (PTH) levels and pulls calcium from bone. Why? The answer has to do with regulation of the body's pH level. pH is a measure of the acid/base balance in the blood. Phosphorus is acid (low pH), while calcium is alkaline (high pH). The body has strict limits on acidity. A high level of acidity initiates calcium draw from bones. The alkaline calcium offsets the acidity, thus restoring the required pH balance. (For more about pH balance in the body, see "pH Balance and Bone Health" on page 61.)

Favorite foods for phosphorus: nuts, peanuts, whole grains, tofu, lima beans

POTASSIUM

Potassium helps the body maintain an alkaline environment, reducing the need to draw calcium from bone. Potassium also helps to limit the osteoclast population and sustain collagen strength. Potassium deficiency increases bone loss by activation of osteoclasts and inhibition of osteoblasts, causing a net loss of calcium from the skeleton and the deterioration of bone microarchitecture.[13]

Favorite foods for potassium: Swiss chard, spinach, avocado, sweet potato, bok choy

SULFUR

Sulfur in the diet forms a compound called methylsulfonylmethane, which inhibits RANKL, osteoclast formation, and bone resorption and suppresses the expression of several genes related to osteoclast growth.[14]

Favorite foods for sulfur: onions and other alliums, cruciferous vegetables such as cabbage and broccoli, legumes

ZINC

Zinc increases osteoblast activity and is necessary for collagen synthesis. It appears that the intake level needed to assist with increased bone mineral density (BMD) in postmenopausal women is higher than the current RDA of 8 milligrams per day; research supports 15 milligrams per day.[15]

Favorite foods for zinc: chickpeas, lentils, seeds, cashews

COPPER

Copper influences bone formation, skeletal mineralization, and collagen scaffold stability. Lysyl oxidase, a copper-containing enzyme, is essential for crosslinking of collagen fibrils, thereby increasing the mechanical strength of bone. Three milligrams per day of copper is associated with greater BMD.[16]

Favorite foods for copper: wheat, oats, mushrooms, cashews, potatoes

MANGANESE

Manganese is a partner in bone matrix formation and is a cofactor (a substance that is essential to enzyme action) for several enzymes in bone tissue. Women with osteoporosis tend to have lower blood manganese levels than women who do not have osteoporosis. Consuming 5 milligrams per day of

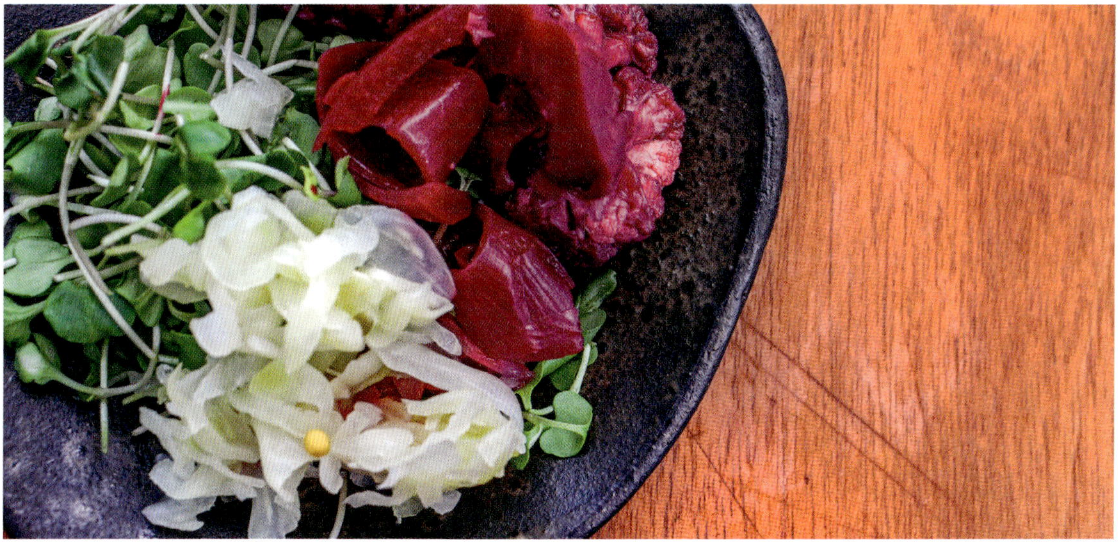

Figure 2.3. Jummee's gorgeous homemade pickles enhance digestion of any food.

Feeding Your Bones

The Selenium Quandary

Magnesium helps calcitonin redirect calcium from blood and body tissue to bones. As such, magnesium is a central player in preventing fractures and protecting bone mineral density.[17] Brazil nuts are a magnesium powerhouse. Since magnesium is elusive in foods, it seems as though eating Brazil nuts daily would be a good choice. However, these buttery, crunchy treats are also a rich selenium store, and that sets up a quandary.

Selenium is an important mineral because it is a component of enzymes and proteins involved in making DNA as well as in metabolism of thyroid hormones. However, selenium is a trace mineral. The body can welcome only tiny amounts, and anything that tips the balance into selenium excess can cause severe digestive distress—and in great excess, even kidney failure or death. Since Brazil nuts are very rich in selenium, and many other plant foods contain trace amounts of selenium as well, a safe level of consumption is up to three—yes, only three—Brazil nuts each day.

A trio of other foods rich in selenium—brown rice, spinach, and cashews—pose their own dilemmas. Brown rice often contains arsenic, so you should keep consumption very modest. Oxalates in spinach protect its nutrient store better than antinutrients in most other greens. Cashews offer an enviable nutrient profile, yet the shells contain a toxin that can leach onto the raw nut and cause both allergic reaction and gastrointestinal distress.

To provide the trace amounts of selenium the body needs, and in some cases magnesium, too, look to sprouted sunflower seeds,

---

manganese, either through food or supplement, is associated with better bone density.[21]

Favorite foods for manganese: hazelnuts, pecans, brown rice, black tea

VITAMIN A

The only form of vitamin A the body can use is called retinol. In plants, vitamin A is found in a group of chemicals called provitamin A carotenoids. Carotenoids alpha (α)-carotene, beta (β)-carotene, and β-cryptoxanthin must be converted to retinol in the body. Lutein and zeaxanthin are carotenoids that are not converted; they are absorbed directly into the macula of the eye to absorb blue light.

Both deficiency and excess of vitamin A negatively impact bone health. A healthy level of vitamin A, in balance with vitamin D, enhances osteoblast differentiation, promoting osteogenesis and suppressing inflammation.[22]

Favorite foods for vitamin A: sweet potatoes, carrots, cantaloupe, squash

VITAMIN D

When you expose your skin to direct sunlight, ultraviolet radiation promotes the formation of a vitamin D precursor called cholecalciferol. That chemical modulates (first via the liver, then the kidneys) to 25-hydroxyvitamin D, which is the immediate precursor to 1α,25-dihydroxyvitamin D, the active form your body tissue and genes need. When this active form binds to vitamin D receptors, which are found in every tissue of the body, it stimulates the

mushrooms, lentils (sprouted where possible), broccoli, and soaked oatmeal.

Correlational studies show that selenium plays an important part in bone health.[18] After controlling for variables, men whose diet included selenium showed higher bone density than men whose diet was deficient in selenium, and women whose diet included selenium developed osteoporosis notably less often than women whose diet did not include selenium.[19] Where this nutrient insinuates itself in bone health—in promoting bone growth, in slowing resorption, or on the vitality of cofactors such as vitamin K2—is under study.

Returning to consideration of Brazil nuts, they are also a top source of strontium, which the body needs in trace amounts, but more can be problematic, as explained in "Strontium," page 36.

So, how do we navigate this dilemma nature presents? Laura advises her patients to:

- Eat a Brazil nut or two each week, but no more than that.
- Always choose roasted cashews, unsalted. Cashews contain a toxic substance called urushiol. Heating breaks down the urushiol and renders it inactive. Typically, even commercially available raw cashews have been heated to weaken the toxic activity.
- Eat sprouted almonds daily, for calcium and also because they help to lower LDL without lowering HDL. (This effect is even more pronounced when you consume the almonds along with dark chocolate.)
- Dark chocolate and sprouted almonds are also a source of magnesium, as are avocados, legumes, and tofu.
- On many days each week, snack on a few hazelnuts and walnuts.[20]

uptake of calcium from the intestines, regulates many pathways, and regulates gene expression.[23]

Vitamin D facilitates calcium absorption in the gut and also coordinates the differentiation of precursor cells to osteoblasts and osteoclasts. With sufficient vitamin D, the system favors a vibrant bone-building population. A healthy level of vitamin D means that more osteoblasts are created.[24]

Calcitriol (1,25-dihydroxyvitamin D) is a hormone that liver and kidney enzymes manufacture from vitamin D. Calcitriol's most important action is to increase intestinal absorption of calcium and phosphorus. Severe vitamin D deficiency leads to a disease of defective mineralization called rickets in children and osteomalacia in adults. Subclinical vitamin D deficiency is found in a large part of the population of the United States as well as in Northern Europe, which experiences the so-called vitamin D winter, because the sun is farther away and the UVB rays are less intense, affecting the body's ability to produce vitamin D.

When your physician tests for vitamin D, the results report on 25-hydroxyvitamin D, which shows the resources for conversion to the final, active form in the kidney. Ideal blood level is 50 to 80 nanograms per milliliter.

Favorite "foods" for vitamin D: sunlight, maitake mushrooms

VITAMIN K2

Vitamin K exists in two forms, K1 and K2. Vitamin K2 is also called menaquinone (MK). Vitamin K2 comprises ten subtypes, MK4 to MK13. Two of these, MK4 and MK7, are the most nourishing for bones. In a healthy gut, vitamin K1 can convert to vitamin K2 (MK4), which activates osteocalcin, which in turn keeps calcium in the bone.[25] Vitamin B6 is a cofactor influencing the vitamin K2 activation of osteocalcin and the deposition of calcium in bone.

Very few foods supply vitamin K2, and few people on a Western diet consume the foods that do. For bone health, a daily supplement of vitamin K2 (MK7) or vitamin K2 (MK7 and MK4) is wise. Some vitamin K2 supplements are synthetic, and some are sourced from food. Laura advises her patients to take one sourced from food, preferably from natto, a fermented soybean product naturally rich in vitamin K2.

Some strains of gut bacteria produce vitamin K2; in addition, the bacteria used to produce Gouda cheese and the bacteria from natto are sources of vitamin K2. Fermented foods that produce lactic acid bacteria such as *Lactococcus lactis* help vitamin K2–producing bacteria thrive in the gut. In natto, the soy is fermented by *Bacillus subtilis*. This produces high levels of the MK7 form of vitamin K2. The average serving of natto itself provides about 350 micrograms of vitamin K2, the general dosage Laura recommends to her patients.

Proper vitamin K intake and transformation into K2 seems to slow or reduce calcium deposits in blood vessels, arterial stiffness, incidence of diabetes and coronary artery disease, and cardiovascular-related mortality.[26] The lower your bone density, the higher the risk of cardiovascular disease.[27] Cardiovascular disease is the number one killer of US women.

Favorite foods for vitamin K: Gouda cheese, natto

POLYPHENOLS

Flavonoid polyphenols—there are 8,000 known types; the most studied is resveratrol—are found in most dietary plants. Flavonoids include three flavonols—quercetin, kaempferol, and myricetin—and two flavones, apigenin and luteolin.[28] These substances exert anti-inflammatory or antioxidative effects, which inhibit RANKL binding, resulting in the suppression of osteoclastogenesis.[29] See also "Quercetin and Other Antioxidants" on page 66.

Favorite foods for polyphenols: blueberries, plums, dark chocolate, black olives, strawberries, cherries, elderberries, coffee

COLLAGEN

Collagen is an integral part of the scaffold that supports the mineral structure of bones, as well as skin and tendons. Collagen is the most abundant protein in the body, and it is unique because it lacks the amino acid tryptophan, which all other known proteins require. Vitamin K2 (MK7 and MK4) not only modulates the deposition of calcium in bone but also increases collagen production and accumulation.[30]

Vitamin C is required for crosslinking collagen fibers in the collagen matrix of bone and stimulates alkaline phosphatase activity, which is a marker for osteoblast formation.

In unhealthy bone, or if bone building takes place when the body is suffering inflammation, the collagen strands will be less random and more uniform, and the final structure will be more vulnerable to impact. If vitamin C and some key trace minerals are missing, then crosslinking for stability will be less effective.

Favorite foods for collagen: Naturally occurring collagen comes from animals, but those on a plants-only diet can boost collagen production by consuming foods rich in vitamin C, such as citrus fruits, beans, and tomatoes.

STRONTIUM

Strontium, a mineral, is present in small amounts in a multitude of plant foods. Like calcium, it can actually attach to the bone's hydroxyapatite scaffold. In a DEXA scan strontium can impersonate calcium—when measuring bone density, the radiologist cannot distinguish calcium from strontium. Strontium-enriched hydroxyapatite may or may not have the same integrity of calcium-rich hydroxyapatite; research is ongoing. There is evidence that strontium has a positive impact on bone turnover, but high levels of strontium in the blood or urine can pose a risk of kidney toxicity.[31] Until research clarifies, limit intake of strontium to bone RDA levels, most of which you can attain via diet.

Favorite foods for strontium: cereals, grains, seafood

FLUORIDE

Fluoride is a trace mineral that is necessary for healthy bones and teeth. Fluoride increases the structural stability of hydroxyapatite and stimulates osteoblasts, thus increasing bone strength and density.

A trace level of intake, such as one part per million in the water supply or 3 to 4 milligrams per day, is optimal. Drinking two cups of black tea provides the full daily requirement for fluoride. Too much fluoride (greater than four parts per million in the water supply or a dose of greater than 50 milligrams per day) appears to increase fracture rate.

TAURINE

Taurine is an atypical amino acid that does not combine with other amino acids to form protein. Taurine was at first thought to play an essential part in bone and connective tissue health. Later, scientists found that taurine is also important to eye health, blood pressure control, thyroid regulation, kidney function, weight control, and mental health. In supplement form, taurine may be a therapy against congestive heart failure[32] and high blood pressure[33] and is under investigation as a mechanism to control plaque formation and deposition.

The human body biosynthesizes taurine from cysteine. When extra supply is required—taurine production declines as the body ages—meat is the primary source; beef, poultry, scallops, octopus, and pastured eggs supply taurine generously. In plant sources, nori seaweed is tops, followed by brewer's yeast, almonds, cashews, hazelnuts, and pine nuts. Speak with a health care provider before supplementing with taurine.

CHOLINE

Although choline is rarely included in conversations about nutrition, it is vital for metabolic health, especially as we age, and is implicated in bone density.[34] Deficiency also causes abnormal fat deposition in the liver, which is a cause of nonalcoholic fatty liver disease, a condition that is significantly increasing in the United States. Choline influences cognitive function, fat transport, neurotransmitter synthesis, and cell signaling, and it is vital for cell membranes in the brain as well as for dopamine (a neurotransmitter) receptors.

Together with several B vitamins—folate, vitamin B6, vitamin B12, and riboflavin—choline is required for the metabolism of nucleic acids, which are the principal component of DNA, and metabolism of amino acids that combine to form protein. This choline-vitamin combination is essential to the breakdown of homocysteine, which is key to some amino acid processes. However, homocysteine accumulation can set off an inflammatory response, which can trigger a loss of bone mineralization.

Favorite foods for choline: Brussels sprouts, shiitake mushrooms, broccoli, eggs

SILICON

There is a correlation between silicon in the diet and connective tissue health, with an important role in synthesis of collagen and mineralizing the

Feeding Your Bones • 37

> **Fulvic and Humic Acid Supplements**
>
> Minerals are naturally present in rock, soil, and water, and plants take up these minerals as they grow. Animals then take in the minerals as they eat plants (or other animals). Over millions of years, as plants and animals die and decompose, minerals have been compressed into layers in the earth. These layers contain fulvic and humic acid compounds, which are mineral compounds containing virtually all the trace minerals body and bone require. This form of mineral is very useful for health and can be used in place of other trace mineral supplements.

hydroxyapatite matrix, strengthening bones, skin, hair, ligaments, and tendons.

Dietary silicon is predominantly found in plant foods. Sufficient silicon (~180 milligrams per day) correlates to higher BMD. Silicon induces expression of gene patterns associated with osteogenesis.[35] This expression functions best in the presence of estrogen, so optimum silicon early in life helps increase BMD before hormones, particularly estrogen, begin to decline. Postmenopause, silicon acts to strengthen connective tissue and collagen synthesis but may not directly increase BMD.[36]

Beer is the best-known source of dietary silicon, but silicon is ubiquitous in the plant kingdom, as plants take up silicon from the soil to strengthen their stems. As such, cereals, vegetables, and fruits offer silicon benefits. On a dry weight basis, oat bran contains the highest amount of silicon; then look to cereal flours, bananas, pineapple, mangoes, green beans, runner beans, spinach, and coriander, with lentils and soy products as runners-up.[37]

Favorite foods for silicon: oat bran, cereals, bananas, beans

BORON

Boron influences the production of sex hormones, thereby assisting in osteogenesis and bone loss prevention. Three milligrams per day is the minimum for maintaining BMD at age 19 and up.[38]

As advanced equipment enables more discrete assessment of chemical effects, scientists have ascertained that this trace mineral plays vital roles in metabolism. These include:

- bone development and regeneration
- reduction of calcium and magnesium excretion
- vitamin D production and metabolism
- enhancement of the body's use of estrogen, testosterone, and vitamin D and increases in serum levels of estradiol, the most potent form of estrogen
- improved magnesium absorption and, to a lesser extent, calcium absorption
- increased levels of antioxidant enzymes that scavenge free radicals such as superoxide dismutase (SOD), catalase, and glutathione peroxidase
- protection against pesticide-induced oxidative stress and heavy-metal toxicity[39] (see "Oxidative Stress and Antioxidants" on page 63 for an explanation of oxidative stress)

Favorite foods for boron: prunes, raisins, peanuts, avocado

CHROMIUM

Chromium is a nutrient the body does not make. Although chromium is ordinarily a concern for pancreatic health and insulin resistance, not bone health, this nutrient is important for people who rely in large part or entirely on plant foods because it plays a central role in breakdown and absorption of carbohydrates, fat, and protein. Vitamins B3 and C improve chromium absorption. If you have insulin resistance, check with your doctor about safely increasing chromium supplementation by up to 200 milligrams per day.

Favorite foods for chromium: grapes, broccoli, Brazil nuts, brewer's yeast

A Resource for Nutrient Data

Few of us could memorize all the nutrients and nutrient levels in the hundreds of consumable plants and fungi available. Fortunately, an excellent and cost-free online source of nutrient information exists: MyFoodData (www.myfooddata.com). MyFoodData offers, cost free, many nutrition tools, including an amino acid calculator for individual foods, for food combinations, and for recipes. On the MyFoodData website you can search by individual foods, by food combinations, by amino acid levels, by ingredients lists, or by recipes. You can store your own information at the site, too, including recipes and your modifications of them. It is a remarkable resource that eases the transition to a plant-forward life and allows us to have great fun testing ingredient combinations that will provide exactly the levels of nutrients we need.

If you rely on a plant-based diet, it is crucial to learn which foods contain protein and which foods can be combined make a complete protein. Another MyFoodData tool, the nutrition calculator, helps with this by reporting the content of calories, vitamins, minerals, protein, fat, carbohydrates, and amino acids in individual foods.

MyFoodData founder Paul House began his career as a data analyst in health care quality improvement in nursing home and home health settings. He became convinced that making healthy nutrition choices was one of the best ways to improve quality of health late in life.

House notes that there are many variations in the nutritional content of foods in nature. MyFoodData uses data from the USDA FoodData Central dataset. The USDA analyzed several samples for each of the commonly eaten fruits, vegetables, grains, and other foods to generate the data.

The data from the USDA is based on samples from the United States. Farming practices such as organic farming and raising livestock on pasture impact the nutritional content of foods in different ways, but it is not possible for the dataset to account for differences in soil quality. Preparation and processing, for example, heating of foods, such as in pasteurization of apple cider and other juices, also has an effect on certain vitamins but not on minerals.

Users may enter their own foods and recipes into MyFoodData as a way of tracking, analyzing, and understanding their diets. MyFoodData will be forever free with unlimited use of the tools, according to House. Users are welcome to add foods, compare foods, sort foods, and build recipes and meals. All the data from the tools is sharable and printable.

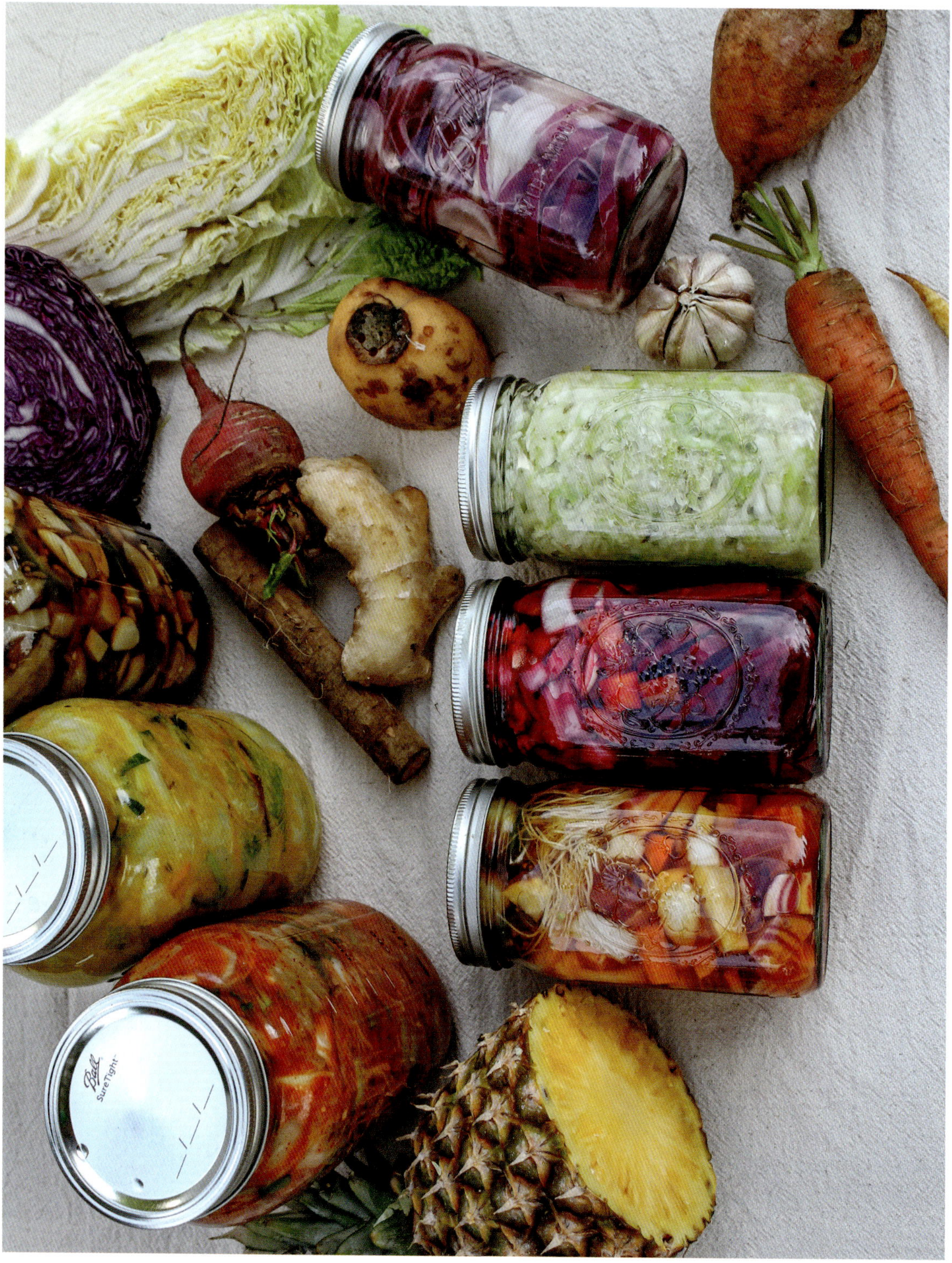

Figure 3.1. Fermenting plant foods powerfully reduces their content of phytates and oxalates.

CHAPTER 3

Managing Antinutrients and Acrylamide

The road to plant-forward eating is lined with opportunities for developing new culinary skills and enjoying delicious food. Yet plant foods are complicated individuals, requiring some time and attention to make them optimally nutritious and a generous contributor to bone health. There are two forces hidden in plain sight that we must rout out lest they thwart our efforts to rely on plant foods, in part or wholly, to nourish body and bone.

Every growing plant contains an army of chemicals that protect it from predators and continue its duties even after the plant is harvested and headed for the digestive tract. These chemicals are called antinutrients because they inhibit or interfere with nutrient absorption and/or irritate gastrointestinal tissue. There are several kinds of antinutrients, including lectins, which you may have heard of as a possible cause of leaky gut. The good news is that it is possible to weaken the effects of antinutrients by preparing plant foods properly before eating them.

The other force we must counteract is a group of chemicals that can form due to some of the ways we cook plant foods. In particular, a substance called acrylamide can compromise or harm health in many parts of the body, including bones.

Meet the Antinutrients

Everything alive has prey and is prey. Simultaneously, everything alive has both defenses to ward off aggressors and internal mechanisms to help ensure survival. Examples of natural defenses are abundant: Roses and hedgehogs have prickles; grasses have serrated edges; and snails have shells. Mosquitoes have the ability to inject blood-thinning substances when they bite their prey, which improves the chances of obtaining a full meal from each bite.

Since plants and fungi cannot hide from the animals and microbes that want to eat or infect them, they have abundant and varied specialized defenses against predation and disease in the form of odors, toxins, bitter-tasting coatings, and chemical signals to warn their neighbors of danger. These chemicals are an integral part of almost all plant foods. Most seeds contain biochemicals that act as strong chemical locks on their nutrients to keep the nutrients safe until the time the seed sprouts and the nutrients are needed to support the new seedling's growth.

There are dozens of such chemicals, and these antinutrient compounds ride in with foods as we consume them. Several types provide important health benefits, such as antioxidant and anti-inflammatory activity, but others can be anywhere from

Table 3.1. Plant Compounds, Food Sources, and Clinical Implications

Antinutrient	Food sources	Suggested clinical implications
Lectins	Legumes, cereal grains, seeds, nuts, fruits, vegetables	Altered gut function; inflammation
Oxalates	Spinach, Swiss chard, sorrel, beet greens, beet root, rhubarb, nuts, legumes, cereal grains, sweet potatoes, potatoes	May inhibit calcium absorption; may increase calcium kidney stone formation
Phytates (IP6)	Legumes, cereal grains, amaranth, quinoa, millet, nuts, seeds	May inhibit absorption of iron, zinc, and calcium; acts as an antioxidant; antineoplastic effects
Goitrogens	Kale, Brussels sprouts, cabbage, turnip greens, Chinese cabbage, broccoli, millet, cassava	Hypothyroidism and/or goiter; inhibit iodine uptake
Phytoestrogens	Soybeans and soy products, flaxseed, hops, maca root	Endocrine disruption; increased risk of estrogen-sensitive cancers
Tannins	Tea, cocoa, grapes, berries, apples, stone fruits, nuts, beans, whole grains	Inhibit iron absorption; negatively impact iron stores

Reprinted with permission. Source: Weston Petroski and Deanna M. Minich, "Is There Such a Thing as 'Anti-Nutrients'? A Narrative Review of Perceived Problematic Plant Compounds," *Nutrients* 12, no. 10 (October 2020): 2929, https://doi.org/10.3390/nu12102929.

mildly disruptive to strongly compromising to well-being and health. Though clinical information is not yet available about the action or impact of some, several have been thoroughly studied and their mechanisms of action are well documented, so we may reliably plan to sidestep some of the negative influence. The name "antinutrients" is a good fit for these substances, because they often bind to nutrients and hold on tight even in the acidic gastrointestinal environment, inhibiting or preventing nutrient absorption. Antinutrients also sometimes irritate or lock on to gut tissue, which can cause perforations in the gut lining, opening two-way traffic and a range of inflammatory responses.

There is evidence that these chemicals can be beneficial, acting as antioxidants, for example, and there are some studies that show higher levels of phytates linked to better bone density. It is likely that those with higher phytate levels consume more healthy plant foods, thereby linking phytates and bone density. We provide all of this information to help you optimize your food, and suggest bringing these preparation methods into your repertoire over time.

In a 2020 article in the journal *Nutrients*, nutritionists Weston Petroski and Deanna M. Minich summarized the cooking methods that weaken specific antinutrients and the cooking methods that can strengthen each one and extend its influence.[1] Tables 3.1 and 3.2 summarize this information.

Glucosinolates and Goitrogens

Glucosinolates and goitrogens are secondary compounds found principally in soy, cassava, and cruciferous vegetables such as mustard and cabbage. Glucosinolates help plants ward off predators, and there are more than 100 kinds, including mustard oil. They interfere with iodine absorption, which may affect thyroid function. Goitrogens actively disrupt the production of thyroid hormones. This triggers the pituitary to release thyroid-stimulating hormone, which then promotes the growth of thyroid tissue, eventually leading to goiter.

How to counteract: Fermentation is especially effective at weakening goitrogens, and seaweed will balance them out by providing iodine.

Table 3.2. Effects of Food Preparation Methods on Antinutrients

Antinutrient	Methods that reduce	Methods that increase
Lectins	Soaking, boiling, autoclaving, sprouting, fermentation	Roasting, baking
Oxalates	Soaking, boiling, steaming, pairing with high-calcium foods	Roasting, grilling, baking
Phytates	Soaking, boiling, sprouting, fermentation	
Tannins	Cooking, peeling skins of fruits and nuts	
Saponins	Washing, fermenting	High-temperature cooking
Phytoestrogens		Boiling, steaming, fermenting (increases aglycone content)
Goitrogens	Steaming, boiling	

Reprinted with permission. Source: Weston Petroski and Deanna M. Minich, "Is There Such a Thing as 'Anti-Nutrients'? A Narrative Review of Perceived Problematic Plant Compounds," *Nutrients* 12, no. 10 (October 2020): 2929, https://doi.org/10.3390/nu12102929.

Lectins

Lectins are proteins that bind to carbohydrates, and they are present in most carbohydrate-rich plant foods, from beans and grains to bananas and potatoes. These substances have some desirable effects, such as stimulating the growth of some bone marrow cells that are osteoblast cell precursors. However, lectins can interfere with absorption of calcium, iron, phosphorus, and zinc. When foods that contain lectins are eaten raw, the lectins can bind to the gut tissue and poke holes in it, causing the condition called leaky gut that can permit toxins to leak out of or into the intestinal tract.

> **How to counteract:** Lectins are water soluble, so the best way to prepare foods that contain lectins is to soak them for several hours or cook them in wet high heat, such as by steaming or boiling them.

Oxalates

These compounds are found in many foods your bones love: leafy green vegetables, tea, beans, nuts, and beets, among others. Oxalates bind tightly to calcium in the kidney such that the calcium cannot be absorbed, and the calcium oxalate joins uric acid to form crystals that can cluster into kidney or gallbladder stones. Ironically, consuming oxalate-rich food with calcium-rich food *reduces* calcium in the body, because the oxalates bind to the calcium in the digestive system and both the oxalates and calcium are then excreted through the stool. If oxalate does not bind to calcium in the gut, it is resorbed, passes into urine, and while in the kidney may bind with calcium and uric acid to form a stone.

Unlike some other antinutrients, oxalates hang on stubbornly in some plant foods, even through steaming or boiling. If you are eating a high-oxalate diet, it is important to be mindful of consuming calcium that remains bioavailable. Broccoli, Brussels sprouts, kale, arugula, mustard greens, and romaine lettuce (and most lettuces) are calcium rich and relatively low in oxalates.

> **How to counteract:** To weaken oxalate's grip, add juice of lemons or any citrus fruit. This is especially effective at weakening the hold oxalates have on calcium. The citric acid binds to calcium in the urine, preventing calcium from binding to the oxalate and thereby preventing the formation of stones. Keep in mind, though, that whether the calcium binds to oxalates or to citrate, the net result is that you lose the calcium.

Phytates

Phytates, also called phytic acid, are agents that bind to minerals in just about every carbohydrate-rich plant food: whole grains, seeds, legumes, and most nuts, especially in the skins. (Macadamia nuts and pistachios are the exceptions.) The role of phytates in nature is to protect nutrients until a seed germinates.

> **How to counteract:** Sprouting is especially effective at weakening phytates because sprouting mimics the conditions for germination and signals the seed to dissipate the phytate, as it is no longer needed. Cooking, soaking (for between two hours and overnight, depending upon the food), fermenting, and pickling break down phytic acid. Some gut bacteria make phytase, the enzyme that breaks down phytic acid.

Saponins

Saponins are plant compounds that act as natural insecticides to protect the plants from pests. They exist principally in legumes and whole grains. Quinoa contains saponins in addition to oxalates and phytates. Solanine, a toxin found in nightshade plant foods, is also a saponin. Solanine is principally found in potatoes but also in tomatoes, capsicum peppers, and eggplant. If you consume moderate amounts of saponin-rich foods, it may help to decrease blood lipid levels and improve insulin sensitivity.[2]

> **How to counteract:** It's easy to weaken the effect of saponins by washing or soaking most types of legumes and grains for fifteen minutes before cooking them. Boiling tomatoes or eggplant does not weaken solanine, but sautéing or frying them does. Solanine increases in potatoes the longer they are stored, whether in a dark place or in the light. If you fry potatoes, keep the temperature low so that, in order to avoid acrylamide formation, the potatoes become golden rather than crunchy.

Tannins

Despite the justified, widely advertised benefits of resveratrol—a polyphenol that is proven to have anti-inflammatory effects in the body—the tannins present in red wine and other foods such as tea, coffee, and legumes can inhibit both heme and non-heme iron absorption. The following foods contain resveratrol but relatively little tannins: peanuts (without the skins), cocoa, blueberries, mulberries, and jackfruit. It appears that a cup of itadori tea (Japanese knotweed) contains as much naturally occurring resveratrol as is in a glass of red wine.

> **How to counteract:** Boiling reduces tannin content.

Overcoming Obstacles

It would be easy to feel overwhelmed about how to overcome these obstacles on a daily basis as you prepare meals. We subscribe to the view of Chinese philosopher Lao Tzu: "The journey of a thousand miles begins with one step."

Germinating (sprouting) seeds and nuts and fermenting are two ways you can prepare foods to weaken and reduce the effect of antinutrients. Once a seed or nut has sprouted, the antinutrients it contains release their hold on nutrients. You can sprout many kinds of beans and seeds (see "Easy Breezy Home Sprouting" on page 198). Try mung beans, adzuki beans, and alfalfa. Once sprouted, beans, nuts, seeds, legumes, and grains offer nutrients in bioavailable form.

Fermentation, a chemical reaction between yeast or bacteria and glucose or other carbohydrate, results in the breakdown of carbohydrates and sugar into lactic acid and alcohol. Fermentation has been used for millennia to preserve food. More recently, science has shown that the reaction also breaks down a compound called phytic acid that is found in many plant foods. Breaking down phytic acid renders other nutrients in a food bioavailable.

Fermenting some plant foods, such as corn, makes iron more bioavailable as well. In a healthy gut, fermented foods support the growth of beneficial bacterial populations. (See chapter 11 for instructions on what and how to ferment.)

For some antinutrients, the solution may be as simple as soaking the food in water. For example, soak rolled or steel-cut oats overnight in warm water with a half teaspoon of vinegar (preferably bone-building vinegar, which is sweet and pleasingly aromatic; see "Dr. Laura's Bone Vinegar" on page 137). In the morning, pour off the soaking water and then rinse the oats through a strainer in warm water. Any remaining vinegar in the oats will be undetectable, and the oats will be free of the antinutrients called phytates. Serve rolled oats immediately; cook steel-cut oats to make porridge.

Acrylamide and Bone Fracture

Some food, when it meets oxygen, turns brown. Think of cut apples left to stand. Typically, this makes the food less than appetizing but not risky to eat. However, another type of browning—the browning that results from applying heat to protein, fats, and sugars—can be detrimental to health. In this case the chemical changes and accompanying odors and tastes that stimulate the production of gastric juices also produce substances called advanced-glycation end products (AGEs). AGEs cause damage to blood vessels, tissues, and DNA, resulting in inflammation, contributing to Alzheimer's disease, heart disease, diabetes (and its complications such as neuropathy), and renal failure. What kinds of foods are we talking about? Think coffee beans, meat on the grill, potatoes in the fry basket, caramelized onions, bread fresh from the oven.

What Is Acrylamide?

The browning of food is called the Maillard reaction, named for an early-twentieth-century French chemist and physicist, Louis-Camille Maillard, who became curious about why food tastes better cooked. He discovered that a host of chemical changes take place when food containing amino acids and certain groups of sugars is heated.

As scientists began to deconstruct the chemical changes in various plant foods that brown and invite us, they found a worrying by-product of the Maillard reaction—a chemical called acrylamide. Acrylamide, once consumed, breaks down into an organic compound called glycidamide. Glycidamide molecules can interact with DNA, damaging it and causing mutations. Recently research has found that glycidamide may arise as an intermediate in the cooking process during the formation of acrylamide.

At first chemists thought that acrylamide formed only in starchy foods cooked at very high temperatures, but ongoing research has found that just about any starchy plant food (including nuts, seeds, and mushrooms) cooked at high temperatures or roasted enough to brown the edges will have a modicum of acrylamide. Acrylamide is a strongly suspected agent

> ## Soldiers for Bone Health
>
> If you include eggs in your diet, try egg on toast—or soldiers, as breakfast toast strips are called in Britain. Be sure to choose pasture-raised eggs, which contain significantly more vitamins D, A, and E than conventional eggs. They also provide carotenoids in a natural matrix with the fats required for vitamin A and E absorption and a healthy ratio of omega-3 to omega-6 fatty acids. By making that toast golden and barely crunchy, not dark, you substantially reduce the acrylamide risk.

of neurotoxicity and strongly implicated in Parkinson's disease, Alzheimer's disease, amyotrophic lateral sclerosis (ALS), and progressive cognitive decline. Furthermore, research suggests that acrylamide can cross the placental barrier and affect a fetus.[3]

In the course of studying the carcinogenic properties of acrylamide, several scientists wondered whether acrylamide could impact bone precursors or bone itself. After eight years following acrylamide consumption among more than 4,000 people, and accounting for key variables, one study had this bottom line: High dietary acrylamide is associated with an increased risk of osteoporotic fractures.[4] Furthermore, there is substantial evidence that acrylamide and all other advanced glycation end products, mediated by oxidative stress, induce cell death across many organs and systems including death of bone marrow cells, where bone cell precursors are born.[5]

Since the appetizing properties of so many nutritious foods would be lost without the Maillard reaction, scientists are searching for a way to foil the acrylamide, to stop it in its tracks during cooking. Scientists are beginning to test the possibility that asparaginase, the enzyme that helps the body digest the amino acid asparagine—which is an essential element in the Maillard reaction—might be used to digest acrylamide before it enters the food source.[6]

Minimizing the Risk

Meanwhile, what can you do to minimize the downside of consuming acrylamide? Should you avoid cooking and baking that produces browning? Not at all. As with most things, it's a matter of moderation and common sense. We recommend that you take care to consume *blackened* foods only sparingly, but don't worry too much about baking bread or other dishes to the golden brown stage.

You can also put your ground coffee into an unbleached paper filter. Acrylamide collects in the oils, and the paper filter catches and holds the oils, so less acrylamide will end up in the coffee itself. Take note that many coffee substitutes, along with most instant coffee products, are higher in acrylamide than ground fresh roasted beans.

Acrylamide forms easily when cooking food that is rich in asparagine (along with other amino acids), food that contains starch, and food that is relatively dry in raw form. Acrylamide forms most easily in tubers such as potatoes and in wheat and oat flours, which are high in asparagine. To reduce the chance of acrylamide forming, before cooking starchy vegetables, soak them in water for half an hour or in water with a half teaspoon of vinegar for a few minutes.

Frying potatoes produces a big acrylamide hit, and potato chips (or vegetable chips) contain about four times more than the raw vegetable. Boiling creamy organic yellow or red potatoes and warming the flavor by adding some good olive oil or cultured butter, perhaps some chives or minced garlic, can easily displace those fries as first choice. So put fries on your *occasionally* list and make roasted vegetables a treat rather than a weekly event.

One final tip: Add a big pinch of fresh or organic dried rosemary to bread dough. Research shows that rosemary oil stops acrylamide formation during baking.[7] Rub the rosemary needles between your

Nachos and Beer?

The deleterious effects of alcohol on bone are known, and acrylamide also has a deleterious effect on many cells including bone. So you might think that nachos and beer is a terrible combination. However, here's some little-known information: Consuming a food high in acrylamide simultaneously with alcohol significantly *reduces* the deleterious effect of alcohol on bone.

palms to release the oil, then drop the leaves into the dough and proceed with kneading.

Small Steps to Start With

Here are some suggestions for specific food combinations that overcome some of the problems antinutrients pose.

- **Spinach and tomatoes.** Try fresh wilted spinach with olive oil, garlic, and sautéed tomatoes. To prepare the wilted spinach, triple wash and soak the spinach for twenty minutes—soaking will be a start toward defanging the very strong hold oxalate has on spinach's impressive calcium store—then sauté in water or olive oil. Although tomato peels and seeds nourish the body with lycopene, they also contain lectins. If lectins affect your digestion, peel and seed the tomatoes before sautéing them. Sautéing reduces the solanine content. Also try our Silky Tofu–Spinach Dip (page 141) or Sweet Potato Boats with Creamy Spinach (page 238).
- **Beets.** Combine beets, watercress, and pistachios with olive oil and lemon juice vinaigrette. The lemon juice reduces the hefty helping of oxalates in beets to a whimper. Watercress, along with kale, is a low-oxalate green. Pistachios are among the lowest phytate edible seeds (called nuts for convenience, they are neither legumes nor nuts but nutrient-dense seeds of the pistachio tree). Try one of our lemon vinaigrette recipes in chapter 10 for a delicious finish.
- **Sweet potatoes.** Boil sweet potatoes to minimize both oxalates and acrylamide. Eat the potato skin and all.
- **Apples and pears.** To reduce tannins, poach instead of roasting or baking these fruits.
- **Nuts.** Almonds, walnuts, and Brazil nuts are among the most nutrient-rich nuts, but they are also highest among nuts in phytic acid. Choose

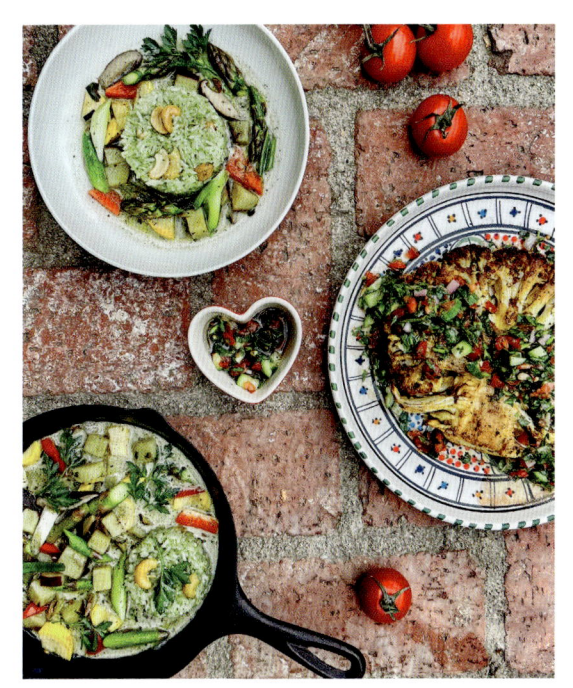

Figure 3.2. Once you learn the preparation methods to counteract antinutrients, you will delight in combining fresh vegetables and other plant foods into salads, soups, and main dishes like these (recipes for all these dishes are in part 2).

sprouted almonds and, where possible, remove the skins. Or sprout your own, following the same method as for sprouting beans (see "Easy Breezy Home Sprouting," page 198).

Soak walnuts and Brazil nuts in water with some salt for at least twelve hours, preferably not refrigerated. Drain them well. Then dehydrate the nuts in a food dehydrator if you have one. If not, spread the well-drained nuts in a single layer on a baking tray and dry them in the oven at 115°F (45°C) for 12 hours.

While soaking is the first step in sprouting any lentil or bean, the question of sprouting nuts is more nuanced. Almonds sprout readily and show a root. After soaking and dehydrating walnuts, pistachios, and Brazil nuts, you will not see a tail, but soaking and dehydrating still may weaken the antinutrients they contain. Hazelnuts need exposure to a long period of cold temperatures to stimulate germination, but they are low in phytates, so most people can eat hazelnuts without any pretreatment. Cashews are not true nuts; botanically speaking a cashew is a drupe, a seed within a fleshy fruit. Commercially available cashews are pretreated to remove the toxin urushiol, so they are no longer viable and will not sprout.

- **Bok choy with mushrooms.** Try bok choy, cilantro/coriander, onion, garlic, and a clutch of mushrooms. Bok choy is among the lowest-oxalate vegetables, and its enviable provision of an antioxidant called quercetin makes it among the best anti-inflammatory vegetables. Cilantro and coriander chelate heavy metals, mushrooms improve metabolic health, onions are prebiotic (your good gut bacteria will thank you), and garlic attends to your blood pressure. If you are pescatarian, add some shrimp. Season with dill for calcium; red pepper flakes are optional.
- **Chocolate.** Nature is perpetually contrary, and nothing shows off this dual nature better than chocolate. Cacao beans are fermented, which helps to defuse tannins, and roasted in order to develop the cacao flavor used to make chocolate. The roasting process can cause high levels of acrylamide to form. Although dark chocolate offers legion health benefits, it contains more acrylamide than products that have a lower cocoa content. So, what about cacao nibs? Those sold as raw are typically fermented but unroasted, and there is strong evidence raw cacao nibs offer the antioxidant anti-inflammatory benefits that are linked to 70 percent or higher dark chocolate along with some suggestion that they help to reduce insulin resistance.[8] We also note that most commercial chocolate is reported to contain some level of heavy metals.
- **Green tea.** A component of green tea, catechins, seems to slow down the growth of osteoclast precursor cells in bone marrow, which helps to right the imbalance in favor of osteoblasts in cases of osteoporosis. However, green tea also contains tannins that can inhibit iron and zinc absorption. The solution is simple: Drink your tea half an hour before or after your meal.
- **Dried fruit.** Let boron-rich prunes be your dried-fruit go-to. For most people, prunes appear to be a bone-protective food, even though prunes develop a small amount of acrylamide during the drying process.[9] Between two and six prunes a day appears to protect bone density. Avoid prune juice, though, because it is strikingly high in acrylamides. You might also enjoy an occasional small handful of dried mulberries. Mulberries are a fine source of calcium, in addition to vitamin K and non-heme iron, but eating more than the occasional handful can actually inhibit mineral absorption.

Learn How to Forage

When considering food choices, the best choice is always ingredients that are locally sourced and in season. In the supermarket or at the farmers market this means your food is fresher, the nutrition is greater, and the carbon footprint is far lower.

Foraging is a great way to eat the freshest foods, so get to know your local wild plants and herbs. Just make sure you have solid knowledge on those plants before you harvest. Depending on where you live, your choices may include cattails, stinging nettles, pine nuts, edible mushrooms, and many more. We strongly advise against foraging without seeking training first. Look for workshops offered at a local nature center or community college, or find an experienced mentor to teach you about the wild edible foods that are available in your area, what season of the year is best for which foods, and where to forage for them. You may find it becomes a wonderful new—and nutritious—pastime!

CHAPTER 4

Healthy Body, Healthy Bones

All life-forms rely on one another for continued existence. Plants rely on us to be stewards of the land, to feed them clean nutrients so they can blossom in good health and reach full productivity. Food animals rely on us to offer them a satisfying, contented life free to live as their natures dictate. A human body's 30 trillion cells coordinate metabolic processes, as long as we supply the body with the vitamins and minerals that it cannot manufacture on its own. If the plants we eat are healthy, if the food animals we choose are healthy, our bodies can be healthy. Our health spans are intertwined. It is a necessary and beautiful partnership.

Because the body is a complex and interconnected system, it makes sense that threats to the health of any part of the body or the body overall could also compromise bone health. These threats might include chronic inflammation or a deficiency of an important nutrient. And following the same reasoning, threats from the surrounding environment, such as heavy metals or air pollution, can damage our overall health, including the health of our bones. It's an unhappy reality: The burden of such environmental threats is increasing, and assessing the risk they pose to any single person depends on the person's genetics plus other variables such as location, water source, local sources of pollutants, and even lifestyle choices.

In this chapter, we explore many aspects of how the health of your body and its systems influence the health of your bones, and we offer tips on nutrition and lifestyle choices you can take to reduce risks. We particularly emphasize gut health because the gut manages nutrient absorption. An impaired, damaged, or inflamed gut lining, or a condition such as irritable bowel syndrome (IBS) or other disturbances, will affect nutrient absorption and directly threaten bone health.

Fortunately, to a greater or lesser degree we can control the negative effects of harmful chemicals or metabolic imbalances and thereby reduce damage and chronic illness.

Emphasizing Positive Influences

Nutrition in the form of organic plants, grown and eaten in season, and food products from organically raised, pastured livestock are the best fuels for a healthy body. The nutrients are freely available for absorption and there are no detours during digestion. Intermittent or seasonal fasting can be another positive influence, as fasting encourages healthy cell turnover and regulation of the inflammatory response.

Getting the Most from Plant Foods

For optimum nutritional benefit from the plants you eat, choose plants that are locally grown in season. We advise *locally grown* because after harvest, nutrients and flavor begin to degrade and continue to degrade over time, and conditions of storage, such as an overly hot warehouse, will exacerbate nutrient degradation further. We advise food plants grown *in season* because when plants grow at their natural time of year, they are at their most nutrient dense. Further, we encourage you to choose those grown organically or by local farmers who use only natural pesticides, because toxic chemical pesticides are inflammatory and cause oxidative stress and free-radical damage. Another reason to buy seasonal foods is that it supports farmers who are practicing crop rotation, which allows the soil to remain nutrient rich.

At cool-weather times of year, look for locally grown asparagus, beets, broccoli, Brussels sprouts, chives, cabbage, carrots, cauliflower, Swiss chard, kale, leeks, lettuce, onions, parsnips, peas, radishes, spinach, and turnips.[1] If you live where winter is long, snowy, and cold, you have fewer local choices. Root vegetables flourish and a good root cellar provides hearty choices. Many growers in cold-winter areas also produce crops in greenhouses and other types of shelters, so winter choices can include kale, carrots, lamb's lettuce, Asian greens (such as pak choi, tatsoi, and mizuna), scallions, spinach, and arugula.

Get started by researching the plants in season where you live and local farms that offer food for sale to the general public. Even one or two local foods will enhance your nutrient balances. You can extend the nutritional benefit most vegetables offer by canning, pickling, or fermenting vegetables you buy in season and then eating those preserved foods during the colder months. Community-supported agriculture (CSA) programs offer local, fresh, in-season food in many areas. Some farmers in cold-winter areas have launched winter CSAs that specialize in providing a weekly share of storage crops and greenhouse-grown cold-hardy greens in the fall and winter months. Contact your state's organic or sustainable farmers organization or visit the Seasonal Food Guide (www.seasonalfoodguide.org) for help in finding a CSA near you.

Managing Turnover

The body's processes of making energy from food—a function of metabolism—and using that energy for activity, growth, and repair—has seasonal rhythms. Two proteins, mTor (which stands for "mammalian target of rapamycin") and AMPK (which stands for 5' "AMP-activated protein kinase"), are the rulers of metabolism. mTor and AMPK are kinases, a type of enzyme that catalyzes the transfer of phosphate groups from ATP (adenosine triphosphate) to other molecules.

mTor senses when there's fuel in the digestive tract; senses the hormones that control appetite and

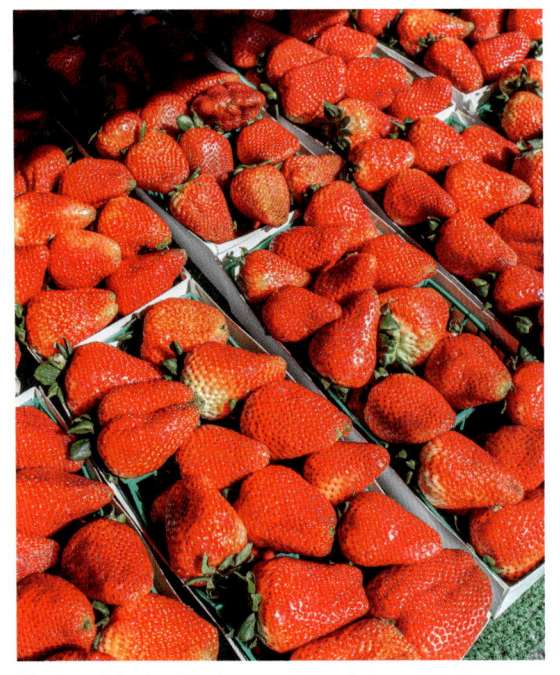

Figure 4.1. A strawberry grown in summer is more nutritious and flavorful than a strawberry grown in midwinter, even locally.

other chemical reactions to the smell, sight, or taste of food; and, very importantly, stimulates the growth of cells. mTor is more active in spring and summer, facilitating protein synthesis and cellular growth in all plants and animals when the environment for growth is optimal.

AMPK acts in two ways to conserve energy. Historically, nutrients were scarcer in winter for humans, although the advent of 24/7 supermarkets has made that anachronistic for most people in the United States. When nutrients are scarce, AMPK slows down metabolic processes that are not fuel-efficient, such as marshaling food and oxygen to make glucose, and can empty cells of stored fat. In the process of autophagy, AMPK triggers recycling of retired cells, the products of cell turnover that, if not excreted, would bulk up and clog the system, causing aging, exhaustion, and sometimes ill health.

Thus, mTor prioritizes growth and activity while AMPK optimizes energy efficiency and clears waste. This is the beauty and importance of nature's seasonal health maintenance routine, but it can be at odds with the typical modern Western diet—big meals, heaps of protein, lots of oxidizing fat, too-quick absorption of processed foods. Such a diet keeps mTor active and arrests AMPK activity, suppressing nature's mechanism for fall and winter energy conservation and housecleaning. This housecleaning mechanism of autophagy is very important to health; animal research shows that healthy autophagy reverses aging.[2]

There are antidotes to imbalance. Exercise and fasting can activate AMPK. In any season, a continuous intake of protein and simple carbs, such as often found in the standard American diet, will activate mTor and impede the housecleaning activities of AMPK.

mTor is directly stimulated by branched-chain amino acids—such as those found in meat—and by insulin. Both prolong the body's time in mTor and the risk of cellular overgrowth. Remaining in the growth cycle without housecleaning creates too much growth, which can play a part in cancer.

Luckily, there is a mini version of the mTor/AMPK cycle that takes place every night: While you sleep, you are not eating, and mTor activity decreases. So, to help balance the mTor/autophagy, don't eat too close to bedtime (Laura suggests a three-hour window) and eat less protein at night.

This is one reason why eating a plant-based meal for dinner can be beneficial. Plant protein does not contain high levels of branched-chain amino acids and keeps mTor stimulation to a minimum.

Spring Fasting

Spring is a time of increased activity and nutrient availability, and beneficial microbiome colonies flourish after the metabolic shift that occurs in winter. Fasting enhances all the metabolic mechanisms that help a body sustain health, by clearing out unwanted cells and waste. Fasting enhances effective detoxification and autophagy (housecleaning) and rebuilds the immune system. Spring fasting is a great way to introduce the art of fasting into your routine. We like Vit-Ra-Tox fasting assistance products because they support the body's cleansing as well as rebuilding processes (you can buy the products online). Fasting also increases insulin sensitivity, suppresses inflammation, and stimulates autophagy (how the body eliminates dead cells). For information on the importance of autophagy, see "Managing Turnover," on page 50. Check with your health care provider to see if fasting is right for you.

Intermittent fasting is one among many popular health promoters; others are inducing a state of ketosis, consuming curcumin, resveratrol, EGCG (from green tea), cruciferous vegetables, genistein (from soy), and caffeine. All inhibit mTor and activate autophagy to benefit health, yet not every intervention is right for everyone. We suggest consulting a nutrition or medical expert who may tailor a regimen.

The Body as Cybernetic System

Let's return to the basic reason why emphasizing positive influences on the body is so important: Each living individual is a cybernetic system—a whole that relies on the interaction of its parts, yet is greater than the sum of its parts. For example, gut health influences the function of the brain's amygdala, which controls mood, emotion, and motivation; depression can disrupt immune response, while social connection can improve immune response.[3]

A perfect example of the cybernetic nature of the human body is the cell danger response—a term for the body's protective response to any chemical, physical, or biological threat. The body gathers chemical, physiological, and neurological responses designed to aid in restoring homeostasis, and that collective response is called inflammation, which, as mentioned in previous chapters, can play an important role in bone health.

Any insult to the body, from a bee sting to a bone fracture—as well as the continuous influx of toxins such as heavy metals in our drinking water and pesticide residues in our food—is a code red signal to mitochondria, the organelles found in almost every type of cell. Mitochondria are responsible for producing energy to power vital cell functions, and they are also sensors that monitor and respond to all conditions within and around the cell. When the mitochondria sense stress, they trigger a series of physiological responses: Cell metabolism changes, cell membranes stiffen, antiviral and microbial chemicals are released, autophagy (cell housekeeping) occurs, and gene expression is altered. These responses alert neighboring cells of danger. The immune system calls up a defense team of immune cells. Histamine production goes up, which widens blood vessels that in turn allow fast transport for immune cells and nutrients. Sleep is suspended. The body's conversion of the inactive to the active form of vitamin D slows down. All of these responses focus the resources of the body on healing. You can see this all in real time when, for example, the area around a skin cut reddens and swells. This shows that the body is on the job.

If this cycle is resolved by management of the stressor, the code red switches off and things return to normal. The cut is cleaned and dressed, and pain subsides. Resolution can also come about if a nutrient deficiency is addressed by a change of diet or by avoidance of foods that contain pesticide residues.

Inflammation and Your Bones

In many cases, it is not so easy to address stress. This is especially true when the body is trying to cope with nutrient deficiency or an imbalance in gut bacteria or of the immune system. An infection can become chronic, and an inflammatory cycle can continue and widen out from the local insult to other areas or to the whole body. When inflammation continues at a low level—say, when one routinely consumes food laden with pesticide residues—inflammation hums in the background, almost invisible. Chronic inflammation is the most potent influence in complex chronic health issues, including osteoporosis. Systemic inflammation can disrupt bone marrow function such that bone marrow overproduces osteoclasts, the cells that degrade bone. Activation of immune cells also directly impacts bone because the activated cells secrete inflammatory signals that are pro-osteoclast, promoting bone loss in chronic inflammatory states such as rheumatoid arthritis.[4]

On the flip side, some anti-inflammatory immune cells secrete the receptor called osteoprotegerin, as described in chapter 1, that interferes with the protein called RANKL and thus stops osteoclast generation.

The takeaway here is that prolonged inflammatory states can directly impact bone via immune system signaling. Fortunately, there are ways to quiet a high-alert immune response that has been triggered by an inflammatory condition (see "Other Strategies for Controlling Inflammation," page 54).

Coping with Food Allergies

There are two types of food allergies. Some are low-level responses called food intolerances. These are subclinical triggers of the immune system that may not be apparent on a daily basis, yet they cause low-level inflammation. Gluten intolerance is one type. Other types of allergies create substantial immune responses. Celiac disease is an example of this powerful type of food allergy.

FOOD INTOLERANCES

To diagnose a food intolerance, doctors may look for a chemical response to a food from either a low-level immune response, the lack of an enzyme, or a sensitivity to a specific chemical either in the food or an additive. Often the response is high release of histamine from mast cells. People can have gluten intolerance that produces digestive discomfort but is not an autoimmune condition. An allergy to wheat triggers strong histamine production without being an autoimmune response. Food allergy testing can reveal foods that may be causing low-level immune response or other symptoms such as rashes or watery eyes.

In her practice, Laura has noted that patients who have undiagnosed food allergies or feel sapped of energy are often eating a set diet including the same foods day after day—foods that may be causing low-level immune response. The good news is that when allergy testing shows low-level immune response and these patients transition to a diet rich in diverse, organic, fresh, local, seasonal foods, often their food allergies subside and energy returns. The adage *fresh is best* holds true, and we contend that *organic is best* holds true, too, as we discuss below.

If you have known food allergies or food intolerances that can create low-level inflammation, always read labels and wherever possible, buy fresh food, free of packaging and added ingredients.

CELIAC DISEASE

Celiac disease is an abnormal autoimmune reaction to gluten. Symptoms may include diarrhea, bloating, abdominal pain, nausea, vomiting, and, if uncontrolled, fatigue and weight loss. This response to gluten results from a genetic disposition. The only known remedy is to strictly eliminate gluten. It's estimated that celiac disease affects about 1 in 100 people worldwide.

Because celiac disease can interfere with nutrient absorption in the digestive system, over time the patient can suffer deficiencies, including of nutrients essential for bone health. People diagnosed with celiac disease must avoid all foods that contain even a smidgen of gluten, including barley, wheat, rye, and some other grains.

If you suspect you may be suffering from celiac disease, it's important to seek testing that will confirm or rule it out, because there are other conditions that can cause similar symptoms but will not be addressed by avoiding gluten. If you are managing an autoimmune condition such as celiac disease, it is also important to know whether you also have food intolerances, because continuous triggering of your immune response by foods or additives can increase the impact of an autoimmune condition.

ADVICE ON GOING GLUTEN-FREE

Chef Jummee uses flours other than wheat flour not only because she has gluten sensitivity herself, but because she wants to ensure everyone can use the recipes in part 2 of the book.

As discussed above, gluten is a protein found in wheat, rye, and barley. Those with celiac disease are unable to eat even the smallest amount because it triggers an immune system response. Some people have gluten sensitivity that is not celiac disease.

There are two issues. First, gluten is a trigger of zonulin in many people. Zonulin is a regulator of intestinal permeability through affecting tight junctions between gut-lining cells, causing a temporary separation of the junction, allowing leaky gut to occur. Increased levels of zonulin over time are correlated with the onset of autoimmune issues.

Second, synthetic chemical herbicides are almost ubiquitously used in large-scale production of wheat in the United States, and these substances are damaging to human health and to the environment. These products turn wheat into a toxic food, and many of these substances are banned in other countries. Many people find they can eat wheat products in Europe without suffering any digestive distress as they would in the United States. The difference is in how wheat is grown and processed in Europe.

Gluten likely triggers a mild inflammatory response in all humans, but if a person has a healthy gut and does not have the genetics for celiac disease, the gut will reset itself with no harm done. Given the chemicals routinely used in US wheat production, we find it safer to simply go gluten-free in our recipes, while leaving the option for use of wheat that is organically and safely produced.

Some people who are gluten intolerant decide to go gluten-free, as do others for various reasons. If you have decided to avoid gluten, keep these points in mind:

- Some widely used plant-based foods are often made with ingredients that contain gluten unless specifically labeled gluten-free: soy sauce, hoisin sauce, teriyaki sauce, some salad dressings, gravies, beer, fried foods, baked goods, crackers, tortillas, barley malt, and more.
- Be mindful that processed foods may contain wheat-based thickeners, flavorings, and stabilizers.
- Flours that do not contain gluten include rice flour, quinoa flour, almond flour, and coconut flour. In chapter 12, Jummee has included recipes calling for gluten-free flours.
- Gluten-free flours may contain some of the antinutrients discussed in chapter 3. Among flours with the lowest antinutrient levels are potato, rice, and tapioca.

Other Strategies for Controlling Inflammation

Some other nutrition-related steps you can take to control inflammation are to eat mushrooms, choose organically grown foods, and eat the rainbow.

EAT MUSHROOMS

One sure way to regulate the immune system is to eat mushrooms. Mushrooms help the immune system stay in balance. It is generally safe to eat some mushrooms each day except in the case of some autoimmune conditions. See chapter 7 for information about medicinal mushrooms.

CHOOSE ORGANIC

Foreign matter is anything that does not occur naturally in the body's own chemistry, with the important exception of foods the body seems built to recognize. (This may explain food allergies and the fact of inflammatory conditions.)

The body reacts to foreign matter as toxic, which triggers inflammation. Glyphosate is the most widely used chemical herbicide and stubbornly remains intact in plant foods even through washing and high-temperature cooking. One of the most rigorous research efforts aiming to test claims that glyphosate causes cancer has confirmed that the herbicide is a cause of non-Hodgkin's lymphoma (NHL).[5]

Organically grown produce is more expensive than conventionally grown produce, and it may seem that buying organic produce would tip the budget balance. Very often it does not. If you'd like to find out how the costs compare where you live, try this little experiment. For one week, write down the cost of every item of processed food and all ready-prepared food that you buy, and tally up the total. The following week, cook at home as much as possible using organically grown or local plant foods. Tally up the costs of those ingredients and compare. In our experience with friends, family, and patients, buying organically grown food and eliminating processed, packaged food actually proves to be a cost savings.

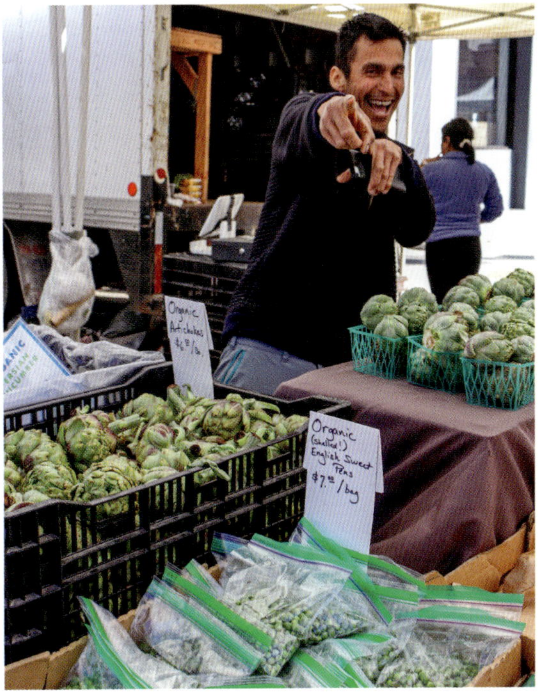

EAT THE RAINBOW

The bright, brilliantly hued phytochemicals in fruits and vegetables are antioxidant, and they are natural inflammation fighters. Fresh organic vegetables are high in vitamins—especially C, A, and K—and abundant in minerals. This is especially true of leafy greens, which are highest in antioxidants and fiber as well. Each colorful pigment produced by plants is linked to a unique contribution to functional health of the immune system, bones, eyesight, heart, and urinary tract. Eating the rainbow may also promote healthy aging and control mutations that lead to cancer by preserving telomere length.

A rainbow of beautifully hued plant foods along with immune-boosting fungi (mushrooms) can keep a body and its bones in excellent health. After all, such foods have been a rich source of vitamins, minerals, and protein-building amino acids for millennia.

Figure 4.2. Consuming organic local food allows you to eat with the seasons.

Consume some raw colors each day. Raw fruits are a treat all on their own. Season your vegetables with cold-pressed olive oil, bone vinegar (see recipe on page 137), and the herbs and seeds of your choice. When you prepare greens, for best nutrient absorption, steam them lightly, add a teaspoon of bone vinegar, and eat them hot or cold.

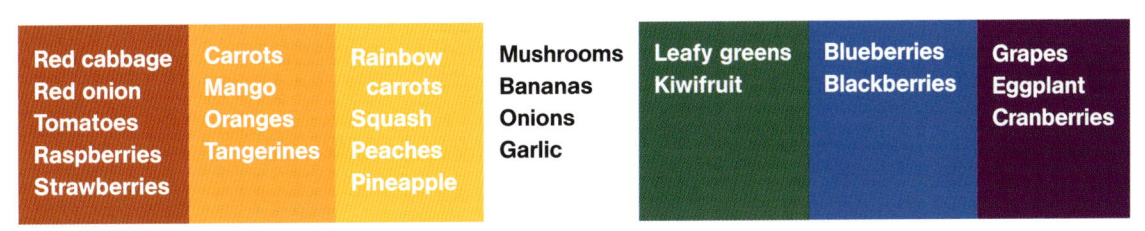

Red cabbage Red onion Tomatoes Raspberries Strawberries	Carrots Mango Oranges Tangerines	Rainbow carrots Squash Peaches Pineapple	Mushrooms Bananas Onions Garlic	Leafy greens Kiwifruit	Blueberries Blackberries	Grapes Eggplant Cranberries

Figure 4.3. Plant pigments are special biochemicals that have lots of health benefits, so eat the rainbow of plant colors!

> ### Astaxanthin
>
> Astaxanthin is a potent carotenoid that research suggests is the most potent antioxidant of all phytochemicals.[6] It is also a powerful inhibitor of the inflammatory response in chronic conditions. Astaxanthin is under investigation as an antidote to various health challenges, including diabetes, male infertility, and the cellular damage caused by smoking. It is the pigment designed by nature that colors lobster, shrimp, krill, crayfish, and salmon. It is also a chemical component of various microalgae and yeast, which are the vegetarian and vegan options for this important chemical.

Hormones and Bone Health

Many of the influences on bones are via hormones: thyroid hormones, insulin, sex hormones, and others.

Thyroid Hormones

Thyroid hormones increase the energy production of all cells, including bone cells; thus, they increase the growth rates of both osteoblasts and osteoclasts. Deficiency of thyroid hormone can impair growth in children, while excessive amounts of thyroid hormone can cause too much bone breakdown and weaken the bones.

Up to 10 percent of the global population has lowered thyroid function. This is referred to as hypothyroidism. Since thyroid medication in excess can lead to a decline in bone density, it is important to take only as much medication as you need. Ask your doctor to monitor the effect by checking your thyroid hormone levels regularly.

CALCIUM-REGULATING HORMONES

The thyroid also produces calcium-regulating hormones, so thyroid health can affect calcium regulation. Bone strength is just one of calcium's functions. It is the key signaling molecule between neurons, and all cells use calcium as a signaling molecule in response to stimuli.

Because of calcium's importance, the body keeps a tight rein on blood calcium levels. When the level falls below the threshold, the body calls on bones to release calcium. When blood calcium level rises above the upper limit, the thyroid releases calcitonin, a hormone that inhibits or arrests the action of osteoclasts and thereby reduces bone resorption and release of calcium into the blood. Calcitonin also inhibits reabsorption of calcium in the kidneys, allowing excess calcium to exit the body through urine. Excesses or deficiencies of calcitonin in adults do not appear to cause problems in maintaining blood calcium concentration or the strength of the bone. Calcitonin is used as a drug for treating some bone diseases.

SEAWEED FOR THYROID HEALTH

The thyroid requires iodine or iodide for healthy function. Unfortunately, the Western diet is almost devoid of iodine—which explains why long ago iodine was added to table salt. Now that natural salts, such as sea salt, have become popular, some people may lack sufficient iodine.

Seaweed is the best possible answer to ensure you take in sufficient iodine, and regularly adding seaweed to your diet provides many and varied benefits. Seaweed is packed with nutrients that are essential for bone health and can contribute to a healthier gut. What's remarkable is that seaweed grows a staggering 300 times faster than land plants do, making it an environmentally friendly food choice as well.

Parathyroid Hormone (PTH)

Parathyroid hormone (PTH) is produced by four small glands adjacent to the thyroid gland. These glands are part of the system that precisely controls the level of calcium in the blood. They are sensitive, and when calcium concentration decreases even slightly, the glands secrete PTH.

PTH acts on the kidney to conserve calcium and to stimulate calcitriol (active vitamin D) production. Vitamin D promotes nutrient absorption and is essential for calcium absorption. PTH also acts on bone to increase movement of calcium from bone to blood. If you have bone loss, one step in determining the cause can be to check your PTH levels.

Magnesium deficiency can also disrupt PTH levels, which disrupts calcium monitoring; this is another reason to identify and consume foods that are rich sources of magnesium.

Excess PTH production is a rare condition called hyperparathyroidism. Over time, this condition leads to mineral density decline.

Interestingly, when a synthetic form of PTH (teriparatide) is administered intermittently, it acts to trigger bone formation. The drug's effect is *opposite* that of PTH secreted by the parathyroid.

PTH circadian rhythm peaks at night, so suppressing this peak by supplementing with magnesium and a small amount of calcium before bed will help manage bone loss.

Insulin

The pancreas, a tiny organ that sits behind the stomach, produces and releases hormones, including insulin, that help to reduce blood sugar levels by stimulating cells to take up glucose. The pancreas also secretes digestive enzymes.

Insulin itself does not impact bones, but elevated blood sugar levels due to insulin resistance or diabetes causes an inflammatory state that affects bone quality, increasing osteoclast (bone breakdown) function and decreasing osteoblast (bone making) function. Any type of diabetes causes inflammation that negatively affects bone strength, bone turnover,

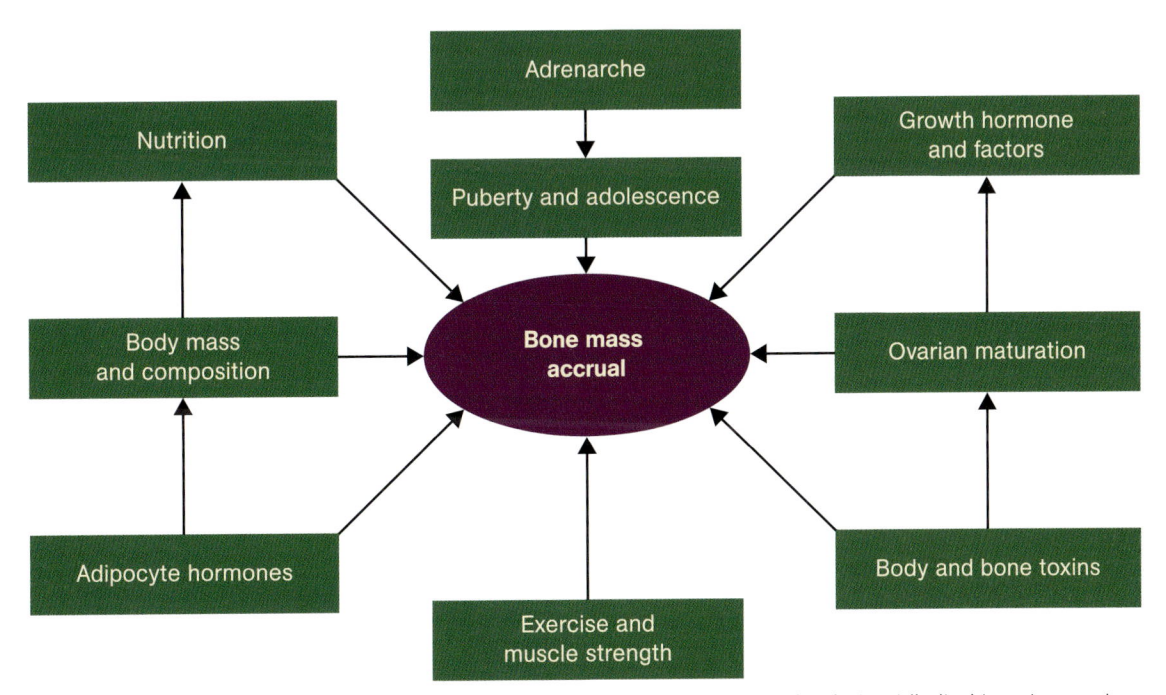

Figure 4.4. Bone turnover relies on the interaction of many hormones, including but not limited to estrogen, testosterone, vitamin D, parathyroid hormone, and thyroid hormone.

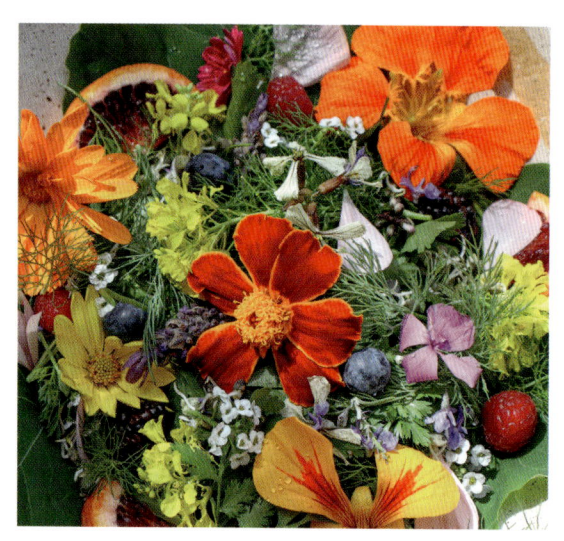

Figure 4.5. Edible flowers from your home garden can be another source of nutrients. Jummee uses them as garnishes for many dishes and as a star ingredient of her Herb and Wildflower Garden Salad (page 203).

and stem cell differentiation. The cumulative result is altered bone mineral density and bone structure.

Pancreatic enzymes affect digestion by helping to ready lipids, carbohydrates, and proteins for absorption. Lipase breaks down fats; insufficient lipase reduces absorption, including of the fat-soluble vitamins A, D, E, and K. Protease helps the body digest protein and destroy harmful intestinal bacteria. Amylase breaks down starches into sugar, the body's first-line source of energy. Over time, the production of pancreatic enzymes may wane, and with this comes waning digestion and nutrient absorption. Some fruits and fermented foods contain digestive enzymes. Among them are pineapple, papaya, mango, avocado, bananas, and kiwifruit; fermented foods like kimchi, miso, and sauerkraut (fermented, not brined), and some spices, like ginger, also contain digestive enzymes. Consume them on an empty stomach.

Sex Hormones

As explained in chapter 1, estrogen and testosterone affect bone turnover in both men and women. Estrogen increases levels of osteoprotegerin, which effectively blocks the activation of osteoclasts, inhibiting bone breakdown.

Testosterone's ability to stimulate muscle growth puts stress on bones and thereby triggers bone formation. Testosterone is also a source of estrogen—it is converted into estrogen in fat cells. This estrogen is important for the bones of men as well as women. In fact, in middle age, men often have higher levels of circulating estrogen than postmenopausal women do, because on average hormone decline among men occurs approximately twenty years later in life than estrogen decline among women.

Plant estrogens exert a weaker but similar effect on bones, as discussed in "The Role of RANKL" on page 16.

Other Hormones

During periods of accelerated growth, the pituitary gland secretes growth hormone, which regulates skeletal growth. Growth hormone stimulates the production of insulin-like growth factor-1 (IGF-1), another hormone produced in the liver and in bone (and less so in other tissue). Decreased production of growth hormone and IGF-1 with age reduces the ability among older individuals to form bone rapidly or to replace bone lost by resorption.

The adrenal gland produces cortisol, an anti-inflammatory hormone whose principal responsibility is modulating the body's ability to respond to stress and injury. Intermittent release of cortisol in response to momentary stress does not cause problems; however, continuous release allows too much cortisol to remain in the blood and reverses the anti-inflammatory effects, causing inflammation that directly weakens bone and the immune system. Physicians prescribe synthetic forms of cortisol called glucocorticoids to treat many inflammatory diseases. However, glucocorticoids decrease function of osteoblasts by inhibiting IGF-1 expression and suppress the function of vitamin D, thereby decreasing calcium absorption. They also decrease calcium channels in the gut. Even mild states of excess glucocorticoids can have a major impact on bone health.[7] If you take glucocorticoids, monitor your bone density and address any decline in bone density as soon as possible.

The Gut and Bone Health

The gut is one of the most potent influences on all body health, including bone health, because it is the screen through which all of our nourishment must pass. The health of the gut is of primary importance to ensure plant nutrition is properly broken down and absorbed. This screen, the gut lining, is guarded by the many and varied bacterial residents that live in our gut, collectively known as the microbiome.

The Microbiome

It's estimated that 100 trillion commensal gut bugs (bacteria beneficial to human health) are present in the gut to help us digest food, create nutrients such as vitamin K2, produce neurotransmitters, manage pathogens, and produce the short-chain fatty acids that feed the cells of our gut lining, helping to keep it intact. Interaction with gut receptors also triggers the secretion of hormones that directly signal the brain, influencing learning, memory, and mood.[8] Thousands of these special commensal bacteria colonize the gut and promote the work of nutrient absorption and digestion.

Since we rely in part on these friendly gut bacteria for health and happiness, we mustn't forget to feed them. The food they like most is an indigestible carbohydrate, called a prebiotic, commonly found attached to plant proteins.

The gut lining is delicate and is only one cell thick. Inflammation, toxins, and a microbiome deficient in beneficial bacteria may cause separation between the cells, leading to a condition known as "leaky gut." Through this leaky gut, bacteria that normally reside only in the gut can infiltrate other parts of the body and may lead to an inflammatory or autoimmune response.

Furthermore, 70 percent of the tissue in the gut is immune system tissue. Why is there so much immune tissue in the gut? Because the gut is a place of contact with the outside world and is the first line of defense protecting the body from inflammatory and other toxic or unwelcome substances. Because gut health and immune system health are linked in this way, the ill health of one can imperil the other. Inflammation in the gut, which has many causes, will affect the immune system. An activated or overactive immune response that can arise in autoimmune diseases can cause inflammatory response in the gut, which can cause systemwide inflammation, thereby affecting the health of the whole body.

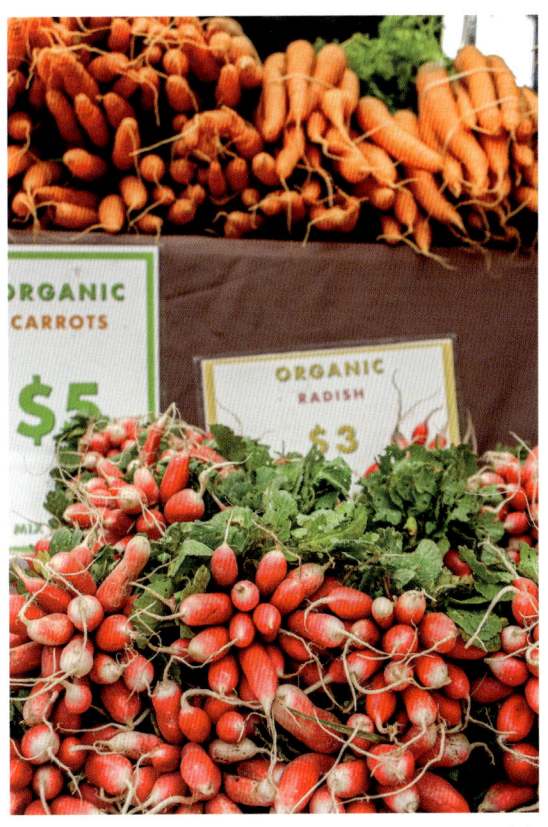

Figure 4.6. Locally grown carrots and radishes are rich sources of beta carotene.

Healthy Body, Healthy Bones

The Gut-Brain Axis

The brain is also directly affected by the health of the gut, in this case via the gut-brain axis. The healthy brain in turn provides proper signaling to the body via hormone and messenger release from the hypothalamus and pituitary primarily. These signals reach glands and organs that further release hormones and signal molecules to manage system health. Ninety percent of serotonin—the neurotransmitter that is responsible for focus, a sense of stability, and happiness—is made in the gut. Communication between the gut and brain appears to be modulated via the vagus nerve, which runs from the brain to the gut. This nerve controls parasympathetic processes such as respiration, heart rate, urination frequency, blood pressure, immune response, and digestion. That means full-body health and brain health are interlinked and interdependent, and perhaps are one and the same.

Keeping the Gut Healthy

A healthy gut is the foundation for all good health and longevity. If you eat food that is fresh off the land and grown without toxic pesticides, and your water and air are clean, your gut lining will be intact and the gut will function seamlessly to absorb nutrients. While this ideal environment is a luxury most of us do not enjoy, there are steps we can take to improve the likelihood that the gut will be healthy and its contribution to body health will be robust.

Which Milk to Drink?

Digestion of milk in the human gut is a fine example of nature helping us take care of health. To wit, commensal gut bacteria produce lactase to help digest the lactose in dairy milk. If that's the case, why does almost 65 percent of the world's adult population report lactose intolerance? Due to factors such as a steady diet of processed food, a diet that isn't varied, certain medications, and toxins in water, among others, a great many of Laura's patients who report lactose intolerance lack a population of the commensal gut bacteria. Furthermore, most of these patients are consuming pasteurized dairy, and the scalding heat of pasteurization destroys the lactase that would otherwise digest the lactose. Unpasteurized milk, often called raw milk, does contain lactase. We love raw milk, and we wrote about the benefits of drinking raw milk for bone health in our first book.

However, many people don't have easy access to raw milk, and there is also a concern about high levels of bovine leukemia virus (BLV) in milk produced in the United States. BLV is a virus that may be implicated in breast cancer. Until this question about US dairy milk is resolved, we are recommending plant-based milks, which are easy to digest and easy to make at home (see chapter 9 for recipes).

We highly recommend homemade plant milks rather than commercial plant-based milks. Typically, suppliers of commercial milks add processed ingredients or unhealthy fat to preserve shelf life, and equally important, the plants are not properly prepared to release nutrients. For example, soybeans and almonds should be sprouted and oats should be sprouted or soaked before making milk.

AVOID HIGHLY PROCESSED FOODS

Highly processed foods are impatient; they do not make it through the full digestion process. Instead, they are absorbed quickly in the upper gut and released into the bloodstream, where they can cause blood sugar levels to spike and raise a variety of false alarms. As a cybernetic system, the body responds, signaling the pancreas, thyroid, parathyroid, and brain. A full-on inflammatory response may endure for all the years one is on a diet of primarily highly processed food.

AVOID GMO FOODS

Some food crops, such as maize (corn), are genetically modified to resist insect pests. Scientists use genetic engineering techniques to insert genes into the plant that themselves produce insecticide. Other major food crops, such as corn and soybeans, have been genetically engineered to be resistant to a specific herbicide, such as glyphosate (Roundup).

So far by appearances it seems that consumption of genetically modified foods does not make humans ill or otherwise affect health. However, we know that genes from the modified foods can be taken up by our gut microflora, and we do not yet know what effect this may have. We do know, though, that the insecticides plants produce as well as the insecticides and herbicides growers apply to crops can affect health.

It is no longer speculation that glyphosate is a carcinogen. It alters the gut microbiome significantly, reduces the synthesis of neurotransmitters, and causes reactive oxygen species to form, which in turn causes oxidative stress and oxidative damage. Glyphosate, which can destroy many commensal gut bacteria species, is linked to IBS.

Laura advises her patients to avoid any foods that have been in contact with glyphosate or any pesticide or insecticide that the body must detoxify, including most conventionally grown wheat. Many wheat growers spray glyphosate on the wheat crop shortly before harvesting it in order to hasten the drying of the grain.

The most reliable way to avoid pesticide residues on food is to start a home food garden and not use any pesticides on it. However, a home garden is not always an option. There is also insurance in choosing organically grown food, as discussed earlier in this chapter.

Since nutrients communicate with genes, it is reasonable to question the effect on genetic expression of unnaturally altered food. For this reason, among others, Laura advises her patients to avoid GMO foods.

pH Balance and Bone Health

As it does with calcium, the body holds to strict pH (acid/alkaline) blood levels. Metabolic acidosis—too much acid—triggers the body to release calcium, which is alkaline, as the body tries to regulate blood pH. PTH senses blood pH and is the primary actor in ensuring the blood pH balance. The acidosis release first will come from circulating calcium; if there is not enough circulating calcium, the body will draw calcium from the bone. The ideal blood pH is between 7.35 and 7.45, which is slightly alkaline. The stomach is typically at a pH of 3.5, which helps food break down properly during the digestion process.

> pH of 0–4 is acidic.
> pH of 7 is neutral.
> pH of 8–9 is alkaline.

Using low-cost paper strips, you can measure your urine pH. Urine pH, as distinct from blood pH, measures the level of acid or alkaline as a system. Look for a urine pH of around 6.5, slightly more acidic than blood pH. You will see your pH change with dietary changes, and fluctuation is normal. If your urine pH is consistently 6 or lower, you can improve and maintain a healthy extracellular pH by consuming more plants and less meat, sugar, and starches, which will help to keep calcium in your bones.

Healthy Body, Healthy Bones

Effects of Commonly Used Medicines

Some common over-the-counter and prescription medications, including prednisone and proton pump inhibitors, can affect bone health.

As noted in "Other Hormones" (page 58), synthetic glucocorticoids such as prednisone can cause bone loss. Bone damage more commonly results from the long-term use of glucocorticoid pills when taken at a dose of 7.5 milligrams (or more) daily for three (or more) months (these do not have to be consecutive months). Glucocorticoid joint injections, inhalers, skin creams, and eye drops have not been shown to increase the risk of osteoporosis. If you must take glucocorticoid pills such as prednisone, be sure to monitor your bone health.

Proton pump inhibitors are a common medication used to relieve acid reflux. Doctors prescribe proton pump inhibitors (PPIs) to about one-fourth of US adults; two-thirds of those adults take high doses. PPIs inhibit nutrient absorption—especially mineral absorption—and may promote dementia. Using proton pump inhibitors long term (for a period of several years) at high doses is associated with increased hip fracture risk in older adults.[9]

When used for contraception, the long-term use of injectable Depo-Provera probably causes a significant reduction in bone mineral density. Discontinuing the drug leads to reversal in most cases.[10]

The antiseizure drugs carbamazepine (Tegretol) and phenytoin (Dilantin) have been associated with a reduction in bone density likely due to low vitamin D and decreased intestinal absorption of calcium.

Other Bone Diseases

Many bone disorders are local, affecting only a small region of the skeleton. Inflammation can lead to bone loss through the production of local resorbing factors by the inflammatory white cells. This process can occur around the affected joints in patients with arthritis. Bacterial infections, such as severe gum inflammation or periodontal disease, can produce loss of the bones around the teeth, and osteomyelitis can produce a loss of bone at the site

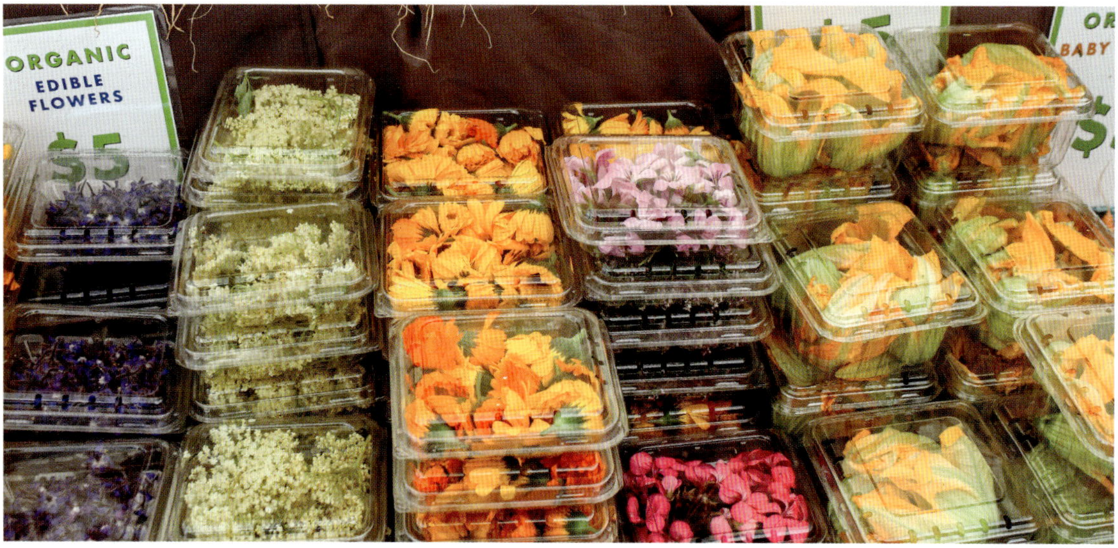

Figure 4.7. Like the squash itself, squash blossoms are bursting with carotenoids, which transform to retinol—the fat-soluble vitamin A. So, for maximum nutrition, sauté them or add them to an oil-rich recipe.

of infection. This type of bone loss is due to the direct damaging effect of bacterial products as well as the production of resorbing factors by white cells.

Paget's disease is a complex condition in which there is formation of large, highly active and unregulated osteoclasts that produce abnormal bone resorption. The precise cause of Paget's disease is not known, but it appears to be the consequence of both genetic factors and environmental factors, possibly a viral infection. The osteoblasts try to repair this damage by increasing bone formation. However, the normal bone architecture has been disrupted, leading to weak bones and the potential for fractures and deformities, even though the bones may appear dense on an X-ray. One reason for this is that the new bone formed is disorderly; it does not have the proper alignment of mineral crystals and collagen matrix. In addition, the new bone may not be in the right place to provide strength.

Osteogenesis imperfecta is caused by abnormalities in the collagen molecule that make the matrix weak and can lead to multiple fractures. In another congenital disorder, osteopetrosis, the bones are too dense because of failure of osteoclast formation or function. This failure of the remodeling process results in persistence of trabecular bone in the marrow space so that the marrow cavity may not be large enough to form red and white blood cells normally. These dense bones cannot remodel well in response to mechanical forces or micro damage and hence may be weaker and subject to fracture even though bone mass is increased.

Oxidative Stress and Antioxidants

Perhaps you have heard the term *free radicals*, that they are powerful agents of aging and illness, and also that antioxidants in food can help to slay these dragons. But what is the source of a free radical's power to threaten health, and how do antioxidants reduce that threat?

The simple answer lies in basic chemistry. Rings of electrons are part of the structure of a molecule. As long as a molecule has all the electrons pairs it is supposed to have in its rings, it functions peacefully. Since in nature, all cells, as all living individuals, strive for stability, if a molecule has an unpaired electron, it will pinch one from any molecule nearby. This activity of pinching electrons is called reactivity. Reactive free radicals can arise in the human body during the processes in cells that produce life-sustaining energy.

As cells combine glucose with oxygen to make energy, the oxygen molecule breaks apart. One part joins the glucose; the other part is left free but with only one electron in its outer ring. This type of scavenger is a free radical. "Free" because it is not part of a complex molecule, such as a protein, nucleic acid, carbohydrate, or fat. And "radical" because chemists call any atom or molecule with an unpaired electron a radical.

As this free radical is driving for stability by scavenging electrons, it is indiscriminate; it will latch onto any matter it encounters: DNA, proteins, lipids, organ tissue, bone tissue. When too many oxygen molecules are scavenging electrons in the body, there may be collateral damage to tissue, and the immune system goes on alert. This latter situation is called oxidative stress.

So, do we have to take this threat as a necessary evil arising from staying alive? Not at all. When we eat foods that contain antioxidants, those antioxidants can donate electrons to scavenging radicals. Can solving the problem be that simple? It is.

The word *antioxidant* has become so overused, so touted by unregulated supplement manufacturers, as to be suspect. But make no mistake: Antioxidants protect health span and life span, and plant foods are the top source. Also, the more unadulterated a food is, the more potent the antioxidants it offers.

Antioxidant deficiency impairs your body's ability to defuse free radicals. A certain amount of oxidative threat can be good, though an explanation of this phenomenon is beyond the scope of this book.

Vitamins C and E, beta-carotene, and flavonoids are antioxidants. Glutathione; vitamins A, E, and C; CoQ10; plant-based antioxidants such as quercetin; and alpha-lipoic acid all help to reduce oxidative stress. Animals free to graze on antioxidant-rich plants retain some antioxidants in their muscle tissue. Lutein and zeaxanthin in pasture-raised eggs are antioxidants. Omega-3 fatty acids in salmon and trout are antioxidants. Sprouts are one of the best sources of nutrition and antioxidant vitamins A, C, and E.

Reducing Oxidative Stress

Toxins can leave behind a population of free radicals when they interact with body tissue. To detoxify, the body produces a peptide, glutathione. Glutathione is the body's master antioxidant and detoxification molecule and is so valuable to the body that it is recycled. Foods high in glutathione detoxify the body of persistent organic pollutants, such as air pollution and environmental chemicals, and protect cells and tissue from damage.[11]

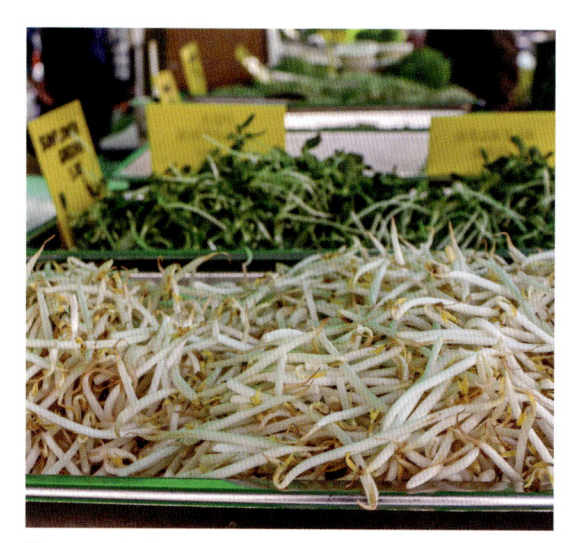

Figure 4.8. Sprout mung beans to release folate and enhance protein availability.

Energy, Aging, and Mitochondrial Health

Looking more closely at how cells produce energy, we find the manufacturing plant in the nucleus, where the mitochondria combine glucose with oxygen to produce energy.

Two events associated with energy production may actually reduce energy. Free radicals left over from energy production may cause damage to the mitochondria themselves. And, with age, the population of mitochondria in the body's cells declines. Less energy created can mean fatigue.

Is this loss of mitochondria inevitable? No. There is a known way to stimulate the body to create new mitochondria: By pushing the body through exercise into an out-of-breath state. Scientists are also investigating intermittent fasting, therapeutic cold exposure, the ketogenic diet, and the use of certain herbs as triggers for mitochondrial growth. For example, *Dan Shen*, the most widely used medicinal herb in China, increases the activity of mitochondrial proteins and generates new mitochondria. It also stabilizes mitochondria in heart cells.[12]

Protein for Glutathione Production

Glutathione is the body's most powerful antioxidant and also the body's most powerful detoxifier. Glutathione is manufactured in the body from the amino acids cysteine, glutamine, and glycine. Foods that support glutathione production are whey, garlic, and onions, all high in cysteine. PPIs and other medications are designed to reduce stomach acid absorption of protein and therefore the body's ability to make glutathione. Also, chronic inflammation can deplete glutathione, so immune system health is also important.

Selenium is required for the function of glutathione enzymes that help protect cells from peroxide and free-radical damage. Foods high in selenium include Brazil nuts, spinach, peas, and beans. Note: When it comes to Brazil nuts, a little goes a very long way. (See "The Selenium Quandary" on page 34.)

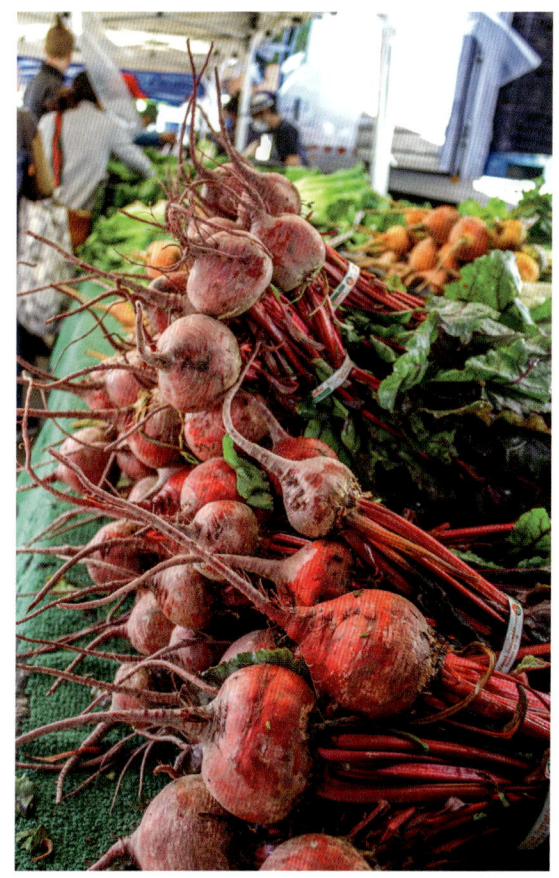

Figure 4.9. Beets are an important source of nitric oxide, yet a stronghold for oxalate antinutrients. Always add some citric acid to beets—perhaps a squeeze of fresh lemon—which will weaken the oxalates.

> ## Grapes for Longevity
>
> Grapes—their flesh, seeds, and skin—are rich in antioxidants, promoting heart health and reducing the risk of chronic diseases. Grape seeds contain compounds that support skin health and may have anti-inflammatory effects. The antioxidants in grapes help us detoxify by regulating reactive oxygen in the liver, assisting cellular metabolism and anti-inflammatory activity in the ovaries and kidneys, and triggering genes to product anti-inflammatory proteins in the colon. Grape skin is a source of resveratrol, known for its potent antioxidant and therefore antiaging and anticancer properties, and for contributing to overall health. Grapes are lovely to behold, and their tangy, sweet flavors make a great addition to salad dressing and salads.[13] Try the Mediterranean Herb and Grape Vinaigrette (page 121), the Green Grape Vinaigrette (page 200), and the Fennel-Radicchio Salad (page 206).

Many plant foods can supply glutathione or help the body generate glutathione and detoxify the body.

- Almonds appear to increase glutathione levels and therefore decrease DNA damage.
- Turmeric increases glutathione levels and improves activity of glutathione enzymes.
- Baru nuts, also called Baru almonds, are a Brazilian legume that are high in omegas and increase glutathione activity.
- Avocado is very high in glutathione and is an excellent choice for detox.
- Okra increases glutathione enzymes and other antioxidant molecules.
- Green asparagus is high in glutathione. (It can be decreased by cooking, so eat your asparagus lightly cooked.)
- Broccoli increases glutathione synthesis in the liver.
- Artichokes can stimulate the production of glutathione in the body.
- Collard greens stimulate glutathione production in the body and also contain alpha-lipoic acid, a powerful antioxidant.

- Beets enhance the liver's ability to make glutathione.
- Spinach is high in glutathione.

Dandelion greens detoxify liver and gallbladder and are included in our recommended bone vinegar herb mix.[14] (See "Dr. Laura's Bone Vinegar," page 137.) The liver detoxifies in three stages, and each stage requires a different set of nutrients. Milk thistle is a potent agent of detoxification; however, there are caveats, so take milk thistle under advisement of a health professional.[15]

Quercetin and Other Antioxidants

Quercetin is a plant flavonoid found in high levels in capers, red onions, and kale. Research has extensively documented its anti-inflammatory effects as well as its status as one of the most powerful antioxidant plant chemicals, protecting cells from oxidative damage. It is good to note that it has the same protective effect on plant cells! Other important plant chemical antioxidants are resveratrol, genistein, lycopene, and curcumin.

Detoxifying Heavy Metals and PFAS

It is estimated that worldwide, 683 pounds of chemicals toxic to animals and plants enter the environment every second. Of these, one-fifth are believed to be carcinogens. Heavy metals, herbicides such as glyphosate, and plastics are all implicated in many severe disease states.[16] And you have likely read recent reports of the dangers of "forever chemicals," such as perfluoroalkyl and polyfluoroalkyl substances (PFAS), that have been found in water supplies, agricultural fields, and consumer products.

Debilitating illness from toxic chemical exposure is not destiny, though, because of the detoxification mechanism in all cells, and the ability of the liver to detoxify the body. The extent to which the body can detoxify depends upon genetics and nutrients consumed. Luckily a number of plants can help the body detoxify; see "Protein for Glutathione Production" on page 64 for a list. And there are steps anyone can take that will greatly reduce the risk of chronic illness, including incessant bone loss and osteoporosis, caused by toxins.

Avoiding PFAS and Other Chemicals

PFAS were first developed in the 1930s for nonstick and waterproof coatings. Now known as "forever chemicals," these substances may be present in public and well water, in the water and soil of Superfund sites, in the air and in the food chain, and in a wide variety of consumer products.

These chemicals invade the body and rampage against health, as shown in figure 4.10. Specifically, PFAS reduce bone mass in children and adolescents—the most important time for building a storehouse of mineral density—and among the general population PFAS reduce the quality of bone, leaving people vulnerable to fracture.[17]

Here are steps you can take to limit exposure to PFAS.

- Wash fruits and vegetables with vinegar and water. (See "How to Clean Vegetables" on page 102.)
- Do not use nonstick cookware. Stainless steel or cast iron are good PFAS-free alternatives. Note: Cookware that says it is PFOA-free and PFOS-free does not mean PFAS free! Cookware that says PFOA- and PFOS-free may still contain newer types of PFAS compounds.
- Reduce or limit the amount of fast food, microwave popcorn, and takeout food you eat. Here's why. In an effort to make them grease resistant, the kind of food packaging used for these foods very often contains high levels of PFAS. (And of course, there are other good reasons to reduce your intake of fast food and microwave popcorn,

including but not limited to the potentially deleterious impact of fast food on digestive health and the unknowns when it comes to GMO corn. See "Avoid GMO Foods" on page 61.)
- Routinely check product labels for ingredients that include the prefix *fluoro-* and the word *perfluoro*, and avoid these whenever possible.

The human body does get rid of PFAS, but slowly. The half-life is four years. That means if you added no more PFAS, in four years half of what exists in your body today will be gone. Limiting your exposure can reduce the levels of PFAS and allow your body to recover.

Heavy Metals in Food

It is well established that all heavy metals can cause cancer.[18] They can bind to and damage DNA and interfere with the production and structure of enzymes and the structure of tissue. Heavy metals engender an abundance of superoxide and peroxide—two devastating types of free radicals—that produce pervasive oxidative stress on a vast scale and thereby engender widespread inflammation. They are harmful to plants as well as to animal tissue.[19]

Heavy metal accumulation is a major cause of inflammation. It also preferentially destroys the cells that make new bone. Heavy metals can accumulate within bone and contribute to osteoporosis.[20]

Though it appears that the risk is from larger amounts of heavy metals than we find in most of our food, the impact is cumulative, as heavy metals accumulate and can stay in the body for weeks and up to lifetimes. There are risks, too, with smaller amounts, such as in some types of fish that harbor concerning amounts of mercury. There is a lesser though notable risk from chocolate, if it contains significant amounts of lead and cadmium. Consumer advocates are aware of this risk and are investigating levels of lead and cadmium in commercially available brands of chocolate.

Neurotoxicity
Disruption of neurotransmission

Endocrine system
Modulation of thyroid and sex-hormone signaling

Immune system
Immunosuppression and chronic inflammation

Liver
Hepatic steatosis and development of nonalcoholic fatty liver disease

Kidney
Kidney cancer

Pancreas
Pancreatic cancer

Male reproductive system
Testicular cancer

Developmental effect
Impacts on birth weight, reduced response to vaccines

Figure 4.10. PFAS have many detrimental effects on human metabolism. There is strong evidence for the effects on the endocrine system, immune system, liver, kidney, and a developing fetus. Evidence is more limited for neurotoxic effects and effects on the pancreas.

It can be alarming to read about all the foods that may contain heavy metals. Leafy green vegetables accumulate more heavy metals than stalk and root vegetables.[21] Lentils accumulate arsenic; soybeans draw cadmium; and sprouted almonds are higher in metals than most nuts.[22]

Cadmium is strongly implicated in some breast cancers, and sunflower seeds and kernels accumulate cadmium.[23] Cadmium can also be present in some soy products and fruit juices. Research reports that corn has the highest level of mercury after

> ### Testing for Heavy Metals and PFAS
>
> Although the human body has some detoxification capacity, the extent of that capability varies depending upon a person's genetics and diet. Each person's heavy metal and PFAS burden will vary. A toxin panel, using blood, urine, hair, or fingernail sampling, can show your individual heavy metal burden.[24] There is a blood test for PFAS burden. Heavy metal and PFAS testing may be available through a health care provider or privately through a commercial testing company.

seafood. Wheat is relatively free of heavy metal toxicity; however, when aluminum is added during the process of making flour, the risks of Alzheimer's disease and cancer go up. Rice, especially brown rice, can carry arsenic in the bran. (Rice from California and Southeast Asia is the lowest in arsenic.)

The lowest risk of heavy metal toxicity is from fruits that we call vegetables—those which contain seeds of the plant, such as squash, tomatoes, cucumber, and eggplant—and melons, yet even these, when consumed as juice (such as tomato juice), can be a source of concentrated heavy metals.[25]

Since many popular plant foods such as leafy green vegetables, grains, and legumes contain some heavy metals, should you avoid a diet of mostly or only plant foods? Not at all. Here again, contrary nature steps in: The solution is to be sure you eat a good share of chelating plant foods. Substances in those foods bind to heavy metals and excrete them in urine, stool, and sweat. Chlorella (a green algae) and wild blueberries top the list of heavy metal chelators.

In addition to their impressive chelating properties, wild blueberries are a powerful antioxidant food renowned for preventing chronic illness.[26] One cup of wild blueberries supplies 13,427 total antioxidant capacity (TAC), due to its content of vitamins A and C, plus flavonoids like quercetin and anthocyanidin. That's about ten times the USDA's daily recommendation, in just one cup. The TAC of cultivated blueberries is 9,019 per cup; they are equally vitamin rich.

Since the state of Maine produces most of the wild blueberries grown in the United States, and most of us don't live in Maine, it's improbable that you'll be able to eat locally grown wild blueberries in season. Helen's solution is to buy a mix of blueberries—the freshest cultivated organic blueberries she can find and flash-frozen wild blueberries from Maine.

Garlic helps to detoxify heavy metals by pulling mercury and lead from body tissue and binding them for excretion. Onion and shallots, eggs, and cruciferous vegetables contain sulfur, which helps these foods to soak up heavy metals. Some vegetables, including broccoli, kale, spinach, and collard greens, are high in calcium, which acts to block the absorption of lead. Spirulina, a blue-green algae, defuses mercury and radionuclides.

Laura recommends routinely consuming antioxidants and chelating plant foods in order to detoxify and fight oxidative stress. It is especially important to include chelating foods if your diet includes brown rice (high in arsenic), mackerel, swordfish, and tuna (high in mercury) and if you eat conventionally grown rather than organically grown plant foods and fungi, because conventionally grown produce has likely been exposed to pesticides that may contain forever chemicals.

CHAPTER 5

Healthy Bones on a Vegan Diet

Whether you are newly fired up about switching to a vegan diet or have been following one for some time, it's good news that plants have the power to protect and strengthen the entire skeleton. In this chapter, we focus on key food practices that will help plants-only consumers both maintain strong bones as their density faces an inexorable decline after age 30 and also keep bone growth ahead of bone loss. We specifically address those bone-health issues—protein levels, iron absorption, B12 and mineral deficiencies—that physicians cite as the challenges plants-only consumers face.

Our bodies are 20 percent protein. A complete protein is twenty amino acids. Of the twenty, our bodies make eleven; the remaining nine—called essential amino acids—we must obtain from food, and that's where this discussion about protein and vegan diets takes center stage. Although complete protein exists in all animal foods, the complete set of amino acids required to make a protein are present only in a few plants. So what's a vegan to do? Using an amino acid calculator to find out the amino acids present in any one plant, and the percent contribution to complete protein, we can combine plants to make up the complement of amino acids we need.

Over time, using a nutrition calculator such as MyFoodData to check plant-food combinations for the completeness of the amino acids they provide becomes routine. A rich diversity of plant foods in your daily diet, such as the recipes in this book provide, will provide you with the whole array of amino acids. As a starting point, we suggest that plants-only consumers become familiar with the plants

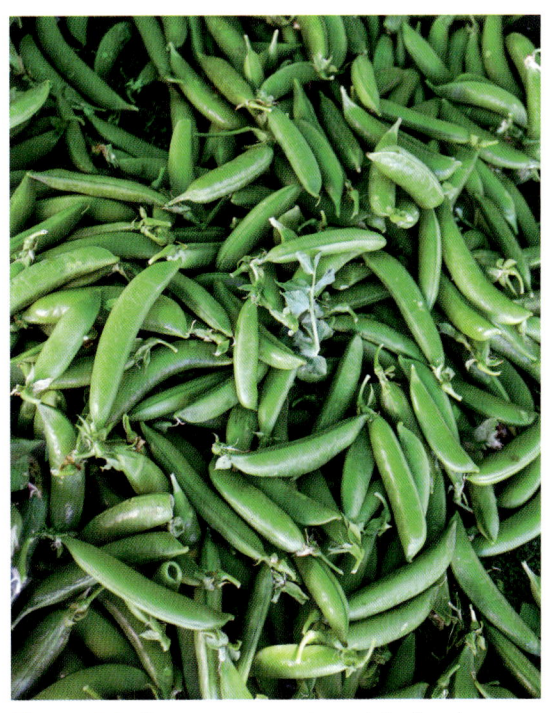

Figure 5.1. Peas are a great contribution to complete protein.

highest in protein as well as some protein-rich combinations they enjoy eating.

Iron absorption can be a challenge for vegans because plant foods contain a form of iron the human body does not readily absorb. There are simple, quick, and effective ways to make it well absorbed.

Vitamin B12 is naturally occurring in all animal foods but rarely in plant foods. Nori, a type of seaweed, is the exception and in fact is an excellent source of this important vitamin.

Mineral deficiency can arise on a vegan diet due to lack of understanding or inattention to the effects of antinutrients. As explained in chapter 3, antinutrients are chemicals that interfere with mineral absorption or cause gut health problems that in turn inhibit absorption.

Protein

Let's start by reviewing the basics: A protein is a complex organic substance composed of a specific set of organic compounds called amino acids. Our bodies have the capacity to manufacture eleven amino acids; these are termed the *nonessential* amino acids. Some of the nonessential amino acids are also termed *conditionally essential*, which means that during times of stress, pregnancy, or illness, we need an increased supply of these amino acids. The other nine are the *essential* amino acids, which we must obtain from food on a daily basis. These are the amino acids we must focus on in depth if we are to ensure we are eating all the amino acids every day—to comprise complete protein, without which the body will not function.

Why Proteins Matter

Proteins matter directly in bone health because they make up the collagen scaffold that holds the hydroxyapatite, the mineral component of bone that is measured by DEXA. Proteins are the fundamental component of all bone tissue.

- Proteins are the building blocks of all tissue in the human body, including the collagen that is a key component in strong bones. Proteins are also involved in the body's every metabolic process, such as digestion, energy production, and DNA replication. Proteins act as enzymes that catalyze chemical reactions in the body.
- Proteins provide structural support for cells, body tissues, and organs.
- Proteins such as hemoglobin transport oxygen and nutrients throughout the body via the bloodstream.
- Specialized proteins called antibodies are crucial to immune support.
- Some proteins are hormones that regulate many biological processes, including growth, metabolism, and reproduction.
- Proteins form some receptors on cell membranes and facilitate signaling and communication. An example is osteoblast and osteoclast communication.
- Proteins form transcription factors, which regulate gene expression.
- In times of extreme nutrient deprivation, the body can break down proteins to supply energy.
- Certain proteins act to prevent blood pH from becoming too acidic or alkaline.
- Certain proteins are essential to blood clotting.
- In animals, a protein called ferritin stores iron and regulates iron metabolism. In plants, organelles called plastids perform much the same function.

Thus, our bodies cannot function properly unless they have a steady supply of all the amino acids needed to make complete proteins.

Meat and other animal foods supply significant amounts of complete proteins, which makes it relatively simple for those who consume meat, dairy, or eggs to keep track of their protein intake. Vegans and those who eat very little animal foods must learn to combine plants that together provide amino

> ## The Amino Acids
>
> The names of amino acids can be hard to keep straight at first; however, as you follow a nutrition plan and work with a resource like MyFoodData's amino acid calculator, these names will become familiar friends.
>
> | Nonessential Amino Acids | Essential Amino Acids |
> |---|---|
> | alanine | histidine |
> | arginine* | isoleucine |
> | asparagine | leucine |
> | aspartic acid | lysine |
> | cysteine* | methionine** |
> | glutamic acid | phenylalanine |
> | glutamine* | threonine |
> | glycine* | tryptophan |
> | proline* | valine |
> | serine* | |
> | tyrosine* | |
>
> * conditionally essential amino acids
> ** Methionine is hard to find in plant foods. We suggest soybean sprouts, lentil sprouts, green peas, spirulina, and lima beans.

> ## Hemp the Wonder Seed
>
> Hemp seed contains all the essential amino acids—and in addition, all the essential fatty acids—our bodies need. Three tablespoons of hemp seeds supply 11 grams of protein. Hemp seed also contains vitamin B6, vitamin C, vitamin D, vitamin E, and sodium. Sixty-five percent of the protein content in hemp seed is edestin, a globulin. Edestin is a form of protein stored by a seed until germination. The body can use hemp seed in its raw state, as edestin is readily digestible. Hemp seed's ratio of omega-6 to omega-3 fatty acids is about 3:1, which is in the range currently considered ideal for the human diet.

acids in the amount and ratios needed to offer a complete protein. And it's important to keep in mind that when you read that a plant food contains protein, the percentage matters. If a plant food contains only 2 percent protein, for example, that means it has a relatively small amino acid content.

Plants with Complete Proteins

Amaranth, buckwheat, hemp seed, quinoa, soy products (including edamame, tofu, and tempeh), and spirulina provide all nine essential amino acids.

We recommend that anyone following a vegan diet include some of these foods every day.

The protein in amaranth is similar in amino acid composition to animal protein, but we'd like to draw your attention to hemp seed protein. It is easy to digest compared to other seed and nut proteins. It has a buttery, nutty, smooth, and soft flavor. Unlike other types of seeds, hemp seeds don't need to be soaked in order to release nutrients, and they don't contain toxins in their hull. Blend hemp seed milk with chai spices (see page 112) to complete your morning energy boost. You can also add medicinal seasonings, such as chaga or reishi mushroom powders, to the mix to boost not only your immune system but also your brain health and help memories and focus for the day.

High-Protein Plant Foods and Fungi

Legumes (such as mung beans, lentils, and chickpeas), nuts and seeds, and grains (including quinoa, rice, and wheat) are good sources of amino acids. By combining these high-protein plant foods strategically, you can supply your body with the building blocks for complete protein. Legumes plus nuts create a complete protein, as do grains plus legumes. As you try different combinations you will learn the amounts of each needed to complete the protein. Try these recipes, too: Sprouted Seeds Bread (page 154); Snap Peas with Tempeh Dust (page 172); and Golden Dal Moringa Khichuri (page 184).

Along with their many other confirmed health benefits, mushrooms are rich in amino acids. This includes shiitake, maitake, oyster, portobello, and porcini mushrooms.

Vegetables generally are low in protein, and fruits offer even lower protein, with a few exceptions, such as bananas.

Chemicals in plants that protect mineral stores and inhibit absorption (see chapter 4) also keep a hold on protein, so the plant foods you combine to make protein will almost always need to be prepared by soaking, fermenting, or sprouting to not only release the minerals but also to make the amino acids fully bioavailable.

The Nature of Proteins

Each protein is unique in the number and types of amino acids it contains, the organization of amino acids in chains, and the way the protein folds into a three-dimensional form as it performs its function. Scientists can identify the function of a protein by its shape. Thus, it is important for a protein to not only include its full sequence of amino acids, but also be folded in its genetically designated shape.

Processing foods through techniques such as pasteurization (exposure to heat) very often destroys the delicate protein folds. Most biological protein substances lose their function when they lose their form. This is called denaturing, and it reduces the nutrient benefits a food provides. For example, pineapple contains bromelain, a powerful digestive enzyme. During pasteurization—all commercially available pineapple juice is pasteurized—the bromelain is destroyed. All plant enzymes are destroyed at temperatures above 104°F (60°C). When a protein or an enzyme is exposed to high heat, it can lose its form. We believe that including sources of fully functioning proteins in your diet is essential.

Easy Recipes for Complete Protein

To get started with combinations for complete protein intake, here are some suggestions from Helen.

OATMEAL WITH MIXED SEEDS

Seeds house the nutrients a plant needs to feed new growth, and most are efficient sources of many bone-health nutrients, including but not limited to protein. For that reason, Laura encourages her patients to eat a variety of organically grown or grown-without-pesticides seeds. Here's a

Mankai Duckweed

Mankai duckweed is a choline- and protein-rich gluten-free plant that grows profusely in Southeast Asia on the surface of clean, still water. Although it is tiny (an entire plant is less than 1/64 of an inch long) the plant contains all the essential amino acids and it is rich in non-heme iron that is well absorbed by the human gut. It is also a rare nonanimal source of vitamin B12.[1] At the time of this writing, it is difficult to find a source of Mankai duckweed in the United States, but there is intense interest globally in overcoming the production and distribution issues that could make this truly super food widely available.

complete protein seed combination Helen developed using MyFoodData. Combine an ounce of each of the following seeds in a bag with a good seal and put it in the freezer. Each week, take out the bag, pour some of the mixture into a jar that you set on your kitchen counter, and eat a teaspoon of the mixture each day.

- Chia seeds
- Hemp seeds
- Sesame seeds (black sesame seeds are more nutritious than white)
- Sprouted pumpkin seeds
- Sprouted sunflower seeds
- Sprouted watermelon seeds
- Dried pine nuts
- Almonds
- Pistachios or dry-roasted peanuts

Add the mixture to one heaping cup of oatmeal (not instant); there you have a ready source of your base of 56 milligrams of protein for each day. For maximum nutrient bioavailability, soak whole oats or steel cut oats (porridge oats) overnight in warm water with ½ teaspoon organic apple cider vinegar; the following morning, pour off the liquid, rinse the oats in warm water, and cook as you wish.

Without the oatmeal you are short only one amino acid: lysine. Lysine is scarce in plant foods but the mighty avocado steps in. With avocado and a big pinch of seeds on a salad, you are rich in complete protein in one dish.

MEXICAN-STYLE DINNER

To make an easy bean dish with Mexican flavors, sauté garlic and onions in olive oil in a saucepan. Add cooked black beans or pinto beans with tomato, oregano, black pepper, and chopped fresh spinach. For a thicker sauce, add a tablespoon of tomato paste. Good accompaniments are sliced avocado on a bed of arugula, yellow sweet or white shoepeg corn, and orange sweet potato. To complete the missing links, eat one of your Brazil nuts with or not long after your meal!

SPROUTS ARE KING

Sprouts top our list of bone-healthy protein-rich foods, even though gram for gram, legumes and beans contain more protein. (Sprouted seeds and nuts contain 4 to 8 grams per quarter cup, while soaked cooked beans contain 7 to 8 grams per half cup.) You may raise a cheer when you see how dense with protein lentils and beans are. However, the sobering fact is that they also contain a panoply of antinutrients that kidnap not only minerals but other nutrients, too, and thus much of the benefit ends up being excreted. Effectively, then, the amount of bioavailable protein in lentils and beans is considerably less than nutrition tools report. Cooking will weaken some antinutrient effect, though the amount of protein available is not predictable. Sprouts, however, are king. Sprouting signals the plant to release its nutrients to be available for the new seedling. The nutrients become bioavailable and thus are readily absorbed.

We highly recommend that you try sprouting some seeds, such as organic peas, mung beans, soybeans, adzuki beans, or any other seeds you can find. (See "Easy Breezy Home Sprouting" on page 198 for instructions.) Use these lovely crunchy sprouts to top appetizers, sandwiches, salads, or just about anything.

Among the protein-rich beans, you should consume them fully cooked. Cooking reduces the antinutrients and also defangs any naturally occurring toxins. When cooked, most of the plant foods in the following list supply about 14 grams of protein per cup.

- fava beans
- black beans
- kidney beans
- great northern beans
- navy beans
- chickpeas

Dry oatmeal, dry roasted soybeans, and hemp seeds contain almost as much protein per cup as the beans listed above. By contrast, a cup of broccoli supplies only about 2 grams of protein, and a cup of zucchini 1.5 grams. One ounce of chia seeds supplies about 4 grams of protein.

Nuts are also excellent sources of protein. Roasting, soaking, or sprouting weakens antinutrients and leaves the desirable nutrients in bioavailable form.

Protein Effects on pH Balance

Many people don't take pH balance very seriously. It has been on the health promotion bandwagon for so long, they dismiss it as just another way to sell books or supplements. But there is good reason to take a close look at pH balance and its effect on human health.

When we refer to pH variations or the effect of food on pH (and measuring urine or saliva pH for purposes of health management), we are referring to the body's relative success in balancing acid and alkaline rather than the pH of the blood. Blood pH does not vary. The human body functions in optimum health when the various pH levels of the body are optimal. (See figure 5.2.)

pH balance is tightly regulated by the kidneys. If the kidneys and circulating calcium are not able to manage the level of acidity, then the body will draw calcium from bones to keep blood at the proper pH of 7.35 to 7.45, with the average at 7.4. Current studies in humans on pH affecting cancer show initial data suggesting that slightly acidic conditions may increase cancer cell growth.

Animal proteins and grains leave an acid residue after digestion, and this is why it's been hypothesized that consuming high-protein diets can cause leaching of calcium from the bones. However, as always, the metabolic story is not that simple. While protein consumption creates metabolic acidity, this does not directly affect your bloodstream in terms of acid/base balance, because the body has many systems in place for keeping this balance stable. The real issue in terms of bone health is that in a continuing highly acidic environment, the body will attempt to stabilize by drawing calcium and other alkaline minerals from the bone. Protein may leave an acid

What Did Early Humans Eat?

People who speculate about what early humans ate hypothesize that the diet was probably a dense intake of protein, calcium, magnesium, and other minerals, with low or no intake of sodium chloride. There were no refined sugars or refined carbohydrates, of course. The California Academy of Sciences reports that, based on tooth analyses, very early humans ate only leaves and fruits from trees, shrubs, and herbs. About 3.5 million years ago, early species started to incorporate animal products into their diets—insects and small animals most likely. Humans adapted to heavier protein intake only relatively recently, about 500,000 years ago, when they began to hunt. It is generally accepted that early diets were alkaline, primarily plants and fruits. The widely reported health outcomes of the Mediterranean diet, which favors plant food and advises reduction of acid-producing meat, suggest that the early diet is still healthful today. But considering that we are generally likely to be living far longer, increasing protein as we age is sound advice as long as healthy levels of calcium and other nutrients are present.

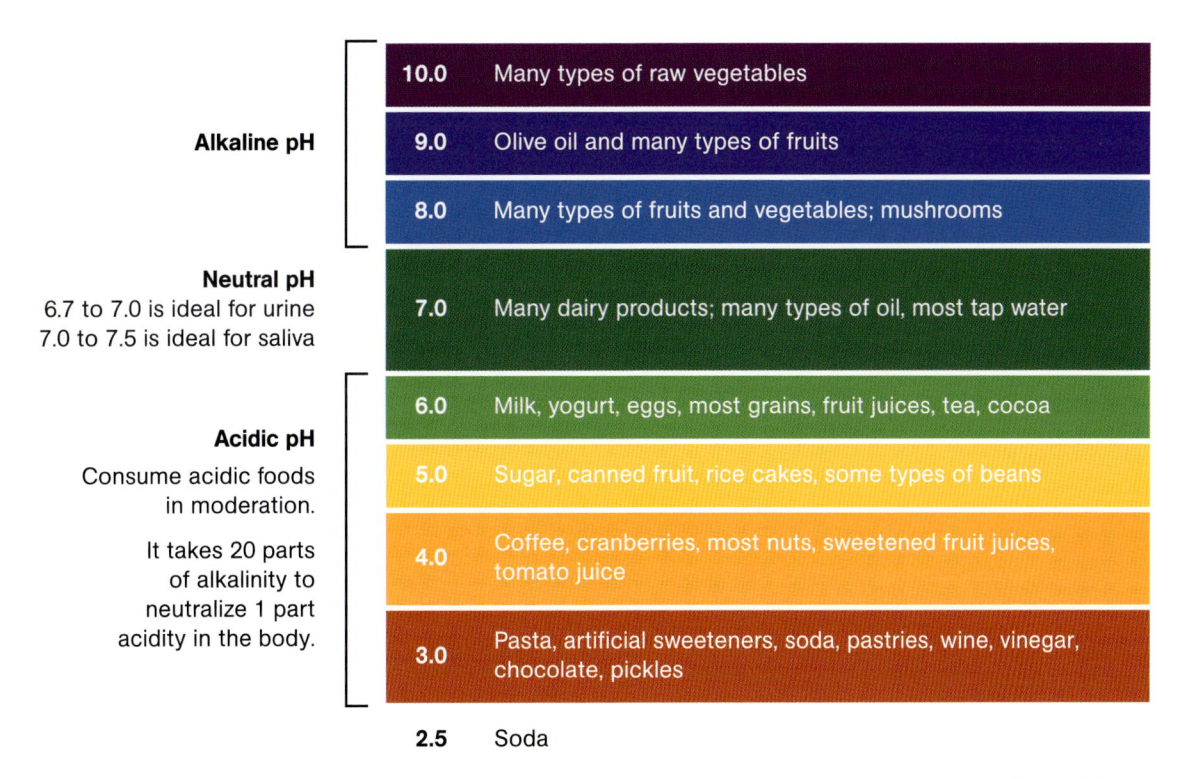

pH	Food
Alkaline pH	
10.0	Many types of raw vegetables
9.0	Olive oil and many types of fruits
8.0	Many types of fruits and vegetables; mushrooms
Neutral pH — 6.7 to 7.0 is ideal for urine; 7.0 to 7.5 is ideal for saliva	
7.0	Many dairy products; many types of oil, most tap water
Acidic pH — Consume acidic foods in moderation. It takes 20 parts of alkalinity to neutralize 1 part acidity in the body.	
6.0	Milk, yogurt, eggs, most grains, fruit juices, tea, cocoa
5.0	Sugar, canned fruit, rice cakes, some types of beans
4.0	Coffee, cranberries, most nuts, sweetened fruit juices, tomato juice
3.0	Pasta, artificial sweeteners, soda, pastries, wine, vinegar, chocolate, pickles
2.5	Soda

Figure 5.2. The pH scale ranges from 0 to 14. The midpoint, 7, is neutral; higher values are alkaline and lower values are acidic.

residue, but if this is balanced by a good intake of vegetables and fruits, your body is likely to have what it needs to keep a healthy acid/base balance.

Ensuring Iron Absorption

Iron is the second most pressing issue for vegans, but not because iron isn't found in plant foods. Your favorite fruits, berries, leafy greens, oyster and white mushrooms, and beans all contain iron. Rather, the issue is iron absorption.

As explained in chapter 2, the iron in animal tissue is called heme iron; the iron in plant foods is called non-heme iron. The human body absorbs heme iron quickly and easily. Heme and non-heme irons are molecularly different, and the heme absorption pathway is more direct than the non-heme absorption pathway. Plant antinutrients strongly inhibit absorption of iron and zinc. Without a boost from other nutrients, non-heme iron is not easily absorbed. Consequently, humans can absorb up to 40 percent of heme iron consumed in animal products, but only just under 5 percent of non-heme iron from plant foods. And this means that iron absorption from plant-based meat substitutes is also limited, despite the authentic-looking meaty red color of these products.

Fortunately, there are three simple ways to promote non-heme iron absorption. Heme iron consumed with non-heme iron promotes non-heme iron absorption, so for readers who include animal food in the diet, the plant iron will have a ready boost. (Note: Egg white slightly inhibits non-heme iron absorption.)

The other ways are to ingest non-heme iron along with either vitamin C or calcium. Let's look at these two vegan options.

Healthy Bones on a Vegan Diet ▪ 75

Vitamin C

Vitamin C (ascorbic acid) is the only nonanimal substance known to promote non-heme iron absorption.[2] Add a vitamin C–rich food—bell peppers, strawberries, broccoli, kiwi, citrus fruit, or any fermented food. Here's why. Ascorbic acid helps to keep iron from binding to other chemicals that render the iron insoluble. It also helps non-heme iron transform into heme iron form. (A note here about grapefruit, which interacts with many pharmaceutical and natural medicines. If you plan to eat grapefruit regularly as a vitamin C source, first check on possible interactions with your medications.)

See the vitamin C and iron lists on page 24 for foods that contain non-heme iron and that are high in vitamin C. Here are some suggestions for tasty combinations from the two lists:

- Lemon vinaigrette with wilted spinach.
- Sprouted beans and chanterelle mushrooms with broccoli.
- White mushrooms with bell pepper, garlic, onion, and fennel.

Calcium

Non-heme iron combines readily with calcium to become insoluble and unavailable for absorption. Does that mean we must set aside calcium-rich plant foods when consuming non-heme iron–rich plant foods?

To get some clarity on this important issue, we asked Holly Batt, a member of the FoodNerd Science Team, about bok choy, which is high in vitamin C yet is among the popular vegetables that contain bioavailable calcium.

Bok choy is a great source of calcium, Batt told us. Most guidelines consider foods with around 20 percent or more of the daily value of calcium per serving as high-calcium foods. This would be roughly equivalent to 200 to 260 milligrams of calcium per serving. In the case of leafy greens, a cup would be one serving. Though the calcium value varies slightly depending on the source, there are approximately 75 to 100 milligrams of calcium per cup of bok choy.

So, what does that mean for the absorption of iron?

The effect of calcium on iron absorption is dose dependent. At lower levels of calcium (less than 40 milligrams of calcium per meal), there appears to be no significant impact on iron absorption. When calcium intake reaches higher levels (above 300 milligrams per meal), the inhibitory effect on iron absorption will be the most significant. Since the calcium content of bok choy is only 75 to 100 milligrams per cup, the inhibitory effects on iron absorption would likely be mild. The exact threshold for this inhibitory effect might vary among individuals based on their overall dietary habits and needs. Other factors such as overall diet and cooking methods also affect the bioavailability of calcium and iron.

Another relevant factor in the calcium-iron absorption relationship is the presence of oxalates, as discussed in chapter 3. Some vegetables, such as spinach and rhubarb, have high levels of oxalic acid. Bok choy contains minimal oxalates (approximately 1 milligram per cup), which reduces the likelihood of it inhibiting the absorption of calcium and non-heme iron. Consequently, bok choy remains a nutritious vegetable choice for those aiming to maintain a balanced diet and obtain essential nutrients without significantly compromising iron absorption.[3]

Foods Rich in Non-Heme Iron

Four top choices for providing non-heme iron are morel mushrooms, dried mulberries, onions, and fennel. Dried morel mushrooms provide 45 percent of the RDA for iron, and for an added bonus, they supply 17 percent of bone RDA for vitamin D. Oyster, maitake, and shiitake mushrooms also contribute to iron requirements. (All other mushrooms provide practically none: 0 to 2 percent.)

Onions have their own vitamin C to help with absorption of their respectable level of iron. Fennel is a high–vitamin C vegetable and also offers some copper and magnesium.

Here are ten runners-up for providing non-heme iron:

- wilted spinach
- lemongrass
- palm hearts
- tomato puree
- asparagus
- lima beans
- Swiss chard
- kimchi
- peas
- cooked chrysanthemum greens

For more choices, see table 2.2 on page 28.

To make a simple iron-rich vegan meal, try a combination that is popular in Mexican cooking, sweet potatoes, morel mushrooms, and guacamole. Here's another: Mushrooms, chile peppers, and pureed tomato with onion, garlic, and oregano is a traditional, simple, delicious combination. This combo is similar to the simple Mexican-style dinner (page 73); you can swap out the black beans for mushrooms. If you invite a mushroom to join in, preferably morel or chanterelle, tomato helps to release its iron store.

Vitamin B12

Vitamin B12 is essential to DNA synthesis, brain health, and blood vessel health, among other life processes. The natural form of vitamin B12 is methylcobalamin; the synthetic form is cyanocobalamin. Vitamin B12 is a cofactor for healthy bone density, and vitamin B12 deficiency suppresses osteoblast function.

Vitamin B12 is water soluble and sourced almost entirely from animal food—milk, eggs, offal, and

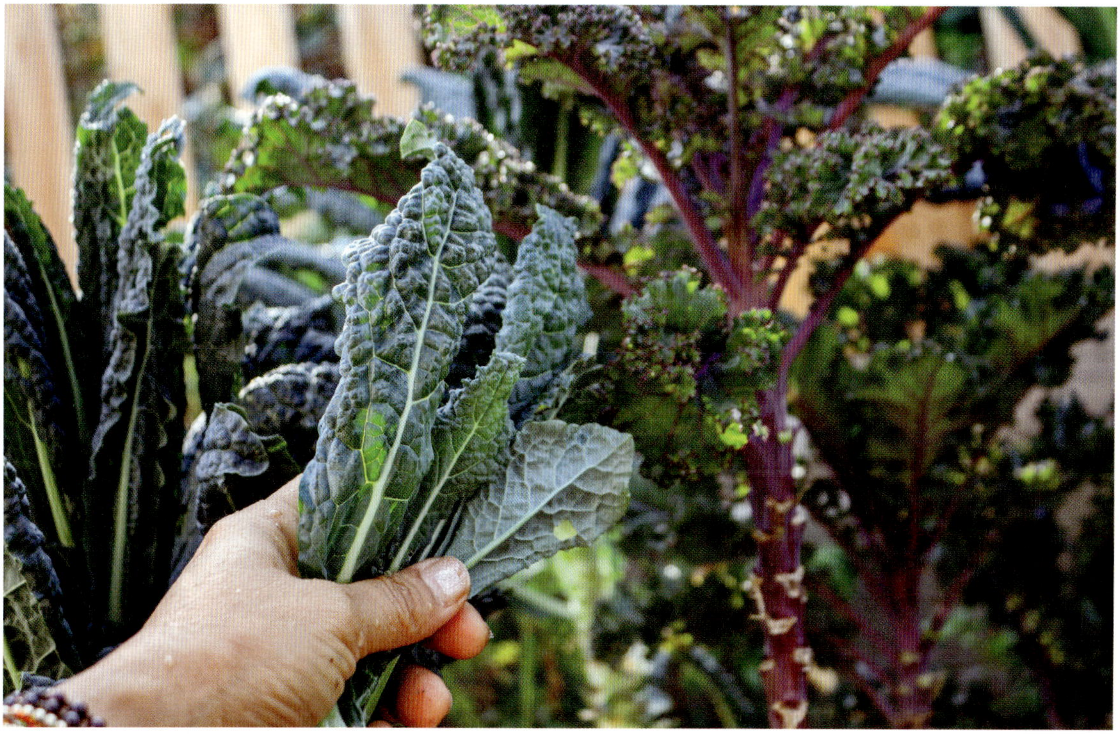

Figure 5.3. Kale has 2 milligrams of iron per 100 grams, along with a complement of antioxidants and enough vitamin C to liberate non-heme iron in mushrooms or other non-heme-iron-rich plants.

meat. A specific strain of bacteria that thrives in mammalian digestive tracts makes vitamin B12. Some types of anaerobic bacteria also produce vitamin B12 in the human gut, and some vegetarian animals eat their feces as a source of vitamin B12. Ancient societies ate insects—crickets are reputed to be rich enough in vitamin B12 to sustain human life.

The good news for vegans and vegetarians is that many plant foods provide small to tiny amounts of natural vitamin B12, and we advise consuming them often, as the body welcomes what is natural.

Fermenting vegetables increases vitamin B12 content because some bacterial strains such as lactic acid bacteria produce vitamin B12. The top choices are dried shiitake mushrooms, lion's mane mushrooms, nori seaweed, algae, Mankai duckweed, and nutritional yeast. Runners-up (but containing only tiny amounts) include hawthorn berries, hops (in beer), bladderwrack (a type of seaweed) primarily as a supplement, and white oak bark as tea.

Vitamin A

As noted in chapter 2, there are two forms of vitamin A: retinol (found in animal foods) and carotenoids (found in plant foods). The measure for vitamin A is retinol activity equivalent (RAE), which represents vitamin A activity as retinol in the human body. It has been determined that 2 micrograms of beta-carotene in oil provided as a supplement could be converted by the body to 1 microgram of retinol. Thus, beta-carotene (as a supplement) has an RAE ratio of 2:1. However, 12 micrograms of beta-carotene from food are required to provide the body with 1 microgram of retinol, giving dietary beta-carotene an RAE ratio of 12:1. Other provitamin A carotenoids in food are less easily absorbed than beta-carotene, resulting in RAE ratios of 24:1. One medium sweet potato offers at least 200 percent of the bone RDA for retinol. One serving—about 1 cup cooked butternut squash—supplies almost 100 percent of the recommended daily requirement. Vitamin A is fat-soluble, so add a half teaspoon of coconut oil or another source of fat.

The BCM01 gene is responsible for this conversion. This gene function can be impaired, so if you are relying on vegetables exclusively as your source of vitamin A, it is important to know the status of your BCM01 function. ("Summing Up Testing Needs" on page 85 discusses arranging for genetic tests.)

Sweet potato is the top choice of vegetable to supply vitamin A. Most varieties contain 3,000 to 16,000 micrograms of beta-carotene per 100 grams, contributing 250 to 1,300 micrograms RAE per 100 grams. Other vegetables that have high conversion to retinol are butternut squash, carrots, kale, turnip greens, red bell peppers, Swiss chard, and dandelion greens.

Choline

Many if not most Americans are deficient in choline, which is important for metabolism of nucleic acids and other functions, as described in chapter 2. Eggs are a main source of choline, but vegans have good choices, too, including legumes, tofu, green vegetables, potatoes, nuts, seeds, grains, and fruit. The goal is to aim for 550 milligrams of choline from the diet on a daily basis. Here are the amounts of choline in some foods.

broccoli	½ cup, cooked	31 mg
Brussels sprouts	½ cup, boiled	32 mg
cauliflower	½ cup, cooked	24 mg
kidney beans	½ cup, cooked	45 mg
peanuts	¼ cup, dry-roasted	24 mg
quinoa	1 cup, cooked	43 mg
red-skinned potato (not russet)	1 large, baked	57 mg
shiitake mushrooms	½ cup, cooked	58 mg
soybeans	½ cup, roasted	107 mg
wheat germ	1 ounce, toasted	51 mg

DHA

DHA is an essential (meaning our bodies can't make it) omega 3 fatty acid that regulates inflammation and brain function. Because DHA is found primarily in fish and fish oil, those on plant-only diets run a risk of DHA deficiency unless supplemented with the proper microalgae. DHA is found as alpha-linolenic acid (ALA) in plants such as flaxseeds, chia and walnuts, and hemp. However, the conversion of ALA to DHA is not efficient, and relying on these sources only may not be sufficient. Hemp seed oil does have a perfect omega ratio and can be a good vegan base for omegas. Testing omega levels is advised. Be aware that it takes 4 months for your body to become replete if you are deficient.

Creatine, Carnosine, and Taurine

Creatine, carnosine, and taurine are nonessential organic compounds found only in animal foods. Although the human body has the capacity to make these substances, plant-based eaters tend to have lower levels of all three, and this often affects muscle mass and performance. Taurine is an amino acid that is not incorporated into proteins, yet it is vital for cellular and cardiovascular health, and supplementation is suggested if testing shows low taurine levels.

Adjusting to Vegan Cooking

Whether or not you are new to vegan cooking, after reading this chapter you may have discovered that vegan cooking for bone health offers the opportunity to build some new skills, and also that there is an up-front learning curve that requires time and patience. For that reason, we have included 100 recipes that are almost all vegan in part 2 of this book. As you cook, the practice will become increasingly part of your everyday life, and we believe the process will become a pleasure. Chapter 19 includes sample meal plans that can help you learn how to eat vegan throughout the week while still providing the nutrients your body needs for healthy bones.

Although Helen is not vegan, she frequently prepares simple meatless meals. Here are a dozen of her no-recipe vegetable and fruit dishes. Choose the ingredients you like, and have fun with the process of putting them together.

1. **Raw salad.** Combine sliced cucumber and rehydrated wakame. Dress with rice vinegar, healthy oil of your choice (we like olive oil plus a little toasted or plain sesame), a fine stream of maple syrup, and showers of sesame seed and cilantro. Optional additions: red pepper flakes, rounds of spring onion, chopped bok choy, thinly sliced broccoli stalks, shaved fennel bulb, red onion, red cabbage, green cabbage. Store in the refrigerator for a week or more. Serving options: Top with a protein you enjoy such as tofu, Gouda, natto, egg, or, if not vegetarian, salmon, shrimp, or leftover roast beef.
2. **Stir-fried green vegetable.** Stir fry chopped garlic; add green beans or any leafy greens plus chickpeas. Sprinkle in some cardamom if you like the taste.
3. **Ratatouille.** Eggplant, tomatoes, zucchini, basil, garlic, and olive oil stewed together make ratatouille. Start by roasting the eggplant and the tomatoes in the skin. Scrape the eggplant from the skin. When the weather is right, barbecue the zucchini by coating in olive oil and turning once on the grill.
4. **Onion soup.** Caramelize a few pounds of onion. Slice white (sweet) or yellow onions very thin, sauté in olive oil until translucent, add a tablespoon of coconut sugar, and sauté until golden. Add caramelized onions to a

rich, dense vegetable (or bone or chicken) broth. Top with baguette croutons. Optional: Top the croutons with vegetarian or Gruyère cheese. Heat in individual soup pots if you have them.

5. **Stir fry.** In any healthy high-temperature oil, such as avocado oil, cook some mung bean sprouts, chopped ginger, minced or finely chopped garlic, pea pods, and sliced asparagus. Optionally include spring onion, lemongrass, or Chinese broccoli.

6. **Pickle.** Steep pearl onions in malt vinegar for 4 to 6 weeks. Use as a relish or pickle.

7. **Roasted root vegetables.** Cut up carrots and parsnips in roughly equally sized pieces. Coat in coconut oil. Roast until soft right through. Optional: Halfway through add turmeric-rich curry powder or ground coriander. Add quartered yellow or halved baby or fingerling potatoes.

8. **Hummus and crudité.** Put 1½ cups cooked chickpeas, ½ cup tahini (ratio 3:1), ⅓ cup olive oil, ground black pepper, and cumin in a mini or regular blender. Whirl. Add more oil to make a soft, thick puree. Slice jicama, celeriac, celery, cucumber, broccoli stalks, or any other crunchy vegetable to scoop up the hummus.

9. **Chocolate banana rounds.** Line a sheet pan with parchment paper. Slice bananas in thick rounds. Use tongs to dip the rounds in melted dark chocolate and set them on the parchment paper. When the tray is full, freeze. Transfer the frozen rounds to a storage container and freeze for up to three months.

10. **Baked apples.** Core apples and place on a baking tray. Into each core opening, put chopped raw or dried figs (for a big calcium boost), cinnamon, coconut sugar or honey, coconut oil or butter. Bake at 350°F (180°C) until a small sharp knife goes all the way through and the apple skins look wrinkled. Options: Substitute chopped dates or raisins for figs; substitute any sugar for coconut sugar or eliminate sweetener altogether.

11. **Fruit ice cream.** Put any plant-based milk (or unpasteurized dairy milk) into a mini blender; add frozen berries or pitted cherries (both stay pliable while frozen). Whirl until you have ice cream.

12. **Your turn.** Make up your own!

CHAPTER 6

Creating a Bone-Health Nutrition Plan

Let's put it all together and then to work for you. Here you will become equipped to create your personalized bone-health nutrition plan—and from there, to select and perhaps create recipes that align with your plan and make the most of foods you love. In this chapter, we set out several examples that model the process of combining foods to meet specific nutritional needs.

Using an Online Nutrient Calculator

As we explained in chapter 2, by using an online nutrient calculator such as MyFoodData you can quickly check foods you like and determine how much of each nutrient is provided in one serving. With that information in hand, you can create appealing food combinations that supply the nutrients your bones need to stay dense and strong.

If you set up a MyFoodData account, you can save the results in your account or print them out for easy reference.

Here's how to use the tools of MyFoodData to search by nutrient.

1. Select the Nutrient Ranking Tool.
2. Select the nutrient, for example "Beta Carotene," and hit Apply. The system will display a list of the plant foods highest in beta-carotene.

Here's how to use MyFoodData to search food groups.

1. Choose the "Food Groups" option.
2. From the dropdown menu, select a food group—for example, Grains and Pasta, Nuts and Seeds, Spices and Herbs, Beans and Lentils, Fruits, or Vegetables.

Here's how to use MyFoodData to build a recipe featuring a specific nutrient.

1. Open the Recipe Nutrition Calculator tool.
2. After putting in the first food, you will be taken to a second page that will allow you to build recipes using the highest-ranking foods for the nutrient you specify.

As a first step, try listing twenty foods you enjoy. Then, using the MyFoodData calculator, note each one's contribution to bone RDA. (A listing of bone RDAs for common foods is in table 2.2 on page 28.) Be sure to note that there can be significant nutritional differences between cooked and raw foods. Can you combine some of the ones you enjoy most to provide bone-health richness? Alternatively, check the nutritional provisions of the ingredients in some of your favorite recipes. You may find you can tweak your favorite recipes to supply the nutrients you need and branch out from there.

Yes, initially it is time-consuming to look up the nutrient contents of food and figure out combinations that meet the levels of bone RDAs, even with the help of the online tools. Fortunately, if you write down or save the combinations you find, in a few weeks you will have a long list of bone-health food combinations to include in dishes you love as well as some substitutions that increase the nutrition of the dish. Exchanging recipes with family or friends may introduce you to new plant foods that you come to love.

Your Personalized Nutrition Plan

How do you make a personalized plan? Create a nutritional profile and address deficiencies, if any. Testing for nutritional deficiencies is available, and Laura recommends such tests to her patients. Many doctors are reluctant to run nutrient profiles, so you may choose to opt for a private test, although it may cost more.

If you show deficiencies despite regular consumption of foods rich in the nutrient that shows up as deficient, you may want to investigate the possibility that there is a genetic cause for deficiency or gut health may be an issue.

Recognizing that routine nutrient testing is in its infancy, Laura created Opal Health, an online platform for personalized bone-health planning. Opal Health provides access to nutritional and genetic testing. The results help you build a complete picture of your own nutritional needs. Opal Health works with Metabolomix from Genova Diagnostics, a testing company that does micronutrient testing; and a genetic test developed at Stanford University for bone density through Axgen.

If you have obtained data from 23andme or Ancestry, then you can use Opal Health to get bone-density genetic results. You can upload your 23andme or Ancestry raw data file to your Opal Health account for recommendations based on your genetics or your genetics plus nutrition test.

Vegan Nutritional Planning

If you are vegan, we suggest you keep a detailed record of plant-food combinations that supply protein, foods that provide vitamins B12 and A, foods that contain non-heme iron, and foods that supply choline. (In chapter 5, we explained the reasons why vegans must pay special attention to these nutrients.) It's also very helpful to keep a list of food combinations that promote iron absorption.

Planning for Protein

Because protein is so fundamental to bone health and overall health, let's start there. The goal is to find foods that in combination supply the body with complete protein (all the essential amino acids). Here are some examples of food combinations that meet that goal, each with the grams of protein it contains:

1 cup cooked lentils (18.9 grams)
+ 1 ounce hemp seeds (9 grams)
+ 1 cup cooked quinoa (8.1 grams)
+ 1 cup cooked spinach (5.3 grams)
+ 1 cup maitake mushrooms (1.5 grams)
+ ¼ cup fresh basil leaves (0.2 grams) =
42 grams protein

1 cup mung beans + 1 cup okra + 1 cup tofu +
1 ounce roasted squash and pumpkin seeds =
68 grams protein

1 cup lentils + 1 cup quinoa + 1 cup tofu =
70 grams protein

1 cup tofu + 1 cup broccoli
+ 1 cup rice + 1 tablespoon soy sauce
+ 3½ ounces shiitake mushrooms =
55 grams protein

1 cup tofu + 1 cup broccoli + 1 cup carrots +
1 cup okra + 1 cup eggplant + 1 ounce shiitake
mushrooms + 1 ounce pumpkin seeds +
1 tablespoon soy sauce =
63 grams protein

Once you've established your basic list of foods to supply protein, you can add other ingredients of your choice to create a tasty meal. Using the first combination above, you could start by mixing together the cooked lentils and quinoa. Then sauté some onion and garlic and add the spinach and mushrooms—and if you include alcohol, a splash of white wine. When they are cooked to your taste, put them over the lentils and quinoa and top with hemp seeds and freshly torn basil leaves.

Planning for Vitamin A

There are several forms of beta-carotene. The conversion of carotene (the form of vitamin A found in plants) to retinol (the active form of vitamin A) varies by carotene and by plant. (See page 78 for detailed information on carotene conversion.) Genes manage this conversion. Therefore, it is possible that one's genetic instruction makes conversion of carotene to vitamin A less efficient. You can find out how efficiently your body manages conversion by taking a nutrition test, and if there is deficiency, by taking a genetic test to find out whether you carry variants on the genes for transformation of carotenes to retinol.

Keep in mind that vitamins A and D work together in the body, so keeping both in the bone RDA range will allow optimum effect.

Here are two examples of tasty combinations that meet the requirement for vitamin A.

1 cup sweet potato + 1 cup tofu + ⅓ cup
shiitake mushrooms + 1 cup Chinese broccoli
+ 1 tablespoon vegan butter =
full RDA of beta-carotene/vitamin A
and complete protein

1 cup cooked mustard greens
+ 1 cup cooked spinach
+ 1 cup cooked collard greens
+ 1 tablespoon vegan butter
+ 1 tablespoon soy sauce =
281% of daily bone RDA for vitamin A
and 50% for iron

Planning for Iron

As explained in chapter 5, the form of iron in plant foods is non-heme iron, which can be more challenging for the body to absorb. If you tend to have low iron levels, it is important to make sure you are consuming plants rich in non-heme iron and ideally combining them with plants that provide vitamin C, which helps boost iron absorption.

The process for doing this is the same as for vitamin A described above, and here is an example we came up with using the MyFoodData tools:

1 cup tofu + 1 cup morel mushrooms
+ 1 cup coconut milk
+ 1 teaspoon lemongrass =
154% of bone RDA for iron,
141% for calcium, and 103% for protein

Another combination we like is to sauté a cup of mustard greens until wilted and add 1 ounce of dried black currants to make Catalan mustard greens. The total vitamin C contribution is 274 percent of bone RDA.

Planning for Choline

People who have folate deficiency have a higher-than-average need for choline. If you are genetically

Creating a Bone-Health Nutrition Plan ▪ 83

impaired in folate transformation to methylfolate, you need to be sure that you are consuming enough choline. The need for choline also increases as you lose estrogen, and choline is vital for liver and brain health. In fact, only 10 percent of Americans meet their need for choline.

Eggs are high in choline, as is salmon. Supplementing with choline is often suggested for vegans, for a total daily intake of 425 milligrams for women and 550 milligrams for men. Too much choline, however, can cause irritability and other effects, so it is important to supplement only when there is a special requirement, such as deficiency.

Here are some examples of food combinations that supply substantial amounts of choline (and protein):

1 cup tofu + 1 cup quinoa + 1 cup broccoli
+ 1 cup cabbage + 1 ounce cashews
+ 1 cup soymilk + 1 cup bok choy =
31% of daily RDA for choline

1 cup roasted edamame
+ 1 cup shiitake mushrooms
+ 1 cup red potato + 1 ounce almonds =
**39% of bone RDA for choline
and 87% for protein**

1 cup mashed cooked lima beans
+ 1 cup mashed cooked chickpeas
+ 1 cup mashed cooked edamame =
**41% of bone RDA for choline
and 115% for protein**

With a little imagination, it's easy to see how you can turn these combinations into a tasty dish. For example, add some olive oil, salt, and cumin or your favorite spices, and the combo of lima beans, chickpeas, and edamame works well for a dip or spread.

Planning for Vitamin B12

Taking in sufficient quantities of vitamin B12 is a well-known challenge for people on a vegan diet. Luckily, fermenting vegetables increases vitamin B12 content, and soy products also contain vitamin B12. A daily cup of soymilk made from sprouted soybeans provides 100 percent of bone RDA for vitamin B12. Mushrooms are also a good source.

1 cup shiitake mushrooms + 1 cup lion's manes
+ 1 cup morels + 1 cup soymilk
+ ½ cup coconut milk =
104% of bone RDA for vitamin B12

Bone Health Testing

Laura recommends to patients that they test nutritional levels and bone density genetics. Even if you are under 30, bone density genetics can alert you to a potential issue later in life and allow you time to build up bone mass. If you are already managing bone loss, additional testing—Ctx and P1NP—can be done between DXA scans, which will allow you to learn more quickly whether your nutritional plan is working, and you can adjust accordingly. General recommendations for health are just that and may or may not apply to each person. Gathering data on your own body is the best way to know what your recovery plan will be. Each will be unique.

Timing of Testing

Most health insurance plans will pay for a DEXA scan every two years. The results of the scan are recorded in a variety of numbers. The easiest for us to use is the T score, which is the difference between your bone mineral density and that of a healthy 30-year-old.

If you are faced with serious bone loss (Laura generally uses a score of −3 as a cutoff, but it varies depending on other health factors) and want to try using nutritional and natural medicine to improve your bone health, it may be advisable for you to discuss medication with your provider.

CTx (and NTx, which is also used as a bone marker) looks at the loss of collagen from the

Summing Up Testing Needs

The single most reliable way to know your unique deficiencies and the health of your gut is to test. Laura uses the Metabolomix micronutrient test from Genova Diagnostics. This is a urine test; looking at blood levels of nutrients does not tell you if or how they are being used by the body. The Metabolomix test is provider-only, so you will not be able to order it directly yourself, but it can be ordered through Opal Health (www.opalhealth.com). Some insurances may cover a portion of the Metabolomix micronutrient test.

Genetics for bone density are not uniform among humans; instead, they are unique to you. For that reason, you will not be able to gauge the impact of your genetics on bone health without testing. Stanford University developed a test that Laura has included in Opal Health's testing. Currently, insurances will not cover the cost of a bone-density genetics test.

CTx and P1NP are conventional lab tests available at Labcorp and Quest Diagnostics. They are provider-only. You can ask your doctor to order the CTx and P1NP, which may be covered by your insurance via your local doctor. You can also order these tests through Opal Health.

Laura also recommends knowing your vitamin D levels and your HbA1c levels. Both should be part of your yearly checkup. If not, you can order tests for these at Opal Health.

If you have been prescribed estrogen or hormone replacement therapy or wish to use hormone supplementation to improve your bone health, Laura strongly suggests that you take a reproductive cancer genetic test, especially if you do not know your parents' history/lineage or if there is a history of cancer in your family. These are through Labcorp and can be tested there or through Opal Health.

If you are using or intend to use estrogen supplementation, Laura suggests that you test your genetics for clotting because of the increased risk of clotting among some people when using estrogen. Clotting genetics are available in the bone-density genetic test available through Opal Health.

How does your body detoxify estrogen? The answer depends on both genetics and diet. An estrogen detoxification test is the best indicator of safe estrogen use. In conventional medicine, typically an estrogen detoxification test is provider-only; however, this test is available at Opal Health.

---

breakdown of bone. P1NP looks at the use of collagen to build bone. CTx and P1NP tests are not readily available to patients without a request from a provider, so there are two ways forward: Your local licensed health care provider can order these for you or you can use a lab test ordering site such as Opal Health. However, physicians often do not or will not order nutrition tests or genetic tests because they do not have experience using them or applying the information gleaned from them.

The CTx and P1NP tests are done as a benchmark before you start your nutritional work. To monitor the effectiveness of the nutritional plan, Laura recommends follow-up testing in three to four months. If there is little or no improvement, then it is likely that underlying factors are affecting bone generation, and further investigation would be advisable. In cases such as this, Laura advises talking with your health care provider and reconsidering whether it is safe for you to rely on nutrition only.

In addition, gut health is vital and at the foundation of all good health and longevity. Laura suggests gut health testing at any time to improve health and longevity. Laura recommends Viome (www.viome.com), a consumer testing company that provides personalized recommendations for foods, herbs, and probiotics. Laura has no relationship with this or any testing company except Opal Health, which was created to provide you with access to the data you need for self-care.

Ensuring good gut health will allow your body to make optimal use of the nutrients in your food so that can truly be your medicine.

Trabecular Bone Score

Although bone-density measurement through DEXA scan is the approved way to gauge fracture risk, it is not the only important piece of fracture risk information. For example, if you are a small-boned person, you are more likely to receive a diagnosis of osteoporosis; however, even if your bones are small, if they are flexible they will not break. There is currently no measure of bone flexibility in medicine, but asking your doctor for a trabecular bone score (TBS) will better help you understand your true risk. Ask your doctor for a TBS at the time you have your next DEXA scan. An Echolight scan is also a good option for assessing bone health.

Assessing Bone Loss

If you are experiencing bone loss, an important first step is to organize your thoughts and consider actions for bone-density improvement. Typically, conventional medicine advises people diagnosed with bone loss to take a pharmaceutical. Laura suggests that one may consider an interim decision to address bone loss naturally via the nutrient route—a decision best taken in concert with a health care provider (see "Talking with Your Doctor" on page 87).

You can adopt the natural medicine approach that Laura has developed in all circumstances, including along with a pharmaceutical remedy. The natural route may take longer to be effective than a pill, so there are some considerations to include in your decision-making process.

Gathering data is an excellent foundation for making an informed decision about your health. First, how severe is your bone loss? Severity of bone loss will tell you how likely you are to experience microfractures, and therefore—in essence—how much time you have to undertake a natural medicine approach. Other factors that play a role are whether you exercise regularly, what the quality of your diet is, and whether there is a history of osteoporosis in your family. If you do not know whether there is a family history of osteoporosis, we strongly suggest a genetic test.

A second important question is, What are your genetics for bone density? Learning this will tell you how easy it should be for your body to regain bone density. Good genetic scores indicate your body's natural ability to have healthy density. Lower genetics scores indicate that regaining density will very likely be more challenging.

Knowing these two data points will help you determine if undertaking a natural medicine approach is wise or if you are already at a point where waiting may endanger your health.

You can also complete the "Worksheet for Scoring Bone Density Loss" on page 87. It can help you determine your next steps.

Talking with Your Doctor

It is useful to plan a conversation with your doctor about testing, because many physicians who practice

WORKSHEET FOR SCORING BONE DENSITY LOSS   POINTS

1. How severe is my bone loss in T-scores? _____ _____

    Scores of less than −3 are a cause for concern: 5 points
    Scores of −2.5 to −2.9: 3 points

2. Is there a history of severe osteoporosis in my family, yes or no? _____ _____

    Yes: 2 points
    No: 0 points, but testing is recommended

3. Do I have a good diet that consists of primarily whole foods with a high intake of properly prepared plant foods, yes or no? _____ _____

    Yes: 0 points
    No: 1 point

4. Do I exercise regularly, yes or no _____ _____

    Yes: 0 points
    No: 1 point

If your overall score is 5 or less, then it is possible you can explore the nutritional approach for at least six months (longer if your score is 0–4).

If your score is 6 or 7, it may be possible for you to undertake the nutritional approach for a short period of time, and this should be discussed with a knowledgeable health care provider.

If your score is 8 or 9, then it is possible that you may need to use pharmaceuticals in concert with nutrition, and this must be discussed with a knowledgeable health care provider.

---

conventional medicine say that one cannot use nutrition to treat bone density loss. For a great majority of us this is not true. However, presenting a plan and inviting discussion gives your physician an opportunity to express pros and cons or reservations and gives you an opportunity to address objections and set out the details of your nutrition plan along with your commitment to closely monitor progress.

If you decide to try a natural medicine remedy for bone density, approach your doctor with a solid plan along with your genetic results for bone density. Invite discussion, welcome the doctor's comments and suggestions, and assure your doctor that you will revisit all suggestions once your agreed-upon period has ended. After this respectful exchange, it is highly likely that your doctor will agree to at least a six-month trial of a natural medicine plan, such as Laura's plan described below. If your density loss isn't too severe, your doctor may agree that you can try the plan for a full year.

Creating a Bone-Health Nutrition Plan

Note that the genetic test for bone density is not widely available and your doctor may not be aware of this test, so be prepared to explain why it is crucial information. If your own doctor declines to order tests, you may order the tests via Opal Health, which is managed by Laura; the test costs will be principally on a private-pay basis.

Laura's Natural Medicine Plan

After working with many patients, Laura developed this protocol to identify the best way forward for each individual.

STEP ONE: GATHER DATA

To begin, gather your nutrition and genetic data through the tests described earlier in this chapter. This information will allow you to identify how to go about reversing bone loss naturally and will help you create protocols to address deficiencies to remove the obstacles. You will also be able to assess your inherent risk for fracture and the state of your gut health and nutrition, which is an important part of making a natural medicine plan.

STEP TWO: MONITOR PROGRESS

As discussed, DEXA scans are usually covered by insurance every two years (in some cases every year); however, some of you will not have a year to try natural medicine. In this case you will need to know more quickly whether what you are doing is helping. Get CTx and P1NP tests (see "Summing Up Testing Needs," page 85). If you have an osteoporosis diagnosis, some insurance companies will cover these tests.

We suggest discussing and using these results in concert with your doctor or other knowledgeable provider.

Your CTx needs to go down. A decrease of 25 percent indicates success. If after three months your score is still increasing, then there are probably impediments to your success with natural medicine, such as impaired gut health, inflammatory conditions, blood sugar issues, or other more complex issues.[1]

Your P1NP needs to go up. A change greater or equal to a 21 percent increase from baseline is considered success.[2] For those taking a bisphosphonate such as Reclast or Fosomax, P1NP levels have been shown to *decrease* up to 70 percent from baseline after six months of therapy due to the drug halting bone turnover. Treatment with conventional hormone replacement therapy can also show a decrease in P1NP levels. Discuss your results with your provider if you are using either of these pharmaceutical interventions.

Tools for Your Recovery Plan

The above data can be put into a plan for improving bone health. This plan will contain some or all of these, depending on your level of bone loss and genetics for bone density:

- Supplements and foods to help remedy any nutritional deficiencies found
- Bone RDA nutrient list
- Therapeutic dosage levels determined by test results
- Use of herbal formulas to increase bone density
- Use of plant hormones to increase bone density

If any of your T scores are less than −3 and if your genetic score is higher than −12 percent, we advise working with a provider who is versed in not only nutrition but the use of herbs for bones.

Sample Bone Health Recovery Plan

Here is a sample bone health recovery plan.

MONTH 1

- Begin personalized nutritional supplementation for bone health. Supplementation might include:
  - Collagen peptides
  - Silica
  - Trace minerals
  - Vitamin K2

- Magnesium
- Vitamin D
- Omega-3s
- Calcium

- Check your vitamin D levels—ensure between 50 and 80 nanograms per milliliter, ideally 60 to 70.
- Take your calcium and magnesium supplements in the evening (see "Make Your Own Calcium Supplement," page 32).
- Take a nutrition test to know what other nutritional work you have to do.
- Take a bone genetic test (use 23andme or Ancestry data if you have it).
- Take CTx and P1NP tests for baseline.
- Start cooking for bone health.

MONTH 2

You will now have your nutrition and genetic data and can either make a plan on your own or work with a provider or Opal Health. Your plan will include any additional supplementation, foods, or further testing that you may need. Your plan will also include the length of time it is advisable for you to use natural medicine, and the likelihood of this effort being short term or long term (which you'll determine based on your genetics and DEXA scores).

- Continue bone-health supplements.
- Adjust supplementation based on your nutrition test results.
- Expand your efforts to cook for bone health.
- Share your plan with your doctor (see "Talking with Your Doctor," page 86).
- If nutritional tests indicate a need to do so, take a gut health test.

MONTH 3

- Continue supplements and cooking for bone health.

MONTH 4

- Retake CTx and P1NP tests.
- Continue supplements and cooking for bone health.

MONTHS 5 AND 6

- Continue supplements and cooking for bone health.

MONTH 7

- Continue supplements and cooking for bone health.
- Retake nutrition test.

MONTH 8

- Adjust nutrition and supplementation according to latest test results.
- Retake CTx and P1NP tests.

MONTHS 9, 10, AND 11

- Continue supplements and cooking for bone health.

MONTH 12

- Get a new DEXA scan, or if not, then retake CTx and P1NP tests.
- Congratulate yourself on the hard work and success.
- If necessary, make a long-term plan for bone care.

Quick-Start Suggestions for Those with Osteoporosis

- Consume calcium-rich foods with your first or second meal of the day.
- Consume at least 1 tablespoon of bone-building vinegar daily.
- Use a splash of plain organic apple cider vinegar with mother on raw or lightly cooked green vegetables. The vinegar helps to release the nutrients.
- Consider boosting a regular bone-building diet with the core trio of supplements: collagen (marine suggested, or pea protein); vitamin K2; and trace minerals, preferably fulvic/humic.

Normal amounts will not interfere with blood-thinning medication, though check with your doctor. Dosing suggestion: 350 micrograms per day.
- If you do not have histamine issues and you are a flexitarian, consume bone broth three times per week for two months. If you have histamine issues, consume bone broth only with advice from a health care professional.
- Prepare foods to weaken phytates, oxalates, and other antinutrients that can lock up minerals and other nutrients in plant foods.
- If your DEXA score is below −3 and nutrition is your sole or primary source of bone health treatment, test CTx and P1NP every three months. If in six months scores do not hold steady or improve, then further investigation such as genetic testing is advised.
- To shed light on your fracture risk, ask your doctor to add a TBS to your DEXA scan.
- Become a regular consumer of phytoestrogen-containing plants, including herbs, or of food-based phytoestrogen supplements.
- If you need extra calcium or wish to supplement, make eggshell calcium supplement powder (see "Make Your Own Calcium Supplement," page 32) and take ½ teaspoon daily, which is about 400 milligrams of calcium, the perfect amount to supplement a calcium-rich diet. Your body absorbs a maximum 500 milligrams of calcium at any one time, so if your supplement requirements are higher than that, spread intake throughout the day.

CHAPTER 7

Ancient Medicine for Bone Health

Zoopharmacognosy is the study and documentation of animals that travel sometimes hundreds of miles to find the plants, insects, and soils that remedy a specific illness. *Zoo* = animal; *pharma* = pharmacology. How the animals know not only which plants, insects, and soil nutrients are antidotes for specific conditions but where those antidotes are found is largely a mystery. That's where *-cognosy* comes in (*cognoscere* is Latin, meaning "to become acquainted with"). We humans do not know how, but the animals know. Not only animals but ancient medical practitioners also knew; they studied and understood the various and differing values and powers of individual plants and the different effects on the human body of the various parts of the same plant—root, stem, and leaf.

Similarly, without the kind of gold-standard study results upon which we rely for evidence-based medicine, ancient peoples used their plant knowledge to practice plant nutrition and plant medicine. Iraqi healers practiced herbal medicine in the Sumerian period, approximately 3000 BCE. In 2600 BCE, the Chinese created the *Huangdi Neijing*, describing how plants can be used as medicine. A millennium later the ancient Egyptians created the Kahun Medical Papyrus and the Ebers Papyrus, describing plant remedies. Three thousand years ago in India, religious healers developed Ayurvedic medicine, detailing combinations of plants that would address and redress a variety of physical and emotional complaints: *ayur* = knowledge; *veda* = life. In about 50 CE, a Greek physician, Pedanius Dioscorides, wrote *On Materia Medica*, a pharmacopeia of 600 medicinal plants and the remedies physicians could draw from them. Ancient healers accurately matched therapeutic plants with conditions and diseases, and they taught and passed along their knowledge in oral and written histories. Today these same practices and remedies are part of the pharmacopeia on which Traditional Chinese Medicine and Ayurvedic physicians rely.

Ancient peoples also knew which plants would not be optimally nutritional or optimally therapeutic until soaked, sprouted, or fermented. Around 10,000 BCE, tribal people allowed milk to ferment into yogurt, and later Louis Pasteur documented the health benefits of dairy fermentation. In the era of the Chu dynasty, physicians discovered the health benefits of fermented vegetables. *Shu-Ching*, written during the Chou dynasty in China (1121 to 256 BCE), refers to the use of *chu*, a fermented grain product.[1] How they knew we do not know, yet clearly ancient peoples, too, had *-cognos*.

The Eternal Bone-Healing Formula

In approximately 500 CE, Shaolin monks in China began advancing the martial arts, developing a new form of kung fu that employed qigong and abdominal breathing to turn their bodies to armor. Their martial practice was intertwined with religious philosophy, the physical and mental a necessary whole—the *Chan* and the *Quan*. They became known as monks with a fighting superpower, and along with this practice they created "fall and strike" medicine as a necessity to treat injuries from practice.

From this ancient medicine, modern herbalists and physicians pull ideas about how to treat bones. We can directly use their methods to heal fractures, but we can also let this treatment guide us on what herbs and methods can be used to help generate bone that has lost density.

The theory of bone in TCM is that optimum bone health relies on the energy of the kidneys as the source of all vitality in the body.

One of these ancient bone formulas was known as "The Eternal Bone-Healing Formula." It originated with the Yi people who came from Tibet to settle in Yunnan province. The Yi were famous for their knowledge of the healing power of plants. This formula is approved based on clinical studies by the National Medical Products Administration, the Chinese government agency that is equivalent to the US Food and Drug Administration, and is officially recommended by the Chinese government to the World Health Organization as a treatment for bone diseases such as osteoporosis.

The Eternal Bone-Healing Formula dates from the Tang dynasty (618 to 907 CE). It includes these herbs:

- Chen Pi—citrus peel
- Hong Hua—saffron
- San Qi—which means "Three Seven," coming from the belief that the herb is more effective when harvested between 3 and 7 years after planting
- Du Zhong—from the Chinese rubber tree
- Ren Shen—ginseng, one of the master herbs of TCM
- Huang Qi—astragalus, the best-known source of telomerase, the enzyme that helps maintain telomere length
- Bie Jia—from the shell of the tortoise; the plant equivalent is Shu Di Huang

To the knowledge of these herbalists and physicians add the knowledge from the Shaolin. Dosages of these would depend on stage of bone loss (DEXA scores) and presence or not of fracture or microfracture.

- Gu Sui Bu
- Du Zhong (do not use if you have an allergy to latex)
- Dan Shen (do not use large doses if you are taking blood thinners)
- Bu Gu Zhi
- Xu Duan
- Dang Gui

Keep in mind that TCM is personalized medicine, so herbal formulas may be adjusted to meet an individual's other needs and constitution.

We use some of these herbs in our herbal vinegar to give it even more bone-health boost (see "Dr. Laura's Bone Vinegar," page 137). Our herbal vinegar is safe for nearly everyone except those who have an allergy to a particular herb. If you are using herbs to heal fracture, we recommend speaking with a knowledgeable provider.

Using the Formula for Fractures

When treating fractures, combining topical and internal treatment always brings the best results. For example, if you are treating a tendon injury, use a topical poultice made from ground herbs mixed with a binding substance such as egg white. Egg white promotes vascularization, stimulating the growth of the vascular endothelium. If using egg white is impractical, you can put the herbs into Vaseline.

The herbs are cooked in a high-proof alcohol and pasted over the fractured area and left in place for two hours or more, a few times a week to start. Use this poultice for extremities but not over the trunk of the body. For ribs and other fractures on the trunk, use remedies taken internally and cover the injury with a light spray of herbs soaked in alcohol (if such a spray is available).

There are multiple stages to injury from both the TCM and Western perspective. The first stage is the inflammation and pain period; the second stage begins after this acute response has gone and the healing process is happening.

STAGE 1

Immediately following injury, trauma usually lasts three to four days but may be longer in higher-force trauma. A fibrin-rich blood clot forms over the area, initiating healing by releasing growth factors. Inflammatory molecules stimulate the origination of new blood vessels and osteoprogenitor cells.

Within hours, a new blood supply emerges, revascularizing the fracture site.

After a few days the blood clot is transformed into new connective tissue called granulation tissue, an intermediary that protects the wound.

STAGE 2

In stage 2, repair begins, with granulation tissue transforming into collagen fibrils and ultimately becoming cartilage. Bone then becomes woven at the fracture site.

STAGE 3

Stage 3 is watching and waiting. It is usually untreated. If stages 1 and 2 occur successfully, then stage 3 will take care of itself. This is the longer process of full bone regrowth and can take 6 to 9 years.

Using the Formula for Bone Loss

Treating bone loss follows the same herbal principles as treating fracture. Not only do we need to provide nutrition specific to bone, but we need to ensure bones have phytoestrogen as well as the right type of fat.

Physicians do not use topical poultices to treat bone loss, unless that bone loss is very severe, and due to the limitations of use over the trunk, we cannot treat the whole skeleton.

Internally we use lower doses of the same herbs used to treat fracture, as they stimulate all aspects of bone health.

Medicinal Mushrooms

The story of fungi is that of a magical kingdom.[2] In this kingdom, edible entities are variously venerated as food, longevity boost, medicinal remedy, and a source of euphoria. The kingdom is vast. The three major groups are molds, fruiting bodies (spore-producing individuals, principally mushrooms and toadstools), and yeasts. Over time, observers have noted nearly 4 million species of fungus and

A Note of Caution

While mycologists—mushroom scientists—reliably recognize edible fungi, when we speak of mushrooms in this book, or include a mushroom in a recipe, we are referring only to those generally accepted as safe to consume. They are routinely available as grocery items or frequently used as over-the-counter medicinal mushroom powders. Do not forage for mushrooms unless you are trained to do so.

described about 150,000 of them. Among those, about 14,000 are species of mushroom, and among the mushrooms, nearly 10,000 are edible.[3] Use of mushrooms goes back millennia. Beginning some 13,000 years ago, people have been celebrating the medicinal power of mushrooms, whose benefits were once ascribed to benevolent gods and more recently to the metabolic action of chemical properties. The current interest in natural medicines has sparked systematic examination of reputed benefits to see which ones, if any, gold-standard research will confirm.

To date there is a body of anecdotal and small-study evidence suggesting the probability that many species of mushrooms, if not all edible mushrooms, can positively affect health.[4] Let us count the ways.

Note: Mushrooms absorb many toxins, including heavy metals, from the soil. Cooking mushrooms with coriander (dried) or cilantro (fresh) helps to reduce risk of heavy-metal damage to DNA.

Immune System Regulators

The skin, gut lining, and nasal passages are barriers, our first lines of defense against gross environmental menace. Behind the scenes, though, the immune system is continuously on alert for the tiniest, even microscopic, barrier breach. A cut to the skin, toxins that escape the gut into the body cavity, bacteria and viruses too small for the nasal passages to trap— each presents a potential threat to health and triggers an immune system response.

The immune system has several branches, each with specialized cells—for example, some for early generalized response, such as to a wound that opens the body to infection or breathing in a toxic fume, and some for memory and tailored response, such as recognition of antibodies from a former infection. The branches communicate with one another in a coordinated effort to attack threat, demolish disease, and restore or maintain life processes. As we have noted, immune system cells are born in bone marrow, and most of them mature there, then travel to settle in predetermined locations, mostly in the lymphatic system, the ideal location from which to carry out their duties.[5]

Every species of edible mushroom, including those used in our recipes, makes a unique biochemical contribution to the health of the immune system. Some help to boost production of immune cells; some support communication among the branches.[6] Some increase the effectiveness of pharmaceuticals such as some chemotherapies. Science points to about 700 species among the approximately 14,000 known mushroom species that have demonstrated pharmacological—that is, medicinal rather than simply nutritional—properties.

Mushrooms, including all those ordinarily consumed fresh, dried, in powder, or as extracts, are antiviral and antifungal due to stimulation of the immune cells that fight these invaders.

Mushrooms can be antimicrobial. For example, a protein, recently discovered, binds to the cell wall of an unwelcome bacterium inhibiting reproduction.[7]

All mushrooms regulate cytokines, which are molecules that regulate the immune system's response. Properly regulated, cytokines will be well balanced between inflammatory and anti-inflammatory responses.

Other Beneficial Effects of Mushrooms

Mushrooms are about 80 percent water. When dried, they retain nearly 100 percent of their nutrients. Almost all edible mushrooms contain most or all essential amino acids. Oyster mushrooms in particular are rich in all nine essential amino acids.

Mushrooms are the only nonanimal source of vitamin D, calcium's absorption partner. Maitake mushrooms grow to full size with a vibrant supply of vitamin D; other mushrooms will produce vitamin D if you leave them in the sun, gills facing up, for 24 to 36 hours, depending upon the size of the mushroom. Then either store in the fridge in a paper bag or mesh vegetable bag and consume within a week, or dry in a dehydrator. Store dehydrated for up to one year. Vitamin D–enhanced mushrooms are a natural vitamin D2 supplement. We prize any nutrient sourced from a natural food matrix, because natural foods do not trigger an immune response; thus, the mushroom as a source of vitamin D is a treasure.

Continuing with our ode to mushrooms, let's consider the reported health benefits to the body in general and some exciting news about benefit to bones specifically. We must, however, note that consuming many types of edible mushrooms appears to lower blood sugar levels and blood pressure and to increase the thinning of the blood. If you take blood pressure medication, diabetes medication, or anti-clotting or blood-thinning pharmaceuticals, you must monitor the effects of consuming large amounts of mushrooms, especially extracts and powders. The amounts of whole-food mushrooms we include in our recipes will be within safe limits.

About 2 percent of an oyster mushroom is lovastatin, a natural cholesterol-lowering remedy. How much is required to have an effect? How effective is it? How much oyster mushroom must one consume to realize the benefit, and how much is safe to consume on a daily basis? As scientists recognize that side effects of pharmaceutical statins are prohibitive for some people, these questions are currently under study.

At this writing, there is exciting news about oyster mushrooms and bone health: The lovastatin in an oyster mushroom promotes osteoblast generation and inhibits osteoclast generation. Because of this, the possibilities of using lovastatin for preventing and treating early bone-density decline are exciting.

Best of the Medicinal Mushrooms

People have been consuming mushrooms as tonics and as medicines for thousands of years. It is beyond the scope of this book to detail the mechanisms of action of each, but we can summarize the impacts of the most thoroughly investigated species. For each we list the name used in common parlance and also the scientific name. Including any or all of these mushrooms in your diet will be a boon to bone health.

REISHI

Reishi mushrooms (*Ganoderma lucidum*), praised as the mushroom of immortality, boost the immune system, lower cholesterol, and treat urinary tract infections and urologic issues. Documentation from China dating to 200 CE shows that reishi was used for medicinal purposes such as tonifying, enhancing vital energy, strengthening cardiac function, increasing memory, and protecting against aging. Current research shows that in mice, reishi arrested tumor cells (bladder, prostate, and leukemia). In humans, reishi modulates the immune system, acts as an antioxidant, and shows antiviral and antibacterial properties.

CHAGA

Chaga (*Inonotus obliquus*) is an edible fungus, though it is not a fruiting body and so not a mushroom. It is shot through with mycelia, tendrils of fungus that act as the root system of most fruiting bodies. It grows on bark. Though edible cooked, chaga is bitter and corklike in texture, so preparing it as a tea is best. Chaga is known to lower blood sugar and have strong antioxidant effects. Chaga has very broad biological activity, including but not limited to anticancer, anti-inflammatory, antiviral, antioxidant, immunomodulatory, hypoglycemic, hypolipidemic, and hepatoprotective. It also counteracts the progression of cancers and diabetes.

SHIITAKE

Eating delicious shiitake mushrooms (*Lentinula edodes*) regularly is a great way to assist with immune system health and general disease prevention. The health benefits attributed to shiitake, a popular culinary mushroom, are legion: antimicrobial, antiviral, anticancer and antitumor, antidiabetic, antihyperlipidemic, LDL cholesterol control, antioxidative, antiaging, hepatoprotective—and importantly, it is an agent of immune system stimulation. Yet until recently, these benefits were the lore of ancient peoples, reported in animal studies or anecdotal, as relatively few gold-standard research studies had conclusively demonstrated these benefits in humans. Happily, evidentiary medicine has undertaken to test claims of many ancient remedies using contemporary guidelines, and research now confirms that regular or daily consumption of shiitake mushroom reduces inflammation and improves human immunity, including gut immunity.[8]

Several clinical trials show that combining shiitake mushrooms with chemotherapy extends survival in patients with stomach, prostate, colorectal, and liver cancers.[9]

MAITAKE

Maitake mushroom (*Grifola frondosa*), also known as hen of the woods, was called the dancing mushroom by ancient peoples who danced each time they were fortunate enough to come upon a maitake mushroom. This species offers naturally occurring vitamin D. Maitake also displays antitumor action, slowing growth of tumors in the colon, lung, stomach, liver, prostate, and brain. The Food and Drug Administration has approved investigational new drug applications for studies on maitake extract to treat advanced breast and prostate cancers.

CORDYCEPS

Recent studies of cordyceps (*Cordyceps sinensis*) have demonstrated that the extracts have multiple pharmacological actions through regulating the immune system—strengthening the response or controlling overactivity. Cordyceps inhibits cancer cell proliferation and inhibits the blood supply within cancer cells and tumors. Notably, cordyceps also provides improvement of insulin resistance and insulin secretion, and positively modulates cardiovascular functions, such as lowering blood pressure and increasing coronary blood flow, among others.[10] In TCM it is used to treat lung and kidney weakness.

LION'S MANE

Lion's mane (*Hericium erinaceus*) targets nerves, including neurons. Lion's mane (shown in Figure 7.1) promotes neuronal survival by stimulating nerve growth factor and brain-derived neurotrophic factor, among other neurotrophins.[11]

AGARICUS BLAZEI

Agaricus blazei is the least commonly known medicinal mushroom in the West but the most studied. Strongly antitumor, its mechanisms are either direct tumor attack or indirect defense via inhibited tumor vascularization and T helper 1 cell immune response. The anti-inflammatory mechanisms are a reduction in both proinflammatory cytokines and oxidative stress and changed gut microbiota.

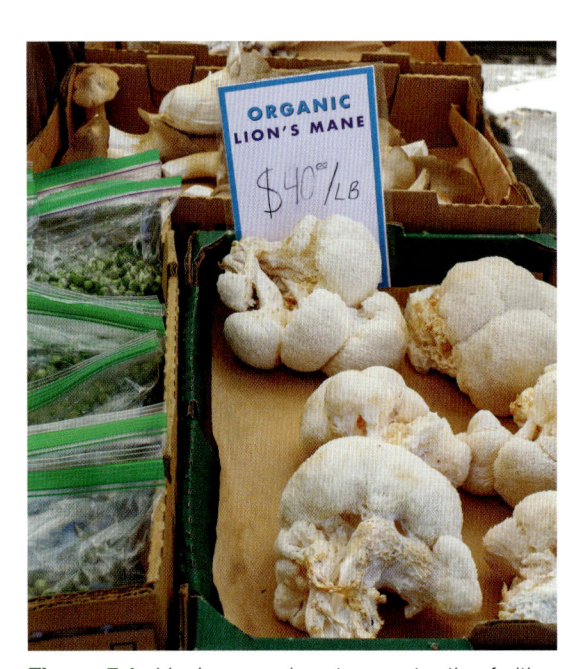

Figure 7.1. Lion's mane has two parts—the fruiting body and the mycelium. Both offer health benefits.

TURKEY TAIL

Turkey tail (*Trametes versicolor*) is a broad-spectrum immunomodulator regulating all aspects of the immune system, so it is a great daily tonic in combination with reishi.

Adaptogens

Adaptogens is a term for plants that are unusual in both the plant world and medicine world, with fascinating effects on the body stemming from direct regulation of the immune system. They literally adapt to the state of the system; that is, they regulate where needed to bring the body into homeostasis. Most plants and especially pharmaceutical medicines work in only one way and do not adapt to the system they are in. It's interesting to note that medicinal mushrooms are also adaptogens.

Studies on animals and isolated neuronal cells have shown that adaptogens exhibit neuroprotective, antifatigue, antidepressive, anxiolytic, nootropic activity. They also stimulate the central nervous system. In addition, clinical trials demonstrate that adaptogens exert an antifatigue effect that increases mental work capacity against a background of stress and fatigue, particularly in tolerance to mental exhaustion and enhanced attention.

Recent pharmacological studies have discovered that the stress-protective activity of adaptogens was associated with regulation of homeostasis via several mechanisms linked to regulation of the hypothalamic-pituitary-adrenal (HPA) axis.[12] The HPA axis is central to the body's homeostasis and stress responses and energy metabolism.

Adaptogens are useful for overall health, yet there are some important guidelines for use. They may react with prescription medications. Speak with your doctor and herbalist if you're taking prescribed medications, to ensure there is no conflict.

Consult your doctor or a knowledgeable health care provider if you are pregnant, breastfeeding, or immunocompromised. The best effects from adaptogens are small doses over long periods of time; in some medicinal systems they are taken daily. Taking larger doses in a single sitting may result in temporary adverse effects, such as nausea or headaches.

Ginseng

Ginseng, a Chinese herbal medicine, is an adaptogen that supports the body's many systems, including endocrine, cardiovascular, and bone. It works in part by helping to manage the inflammatory response, which in turn affects the whole body. Ginseng has been used safely for thousands of years. Recently, in research among women with osteopenia who included ginseng, bone generation markers increased.[13] Ginseng has a mild stimulatory effect and can help with focus.

Ashwagandha

Ashwagandha is another well-known adaptogen from the Ayurvedic medical system of India; ashwagandha works similarly to ginseng in affecting multiple systems and managing inflammation. Ashwagandha also acts as a phytoestrogen, so it can aid in managing bone loss. In research it has been shown to reverse the age-related changes in bone structure in rats.[14] Note that this plant is in the nightshade family, so may not be suitable for those with an autoimmune condition.

Tulsi

Tulsi, also known as holy basil, is another plant commonly used in Ayurvedic medicines. Practitioners say that tulsi promotes focus and alleviates anxiety. One clinical trial found it significantly diminished generalized anxiety disorder in patients, as well as their associated stress and depression.

Rhodiola

Rhodiola (*Rhodiola rosea*) grows in European, Asian, and North American high-altitude climates.

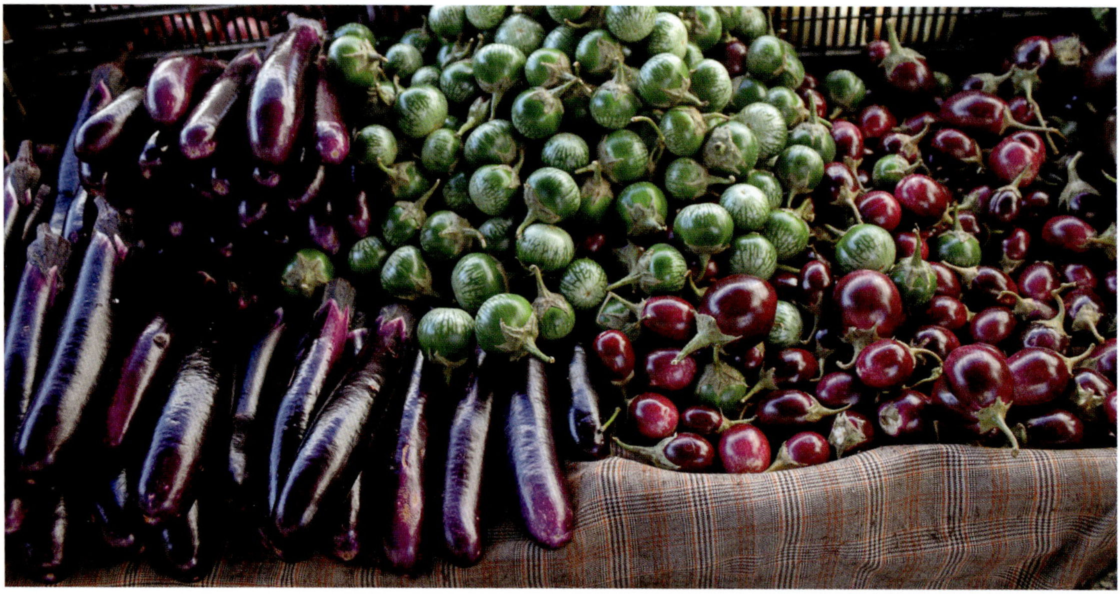

Figure 7.2. Eggplants are a yin food, with a cooling nature, regulating blood circulation and clearing heat from the body.

In two separate preliminary studies, doctors on night duty and students taking exams took rhodiola. The results suggest rhodiola can significantly reduce fatigue when compared to placebos.

Plants as Personalities

In Traditional Chinese Medicine each plant has a personality. This personality can be described as hot, such as a chile pepper, because it produces heat in your body; or it can be described as cold, such as a bamboo shoot, because it cools your system. This dichotomy can also be described as yin and yang, with yin foods being refreshing (green vegetables generally fall into this category) or salty. Meat, fatty cheese, sugar, and chocolate are yang foods.

Each cooking method also is either yin, such as boiling or steaming, or yang, such as grilling or frying. Raw and fermented foods are strongly yin.

You have a type, too, which can be predominantly yin or yang. Your constitution and body type contribute, as well as your mental type. Yin type tends to be thin and paler, introverted. A yang type is muscled, robust, extroverted. A step deeper, we find each of us is also composed of different ratios of the Five Elements of Wood, Water, Earth, Air, and Fire, as are our foods.

Foods also have a taste as part of their personality, and there are five basic tastes: sour, bitter, sweet, pungent, and salty. Each taste has affinity for different organ systems, so if you are managing health, knowing which organs need assistance can help you choose foods to assist.

Yes, there is a bounty of information that can inform your food and cooking choices, and we encourage you to explore and identify your preferences and body's needs. Luckily, our bodies are often aware of what we need, and if we are listening, we intuitively reach for the food that will meet the need.

Once you understand your constitution (from your own monitoring or from working with a professional nutritionist or physician), the season, and the nature of food, you can open up to another level of eating in harmony with your body, the foods, and nature itself.

PART II
Creative Cooking for Healthy Bones

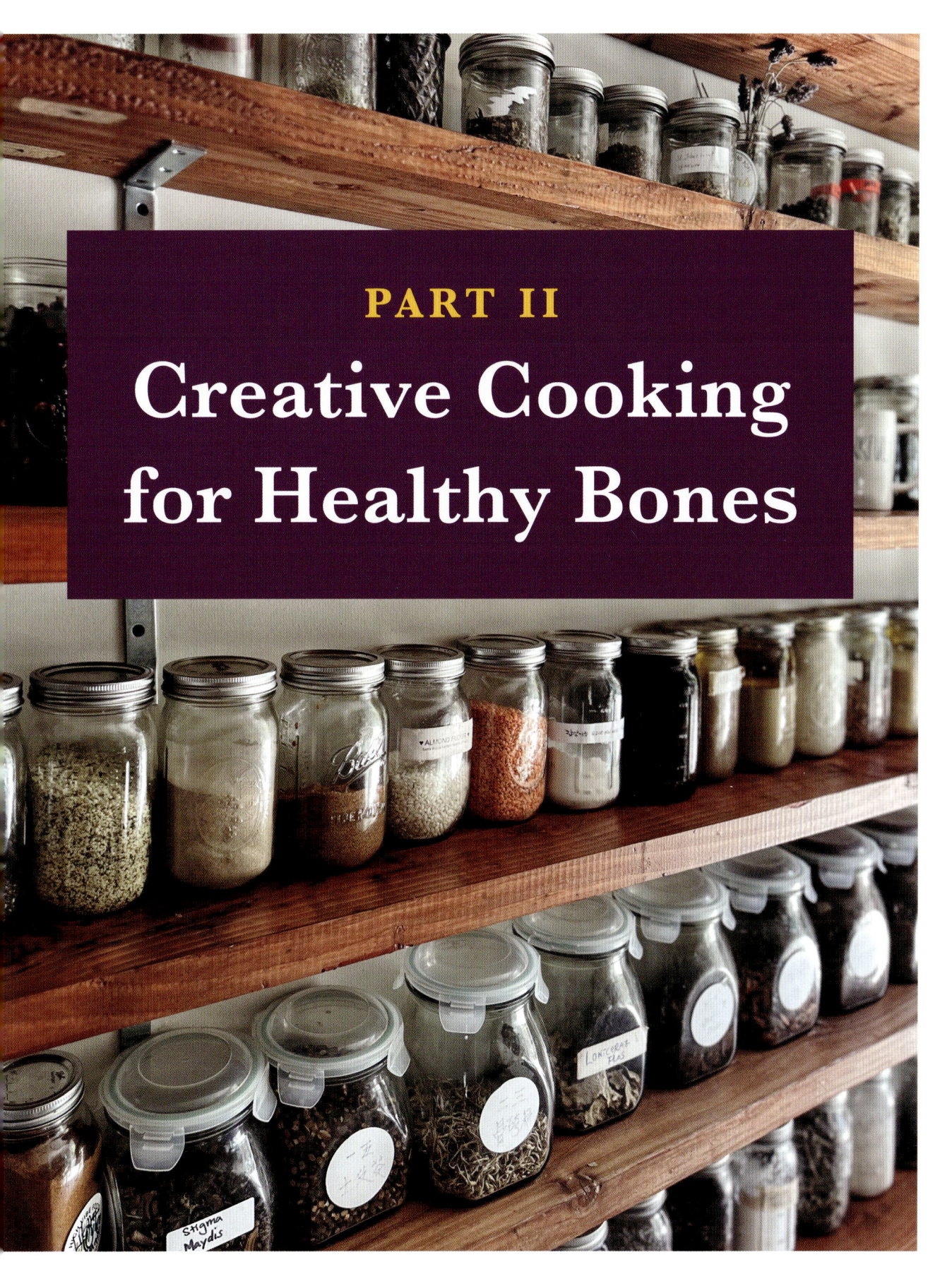

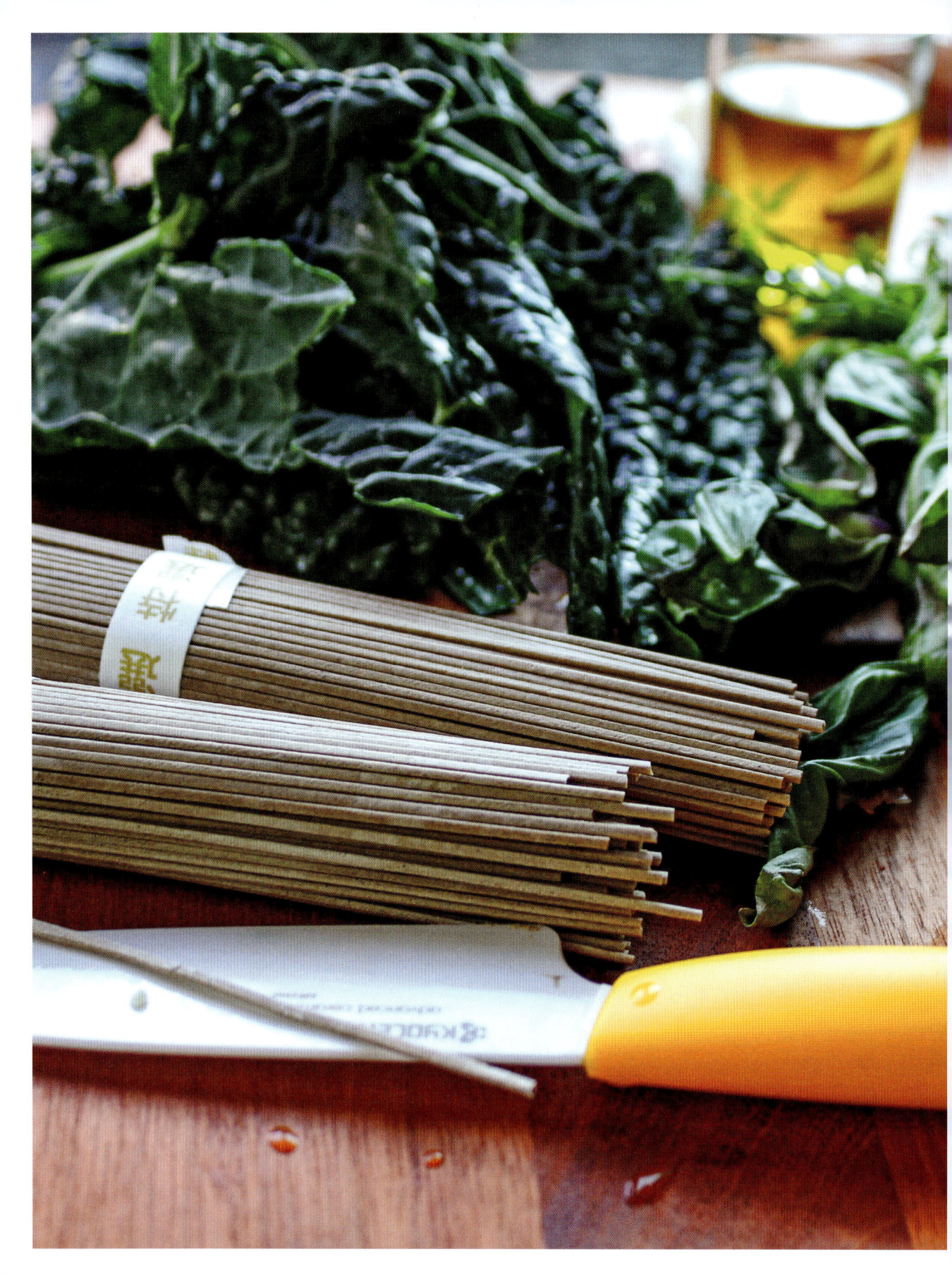

CHAPTER 8

Jump-Start Your Kitchen

Through the recipes in this book, I (Jummee) hope you will discover the pivotal role that cooking can play in unlocking your full potential. Cooking is not just a creative process; it empowers you and nourishes you as a whole. Whether you are seeking meaning and your heart's passion or are curious about how to unleash your inner superhuman, come back home to the kitchen. Peel the vegetables, clean them with gratitude, chop and cook foods you adore. Plate your dish with such beauty that it inspires you to relish it. Cherish that moment when you realize how much the food loves you, extending an invitation to a journey of self-discovery, and perhaps even the doorway to enlightenment.

In this chapter I guide you through some basic kitchen skills that you'll put into play as you prepare the recipes, from how to wash fresh produce and soak grains and beans to how to season foods to taste. I offer advice on what equipment you might want to add to your kitchen and how to stock your pantry so you are ready for cooking a bounty of colorful, flavorful, creative vegetarian and vegan dishes that will help you support your bone health and feel more energized and alive.

Cooking Basics and Tips

Whether you're an experienced cook or just dipping your toes into cooking for the first time, mastering the basics is essential. The kitchen is a creative sanctuary, but using tools like knives and fire requires mindfulness. Here, I share my best advice and tips to set the stage for breezy and soul-soothing cooking. With practice, you'll transition effortlessly into kitchen mastery, making each meal a serene and mindful experience.

Let's Start with Water

The human body is composed of over 70 percent water, and consuming high-quality water is critical for optimal health. Unfortunately, tap water in many urban and suburban areas may contain heavy metals and substances, such as pesticides and fluoride, that can negatively impact bone density and pose serious health risks when consumed over the long term. Despite that risk, I prefer fresh tap water over commercial bottled water. The "spring water" in plastic bottles from the store may not be genuine spring water; the exact source of the water is often not stated. Also, it's possible the water may have been stored in warehouses (so it is not fresh) and in plastic containers that have been exposed to sunlight, which may lead to leaching of heavy metals from the plastic into the water.

The ideal way to ensure a clean water supply for drinking and cooking is to install a comprehensive water filtration system for the entire house, which will remove potential toxins that may be present in the municipal water supply. Alternatively, a practical option is installing a simple filter system on your sink.

Natural spring water from underground is the top choice due to its potential content of beneficial minerals. However, this is not available to everyone. If you have a source of natural spring water from an underground source, it's advisable to test that water before consumption, even if it is a trusted source. Many options of home water testing kits are available online.

To boost water vitality, pour clean water into a 2-quart (2 L) glass jar, add 1 teaspoon sea salt, shake well, and let sit for a few hours near a window exposed to the sun from morning to midday. This process allows the transfer of energy from the sunlight to the water. If left in the sun for a longer period (up to 48 hours), the UV radiation from sunlight can kill pathogens and bacteria in the water.

How to Clean Vegetables and Fruits

I recommend keeping things simple and natural when cleaning vegetables and fruit. Clean your sink well to start. Then plug the sink, fill it halfway with cold water (using cold water helps to keep the vegetables fresh), and add a tablespoon each of baking soda and white distilled vinegar. Mix it up, and then plunge your vegetables into the water. Leave them to soak for about 5 minutes; you may see loose dirt settle to the bottom. Then drain the water and rinse the vegetables under running water. Dry them thoroughly—either with a cotton cloth or a salad spinner if you're prepping for a salad.

Storing Fresh Herbs and Vegetables

Preserving the freshness of your greens is a gamechanger. Gently wash herb sprigs and pat them well with a damp cotton cloth. Add about ¼ cup (60 ml) of water to a glass jar, stick the cut stems of the herbs into the water, and store the jar in the refrigerator. For cabbage and leafy greens, after cleaning them and draining the water, there's no need to dry them; simply wrap them in a damp cotton cloth and refrigerate.

For root vegetables, remove loose dirt before washing them as described above. After washing, trim the tips, and store them in the vegetable section of the fridge covered with a wet cloth to keep them hydrated and fresh for longer.

Soaking Grains and Beans

In chapter 3, you learned that that although grains and beans can be excellent sources of nutrients, they also contain antinutrients, including lectins. Because of that, we need to take steps to neutralize or eliminate the antinutrients before using grains and beans in cooking. Fortunately, it's not hard to do. These harmful substances can be eliminated by soaking overnight, which will draw most of the toxins into the water. Removing these toxins aids digestion, reducing gas and enabling your body to break down and absorb nutrients effectively.

Presprouting and fermenting are also effective techniques for disarming antinutrients in plant foods. These techniques are more involved than simply soaking the food, but they are easy to learn and the results will enrich and invigorate your cooking on many levels. Chapter 11 explains fermentation in detail, and you'll find step-by-step instructions for sprouting on page 199.

A SIMPLE SOAKING METHOD

Here's a technique for soaking dry beans and hard grains such as barley, sorghum, and brown rice. Keep in mind that longer soaking times allow more natural toxins to dissolve, and those toxins can then be washed away by rinsing the soaked beans or grains. If you can't soak for the full amount of time, even a few hours is better than nothing.

1. Place the grains or beans in a large pot or bowl, wash them under running water, and drain well. I like to express gratitude by saying "Thank you, rice and farmers" or "Thank you, beans and farmers" as I do this.

2. By volume, add three times more clean, filtered water than dry goods to the pot, and leave the pot on the counter to soak.
3. After one to two days, pour off the soaking water and refill the pot with twice the volume of water than the beans or grains. Leave them to soak for another one to two days.
4. Pour off the soaking water again. Rinse the beans or grains a final time and drain them before cooking.
5. If you aren't ready to cook the soaked beans or grains right away, cover them again with clean water and store them in the refrigerator for up to a week.

Soaking Dried Fruits and Seeds

Store-bought dried seeds (such as sesame and sunflower seeds) and dried fruits may contain preservatives such as sulfur dioxide. Soaking seeds and fruits for at least an hour helps reduce and eliminate most harmful chemicals, making them easier to digest. Soaking up to 3 hours can be beneficial.

The Art of Seasoning

First, let's be clear what seasoning a dish means. It is not adding spices, although spices do add flavor. To be precise, seasoning is the art of adding salt. When added properly, salt elevates all other flavors.

If you have been in the habit of sticking strictly to the precise amounts of salt specified in a recipe, it's liberating to let go. Various salts have different levels of saltiness, and blindly following a fixed ratio won't do the trick. Here's the secret: Start with a tiny bit of salt in the initial seasoning. Gradually add more in three or four increments, tasting each time. This way, you'll discover the perfect level of seasoning without risking oversalting. Remember, tread lightly and build up to that ideal taste.

I often choose high-quality, unprocessed sea salt for its mineral content and complex of sea microbes. These microbes can improve your gut health by enhancing the diversity of beneficial bacteria in your digestive system. I also use lava salt and pink Himalayan salt.

Using freshly ground black pepper also makes a world of difference compared to a packaged preground black pepper. I recommend buying whole peppercorns and grinding them fresh to add to recipes.

Choosing Kitchen Tools and Appliances

You don't need a kitchen filled with fancy equipment to be a great cook. You just need equipment that does the job well and is built to last. Here are my recommendations for kitchen tools and appliances I use the most.

Pots and Pans

Ever since I started using cast-iron skillets and pots, there's no turning back for me. From perfectly crispy pancakes to even heat distribution and a steady simmer for flavorful soups, these pans deliver, regardless of stove irregularities. I can't emphasize enough how worthwhile the initial investment and simple maintenance are. One or two will last a lifetime. For beginners, start with a versatile 8-inch (20 cm) cast-iron skillet; it's robust, nontoxic, and beats other nonstick alternatives that may harbor harmful chemicals.

I am also a huge fan of glass baking dishes (versus metal pans) for oven use. Glass pans hold heat more consistently than metal pans do, and thus provide a slower, more consistent bake. It's helpful to have a 9- by 13-inch (23 × 33 cm) baking dish and one or two 8-inch (20 cm) round cake pans.

Here's a quick guide to different pans for different purposes:

Cast-iron skillets and Dutch ovens: Ideal for baking nonacidic foods like biscuits, rolls, cornbread, and fruit crumbles. Withstanding high and low

How to Clean Cast-Iron Cookware

Cast-iron pans and pots need a little TLC. Skip the soaps and chemicals. The flavor of the soap will stay and literally bake into the pan. Clean the pan with kosher salt instead, using a soft, dry cloth and a wooden spatula as a scraper. After the scraping is done, clean the pan with a warm, wet cloth; drizzle on a little vegetable oil; and wipe it around the skillet to coat the surface so it won't rust.

temperatures, cast iron is versatile for both baking and cooking.

Ceramic baking dishes: Similar to glass pans, ceramic dishes are perfect for casseroles such as bread pudding, baked French toast, and pasta dishes.

Glass baking dishes: Opt for glass dishes for low-temperature, long-baking baked goods like banana bread, fruit pies, coffee cake, and extended-bake pasta dishes.

Metal pans: Use metal pans for high-temperature, short-baking foods such as roasted vegetables, brownies, cakes, and cookies. Due to metal's heat conductivity, these pans are recommended for items needing quick cooling.

Everyday Tools

I like to display the tools I use every day right by my stove or store them in a nearby drawer.

- A granite mortar and pestle, 3- to 5-cup capacity, is a great tool to make pesto or dressing.
- A mandoline works well to slice food thin in consistent shapes.
- Tongs, wooden spoons, and all-purpose spatulas are handy for serving.
- A silicone spatula is a great tool for mixing and scraping batters and doughs.
- A whisk handles many mixing tasks without the fuss of an electric mixer or immersion blender.
- Keep parchment paper on hand to use in place of aluminum foil. Foil and plastic wrap seal out air, but parchment paper lets food breathe a bit when wrapped. When used in baking, this helps maintain crispness in exterior crusts instead of making them soggy. Parchment also saves time on cleanup.
- A set of three glass measuring cups with 1-cup, 2-cup, and 4-cup capacity is very useful. Smaller metal measuring cups for quantities from ¼ cup to 1 cup are essential for dry ingredients. A set of measuring spoons is also a must-have.
- Zester: This tool saves my life. It is so handy to use for grating garlic and cheese and zesting citrus. It is easy to handle and simple to clean.

Small Appliances

My four favorite small appliances are a food processor, a mini blender, a large blender, and a cold-press juicer.

Food Processor: Use this versatile tool for mashing, making doughs or batters for baking, or any dishes where you want a smooth texture.

Mini Blender: With its 16-ounce capacity, smoothies and dressings are so easy and quick to make in small amounts.

Large Blender: Look for a blender with a 64-ounce capacity. Use it for making creamy soups, silky plant-based milk, large batches of pesto, and lemonade.

Cold-Press Juicer: Unlike motor-based high-speed juicers, which damage fiber and minerals due to their speed, the cold-press juicer retains most of the fiber and vitamins. It's a must-have appliance for making morning green juice, vegetable juices, and fruit juices.

How to Use and Care for Knives

For cutting and chopping, I like using a Global Chef brand knife with an 8-inch (20 cm) blade. If you have small hands, you might prefer a 6-inch (15 cm) chef's knife. From there you might decide you also want one to two specialty knives.

A ceramic paring knife with a 3-inch (8 cm) blade is very handy for cutting up smaller veggies and for peeling garlic and fruit.

A 10- or 11-inch (25 or 28 cm) whetstone sharpener is a tool that is quite effective and safe to use to sharpen knives.

Mastering knife skills can transform your cooking experience, making it not only safe and secure but also remarkably effective.

Honing a Knife

Your knives deserve a spa day. Regular honing is key; hone knives weekly to keep your blades at their best. Use a knife steel at a 20-degree angle, and voilà—your knives will sing with joy! If you are not familiar with a knife steel, use a whetstone. In running water, place the whetstone on the sink. Position the blade on top of the stone at a 15- to 20-degree angle, facing toward you. Maintain a consistent blade angle during sharpening to prevent accidental damage to your knife. Apply gentle pressure. After using the finest grit, use a leather or felt strop to eliminate any remaining burrs and polish the edge.

My Pantry to Yours

Here's my pantry list. These items are my core shelf-stable ingredients that enhance my cooking and save time. They are basic, versatile, and highly nutritious ingredients I use in all my recipes to help promote longevity and balanced nutrition for healthy bones based on organic, vegetarian or vegan, gluten-free, chemical-free, nonprocessed, non-GMO choices. If you're eating gluten-free, be sure to read labels. You may find gluten in surprising places. For example, most store-bought brands of liquid aminos contain wheat gluten, which is often GMO-derived unless labeled non-GMO. (For more about hidden gluten in foods, refer to "Advice on Going Gluten-Free" on page 53.)

Many of these items will be familiar to you, but some may be new, such as superfood powders. These powders—reishi mushroom, bee pollen, moringa, and wheatgrass powder—incorporated into your daily cooking will enhance a dish's

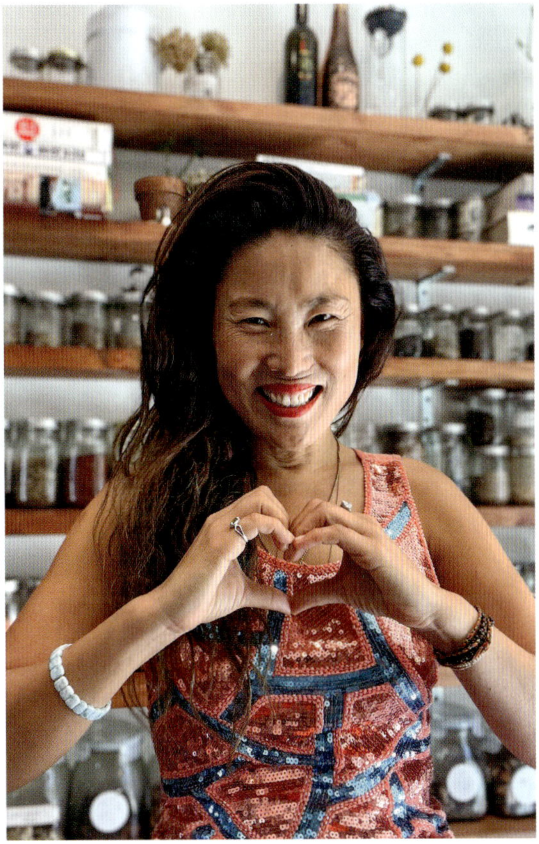

Figure 8.1. Organizing the shelves of my pantry is one of my delights.

nutritional balance and turn ordinary food like rice into a flavorful superfood.

There's no need to stock your pantry all at once! Trying to do so might be overwhelming and discourage you from cooking. Start with the ingredients that you need in order to prepare one of my recipes that has caught your eye. Add more items gradually, and in three to six months, you will see your pantry is fully ready to rock and roll. Keep in mind that my lists reflect my personal preferences, which might be different from your tastes and cooking style. Adjust these lists based on your favorite things to cook.

Spices, seasonings, and dried herbs: basil, bay leaves, cardamom, cinnamon, cloves, curry powder, dill, hibiscus, holy basil, licorice, nutmeg, rose petals, rosemary, saffron, thyme, truffles, turmeric, umami powder

Oils and fats: avocado oil, coconut oil, extra-virgin olive oil, cold-pressed black sesame oil, flaxseed oil, ghee, hemp seed oil, MCT (medium-chain triglycerides) oil, sunflower oil, walnut oil

Gluten-free flours and meals: amaranth flour, arrowroot powder, almond meal, brown rice flour, buckwheat flour, cassava flour, flaxseed meal, gluten-free flour blend, oat flour, quinoa flour, sorghum flour

Vinegars: apple cider, brown rice, plum, yuzu

Liquid seasonings: coconut soy sauce, gluten-free soy sauce, liquid aminos (coconut aminos are soy-free)

Sweet liquids: date syrup, honey, maple syrup, molasses

Pastes: aged miso paste, black bean paste, sweet chili paste (gochujang)

Salts: green salt, Himalayan salt, lava salt, unfiltered sea salt

Noodles: black bean noodles, buckwheat noodles, mung bean noodles, mushroom noodles, pasta, rice noodles, sweet potato noodles

Superfood powders: acai, bee pollen, beet, burdock root, cacao, chaga/reishi mushroom, dandelion root, lion's mane mushroom, maca, matcha, moringa, pine pollen, wheatgrass

Dried beans: black beans, edamame, mung beans, red beans, white beans

Rice and grains: basmati rice, brown rice, forbidden rice, quinoa, sticky brown rice, white sushi rice, wild rice

Nuts: Brazil nuts, cashews, macadamias, pine nuts, walnuts

Seeds: black and golden sesame seeds, chia seeds, pumpkin seeds, sunflower seeds

Canned and bottled goods: artichoke hearts, coconut milk, roasted red peppers, tahini, tomato sauce, tomato paste

Beyond Store-Bought Staples

I vividly recall the moment I made my first batch of hemp milk, surrounded by health-conscious folks and the beauty of the California environment. The nutty flavors and silky textures of the milk amazed me. It was not only easy but also cost-effective and eco-friendly. This ignited my confidence and a deep connection with my food.

Learning how to make some of your own essential kitchen staples that simplify cooking is empowering. As you stock your pantry, keep in mind that there are many staple foods that are reasonably simple to make yourself.

Whether it's whipping up plant-based milk for a nutritious breakfast, fermenting kimchi and pickles, sprouting seeds, creating sensational dressings and pesto, or baking delicious seeded quinoa bread, making your own instead of relying on store-bought liberates you from sourcing items with no connection to you.

You'll find recipes for such staples throughout the chapters that follow, where you'll also learn methods, tools, and formulas focused on bone health, inflammation reduction, robust brain health, and high antioxidants.

CHAPTER 9

Juices, Lattes, Milks, and Smoothies

Juicing can be a fast way to improve your metabolic health or cleanse your body to reset for better digestion. Juicing facilitates easy nutrient absorption and enhances vitamin and mineral intake. In contrast to a traditional heavy breakfast that demands your digestive system's full attention early in the morning, potentially leaving your body feeling tired instead of energized to kick off the day, juicing allows for quicker nutrient assimilation. Consequently, your body conserves a significant amount of energy.

As for lattes, can you believe that Americans consume about 146 billion cups of coffee every year? It's quite the coffee craziness! My intention in offering caffeine-free coffeeless latte recipes is to help people make a smooth transition from coffee addiction to healthier energy-boosting drinks. My latte recipes depend on plant-based milks, and I highly recommend making those milks from scratch. Sure, picking up a carton of plant-based milk at the store is convenient, but once you've tasted my recipe for Cashew-Goji-Vanilla Milk (page 112) or Pistachio-Mint Milk (page 112), you'll know that it's worth the effort to make your own. You'll love making up your own blends, not to mention its cost-effective freshness! As you'll see in the recipes for plant-based milks in this chapter, water is a major ingredient. Because of that, using filtered water or clean spring water is especially important.

Smoothies are the ultimate combo of health and deliciousness. What could be better than a nutritious smoothie in the midst of a busy morning? Packed with fruits, veggies, and protein, they provide an instant energy boost. These recipes can also help improve digestion and boost immunity. Smoothies curb your hunger, helping you sail through the day without feeling the urge to reach for a sugary snack.

Basic Juice Formula

MAKES 6 TO 8 OUNCES (180–240 ML) FRESH JUICE EXTRACT

Here's my basic formula and method for making a juice extract, plus ingredient lists for five of my favorite juice extract blends. Note that in addition to the water listed as an ingredient for several of the recipes below, I always add water to a fresh juice extract before drinking it. Juices are rich in minerals and vitamins, and the body has a limited capacity to absorb these nutrients within a short period. Diluting juice with water can aid your body in absorbing the nutrients.

I recommend drinking a 16-ounce (500 ml) glass of diluted juice extract in the morning between 7:00 and 9:00 a.m. Drink part of the juice, wait 30 minutes, then drink some more. This gives your body time to digest.

If you are doing a liquid-fasting routine, drink the contents of two 1-quart (1 L) jars of diluted juice between 7:00 a.m. and noon, drinking 8 ounces (250 ml) an hour. Then you can repeat between 1:00 and 4:00 p.m.

I use a cold-press juice machine that extracts the juice fully. If you don't have a juice machine, you can use a large Vitamix or other high-speed blender.

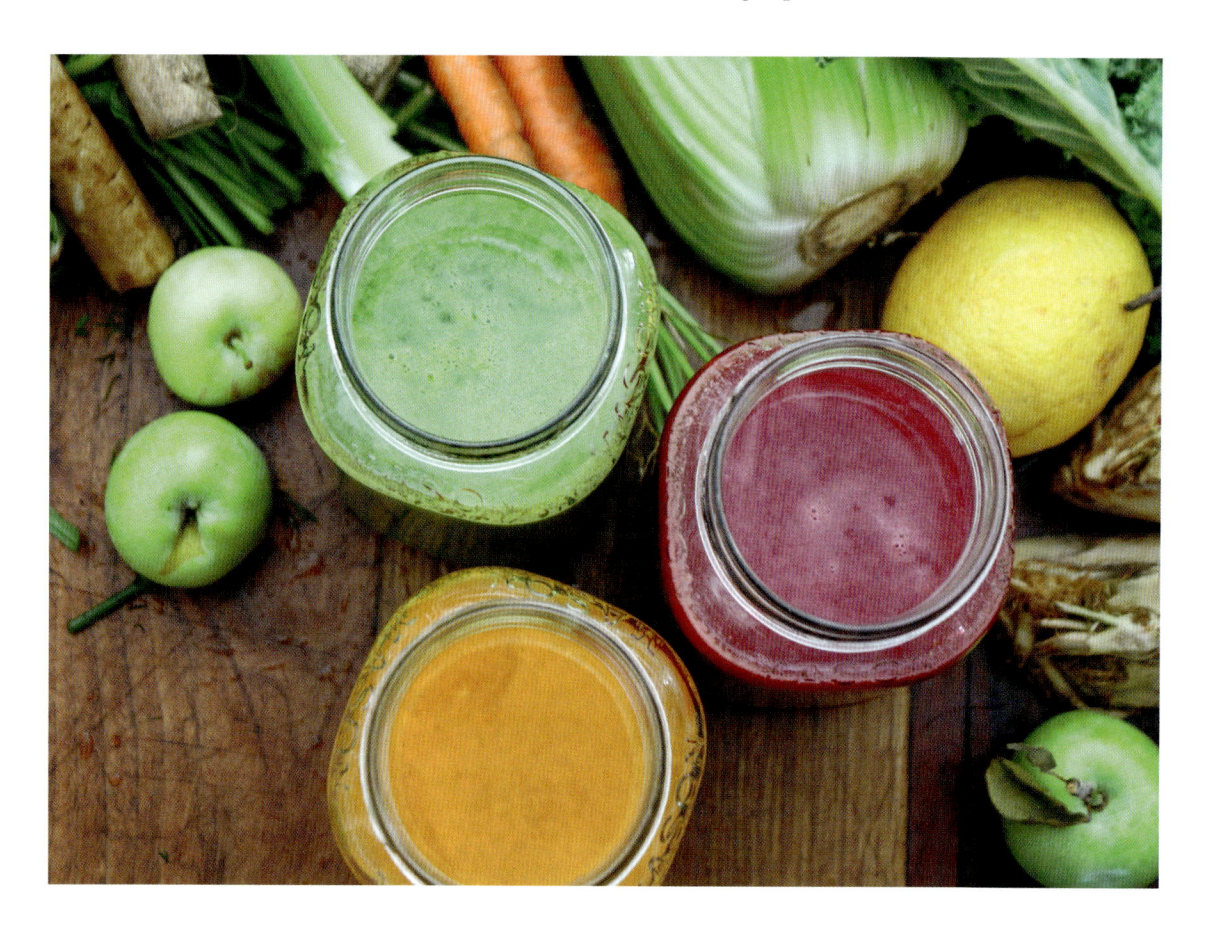

1. Clean the ingredients properly (see page 102). Since we use the vegetables and fruits whole, skin and all, thorough cleaning is important.
2. Cut the ingredients into 2-inch (5 cm) or smaller cubes, depending on the capacity of your juice machine.
3. Put the ingredients in the juice machine slowly, avoiding clogging, and process them. If you don't have a cold-press juicer, use a high-speed blender: add the ingredients and an equal amount of water, blend them well together, then filter the blended liquid through cheesecloth or a fine-mesh strainer to remove fibrous material.
4. Measure the quantity of juice extract you've made, and dilute the extract with three times that amount of water.

Basic Green Juice

Choices of leafy greens and green vegetables for this blend include celery (ribs and leaves), wheatgrass, spinach, kale, Swiss chard, dandelion greens, collard greens, cabbage, fennel (fronds and stems), arugula, parsley, cilantro, mint, dill, chives, radish greens, cucumber, or broccoli (including leaves and stem). To make this extract for use as a cleansing drink, add 4 ribs of celery.

4 stalks any leafy greens, hard stems removed
1 parsley sprig
½ medium green apple, cored
¼ medium citrus fruit (such as lemon, grapefruit, or orange)
1 tablespoon grated fresh ginger

Beet to Beat Juice

This recipe features beets. Other root vegetables that supply bone-health nutrients include celery root, carrot, jicama, turnip, parsnip, sweet potato, and radish.

1 cup (240 ml) filtered water
5 dill sprigs
2 celery ribs
1 medium beet
½ medium apple, cored
¼ medium lemon
1 tablespoon grated fresh ginger

Follow Your Gut Juice

This juice is a powerful general tonic for the whole body.

1 cup (240 ml) filtered water
Four 6-inch (15 cm) pieces burdock root or 1 parsnip
4 dandelion leaves
¼ cup (30 g) white radish
5 parsley sprigs
5 cilantro sprigs
¼ medium lemon
½ medium green apple, cored
1 tablespoon grated fresh ginger

Morning Ritual Green Juice

For a revitalizing variation on this anti-inflammatory, detoxifying blend, add 5 cilantro sprigs and 4 dandelion leaves and reduce to 2 celery ribs and 2 kale leaves.

1 cup (240 ml) filtered water
5 kale leaves
5 parsley sprigs
3 celery ribs
½ medium apple, cored
¼ medium lemon
1 tablespoon grated fresh ginger

Sunny Carrot Juice

This blend supplies carotene, which can support eye and skin health and reduce the risk of some chronic diseases.

1 cup (240 ml) filtered water
5 dill sprigs
2 large or 4 medium carrots
2 celery ribs
½ medium apple, cored
¼ medium orange
1 tablespoon grated fresh ginger

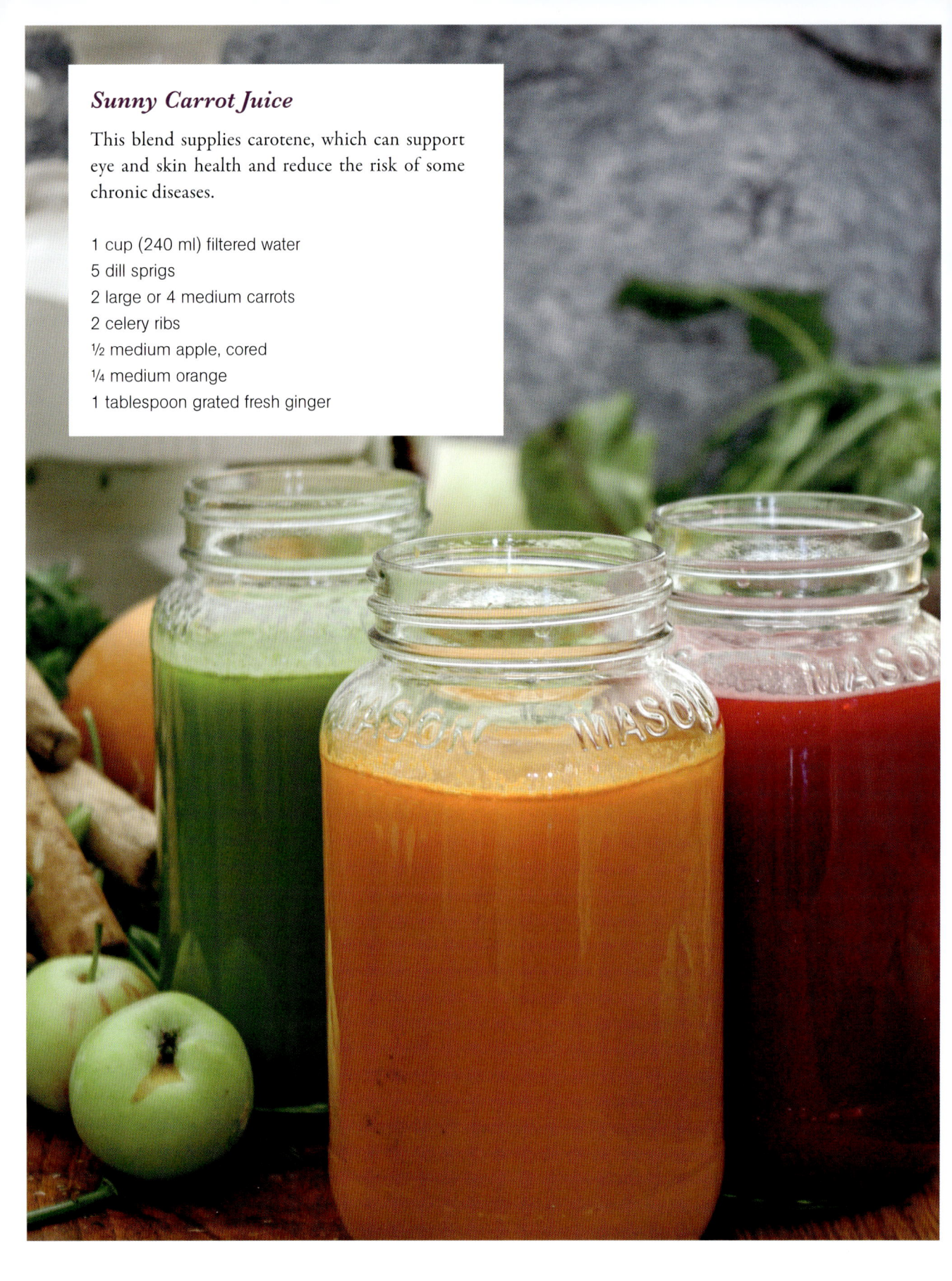

Plant-Based Milk 101

MAKES 6 CUPS (1.4 L)

I am excited to share this basic formula and sample variations for homemade plant-based milk. In a few steps, you can make various types based on the golden ratio by the following volume:

1 part protein : 6 parts water : ⅛ part flavor ingredient

Only a minimal portion of nuts and seeds is needed to make a large amount of milk, which means drinking plant-based milk is less likely to trouble your digestive system than consuming a large amount of raw nuts and seeds might. So, try drinking nuts and seeds instead of snacking on them! It is easy, fun, and simple.

You will need a nut milk bag and a full-size, powerful blender for this recipe. I suggest storing plant milk in glass jars. It will keep in the refrigerator for a week or two. A high-speed blender also works best for making the special milk recipes below. Simply add all ingredients to the blender and blend until smooth.

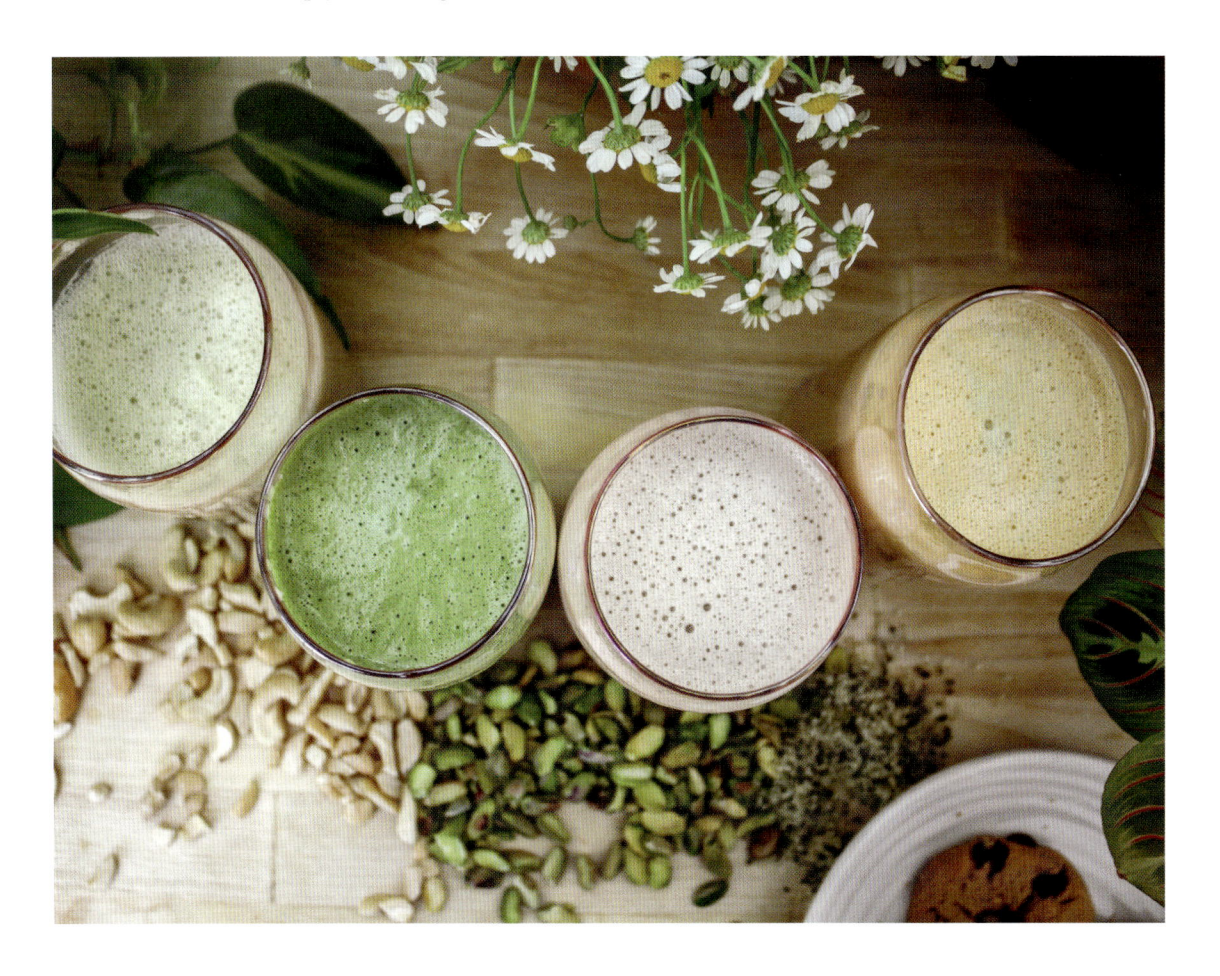

1 cup protein ingredient of your choice
6 cups (1.4 L) filtered water
2 tablespoons flavor ingredient(s) of your choice
Sea salt
Fresh lemon juice (see Tip)

PROTEIN OPTIONS

Nuts: almonds, Brazil nuts, cashews, hazelnuts, macadamias, walnuts

Grains and seeds: brown rice (cooked, not raw), hemp seeds, oats, pine nuts, pumpkin seeds, sesame seeds, sunflower seeds

HIGH-NUTRITION, IMMUNITY-PACKED FLAVOR OPTIONS

Savory: chaga powder, coconut oil, cordyceps mushroom powder, ghee, maca powder, matcha powder, MCT oil, mushroom powder, pine pollen, reishi powder, spirulina, wheatgrass powder

Sweet: beet powder, cacao powder, chai tea powder, goji berry powder, hibiscus tea broth, honey, maple syrup, mint leaves, monk fruit sweetener, pitted dates, pomegranate powder, vanilla extract

Spices: ground anise seed, ground cardamom, ground cinnamon, ground cloves, ground ginger, ground nutmeg, saffron

1. Soak the nuts, grains, or seeds for at least 30 minutes and up to one day. Drain.
2. Add the soaked protein and the water to the blender. Do not fill the cup more than 80 percent full to avoid bubbles and spills (process in batches if necessary). Blend on the slowest speed, gradually increasing up to the maximum speed up for 8 to 10 minutes, until the milk becomes consistent and has a very silky texture. You don't want lumps. Add the flavor ingredient(s), a pinch of salt, and a few drops of lemon juice and blend just to combine.
3. Strain the milk through a nut milk bag or cotton cloth into a bowl and squeeze the bag to extract all the liquid. Pour the milk into jars and store in the refrigerator.

TIP

Adding just a hint of lemon is so important. It protects from enzymatic browning and removes any dull nut flavor. You will not taste any acidic flavor from the lemon juice at all.

Cashew-Goji-Vanilla Milk

1⅔ cups (400 ml) homemade cashew milk (see page 111)
2 tablespoons goji berry powder
1 teaspoon maple syrup or honey
⅛ teaspoon ground ginger
⅛ teaspoon fresh lemon juice
⅛ teaspoon freshly grated nutmeg
⅛ teaspoon vanilla extract

Hemp Seed Chai

1½ cups (360 ml) homemade hemp milk (see page 111)
¼ cup (60 ml) brewed chai tea, cooled
1 teaspoon maple syrup or honey
½ teaspoon coconut oil
⅛ teaspoon ground cinnamon
⅛ teaspoon freshly grated nutmeg
⅛ teaspoon vanilla extract

Pistachio-Mint Milk

1⅔ cups (400 ml) homemade pistachio milk (see page 111)
5 or 6 mint leaves or 2 tablespoons brewed mint tea, cooled
1 tablespoon shelled raw pistachios, soaked
1 teaspoon maple syrup or honey
⅛ teaspoon ground cinnamon
⅛ teaspoon freshly grated nutmeg
⅛ teaspoon vanilla extract

Coffeeless Lattes 101

Making coffeeless lattes is loads of fun. I offer five delicious choices, each carefully crafted to provide a well-balanced blend of ingredients, including anti-inflammatory compounds to ease joint pain, support digestion, boost the immune system, and enhance nutrient absorption—all while helping you maintain a calm focus throughout the day, without relying on caffeine.

The key to making foamy, consistently flavorful lattes is to use a powerful blender. If you can warm the milk before blending, it enhances the flavor, although this is not necessary.

1. Warm the milk (optional).
2. Add all ingredients to the blender.
3. Blend, starting on low and increasing the speed to high, 3 to 5 minutes.

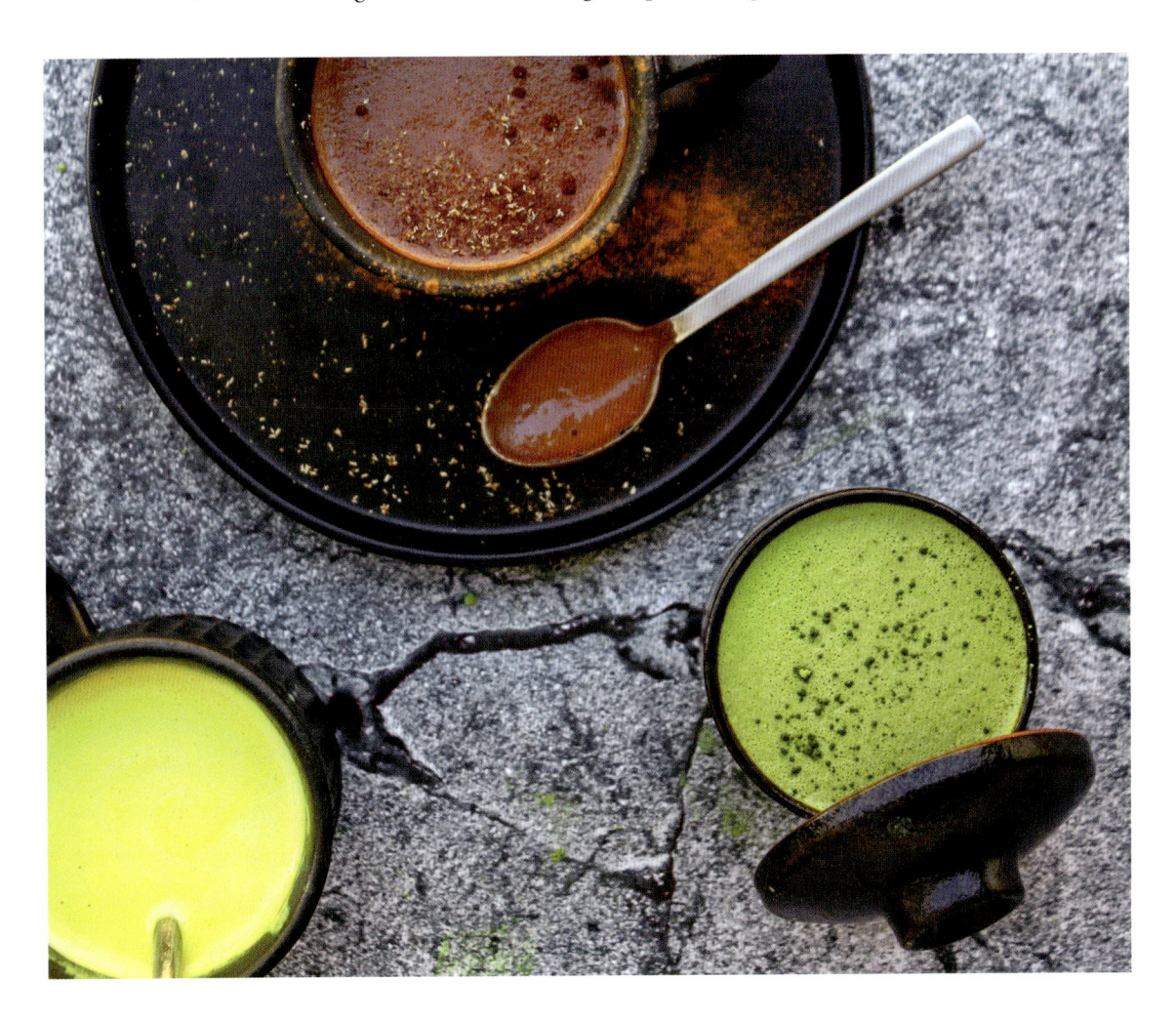

Juices, Lattes, Milks, and Smoothies

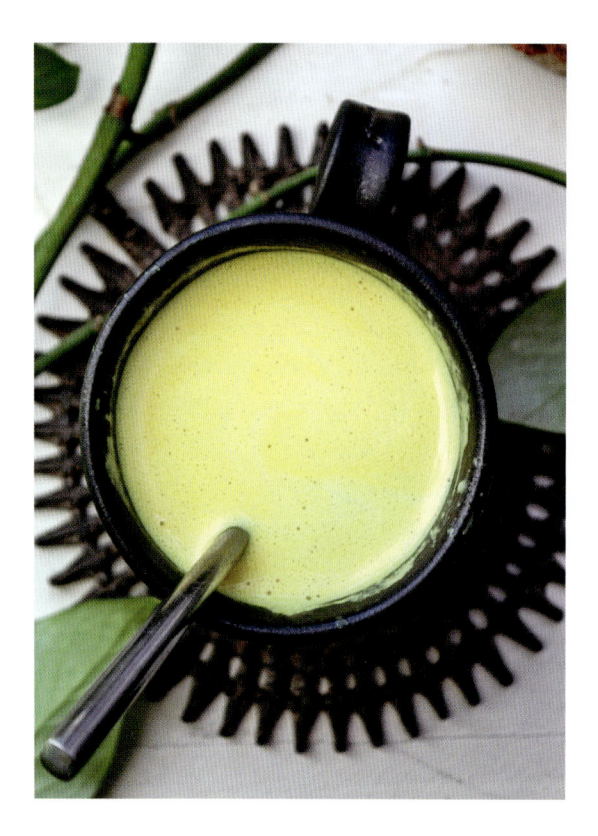

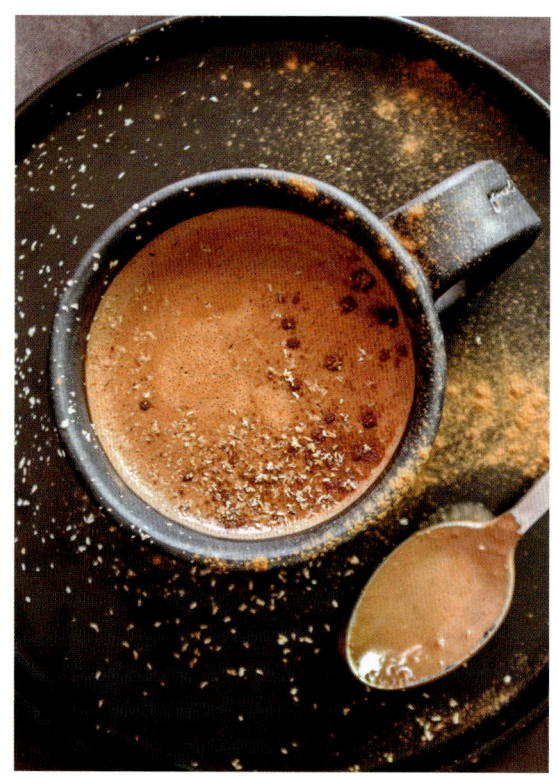

C-Packed Pink Latte

1½ cups (360 ml) homemade cashew milk
   (see page 111)
⅓ cup (40 g) beetroot, maca, or goji berry powder
4 teaspoons ground ginger
2 teaspoons maple syrup or honey
2 teaspoons ground cardamom
1 teaspoon ground cinnamon
1 teaspoon fresh orange juice
⅛ teaspoon ground cloves

Golden Milk Latte

1½ cups (360 ml) homemade cashew milk
   (see page 111)
3 tablespoons coconut milk
2 teaspoons maple syrup or date syrup
½ teaspoon ground turmeric
½ teaspoon MCT oil or coconut oil
¼ teaspoon ground ginger
⅛ teaspoon ground cardamom
⅛ teaspoon fresh orange juice
⅛ teaspoon vanilla extract
Pinch salt

Hearty Cacao Latte

1½ cups (360 ml) homemade almond milk
   (see page 111)
¼ cup (60 ml) coconut milk
2 pitted dates or ¼ cup (60 ml) date syrup
3 tablespoons (22 g) cacao powder
1 teaspoon dandelion root powder
1 teaspoon reishi or chaga mushroom powder
¼ teaspoon ground cinnamon
⅛ teaspoon fresh lemon juice
⅛ teaspoon vanilla extract
Pinch freshly grated nutmeg, for garnish

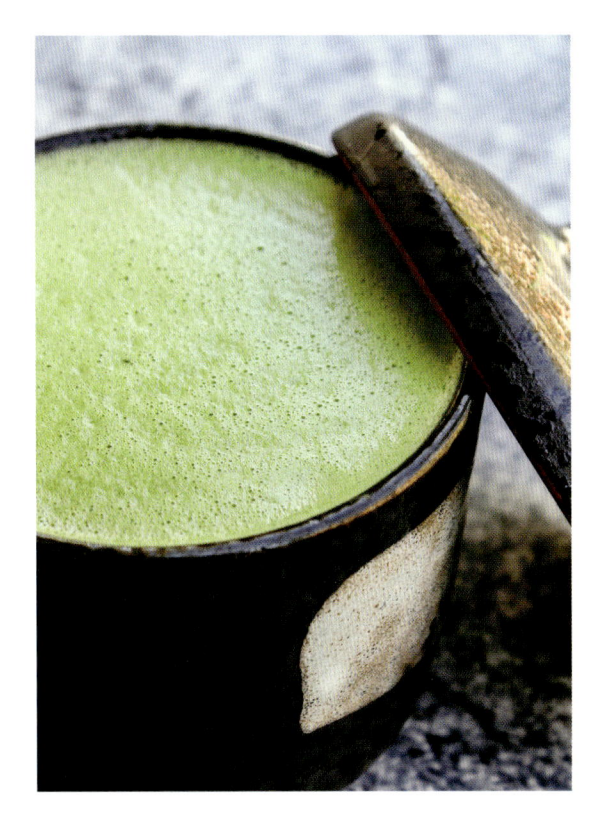

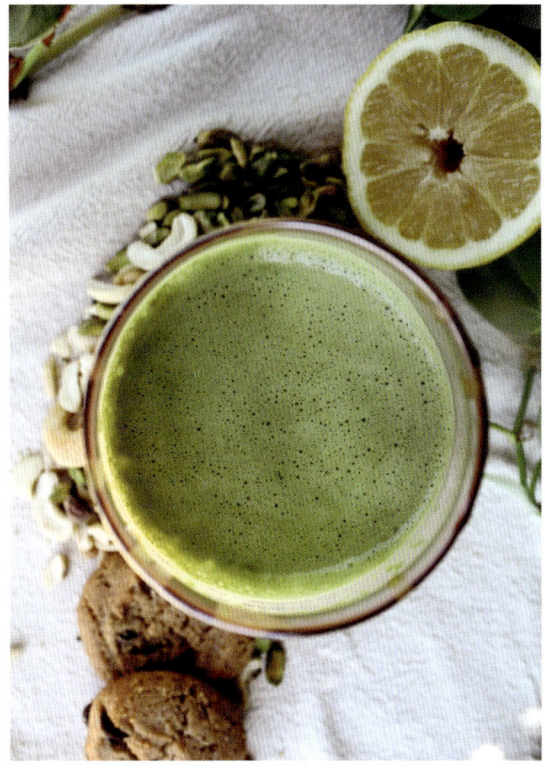

Morning March Matcha Latte

1½ cups (360 ml) homemade oat milk (see page 111), warm or hot
¼ cup (60 ml) coconut milk or plant-based yogurt or kefir
2 tablespoons maple syrup or date syrup
2 teaspoons matcha powder
1 teaspoon wheatgrass powder
½ teaspoon MCT oil
¼ teaspoon fresh lemon juice
⅛ teaspoon ground cinnamon

Pine Nut–Matcha Latte

1⅔ cups (400 ml) pine nut milk (see page 111)
1 tablespoon maple syrup or honey
¼ teaspoon matcha powder
⅛ teaspoon ground cardamom
⅛ teaspoon freshly grated nutmeg
⅛ teaspoon vanilla extract

Juices, Lattes, Milks, and Smoothies

Smoothies 101

MAKES ABOUT 2 CUPS (475 ML)

If time is one of your most precious commodities, you'll appreciate that the prep time for a smoothie is 5 minutes or less. It's a quick, tasty way to sneak in essential nutrients and antioxidants.

1. Wash ingredients, dry them, and cut into pieces.
2. Place all ingredients in a blender, and blend, starting at low speed and gradually increasing to high speed, for 2 to 3 minutes total, until smooth.
3. Serve with your favorite toppings, such as nuts, seeds, or fruits.

Awakening Golden Smoothie

Mango and pineapple join forces in this smoothie to deliver a wave of vitamins and tropical delight. Tahini adds a creamy texture and heart-healthy fats.

- 1 cup (240 ml) homemade cashew milk or almond milk (see page 111)
- 1 orange, unpeeled, sliced
- ½ cup peeled and roughly chopped mango (85 g) or papaya (70 g)
- ½ cup (85 g) peeled and roughly chopped pineapple
- 2 tablespoons tahini
- 1 tablespoon maple syrup or date syrup (optional)
- 1 teaspoon coconut oil or MCT oil
- ¼ teaspoon ground turmeric
- ⅛ teaspoon ground ginger
- ⅛ teaspoon pine pollen
- ⅛ teaspoon lion's mane mushroom powder

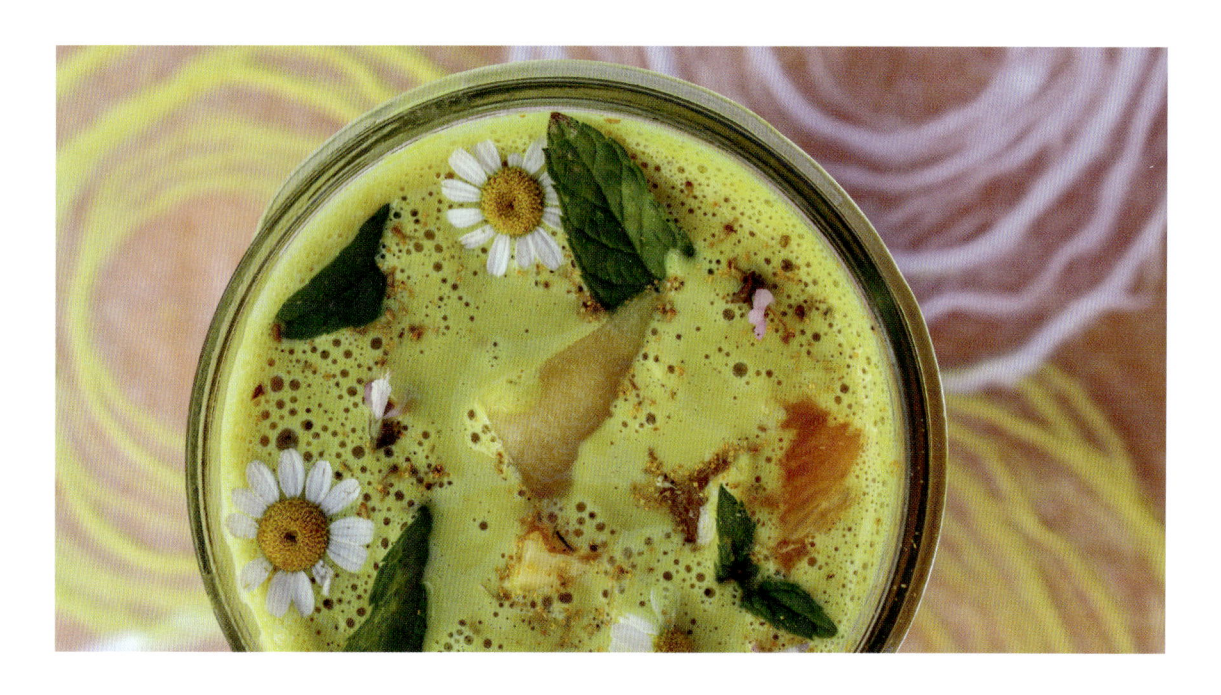

Berry Paradise Smoothie

Fresh berries are nutritional superheroes, loaded with antioxidants, vitamins, and fiber. For strong bones, toss in some hemp seeds, sliced blanched almonds, or crushed pistachios for good protein and omega-3 fatty acids.

1 cup (240 ml) homemade hemp milk (see page 111)
8 to 10 raspberries
5 medium strawberries or blueberries
½ medium banana
1 teaspoon fresh lemon juice
⅛ teaspoon ground cinnamon

Green Shield Smoothie

When you're on the brink of getting sick or recovering from a hangover, this is the smoothie to turn to. The ingredients provide high vitamin and mineral nutrition, and help fight inflammation, promote strong bone health, and support smooth digestion. If you wish, garnish this superb smoothie with crushed pistachios, macadamias, or Brazil nuts; dried rose petals; or a cinnamon stick.

1 cup (240 ml) homemade hemp milk (see page 111)
¼ cup (60 ml) aloe vera juice
¼ cup (30 g) roughly chopped Granny Smith or any tangy apple, with skin
1 kale leaf
½ medium-sized ripe avocado
1 tablespoon spirulina powder or wheatgrass powder
1 tablespoon maple syrup or honey
¼ teaspoon fresh lemon juice
2 mint leaves

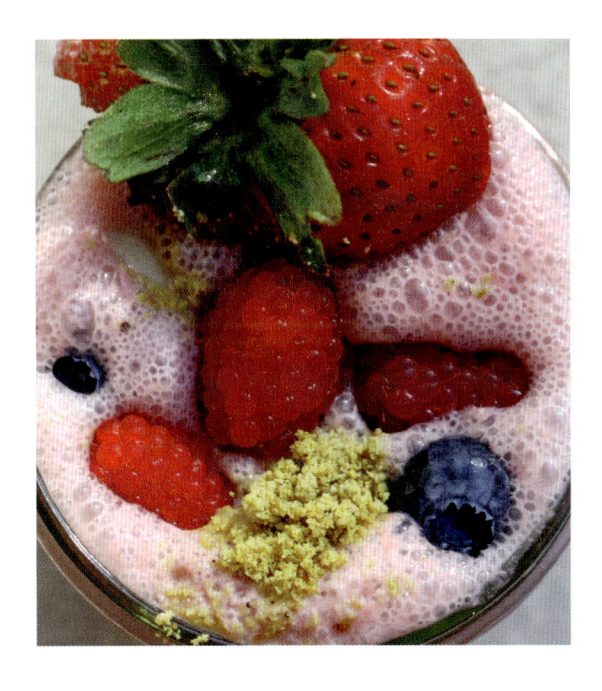

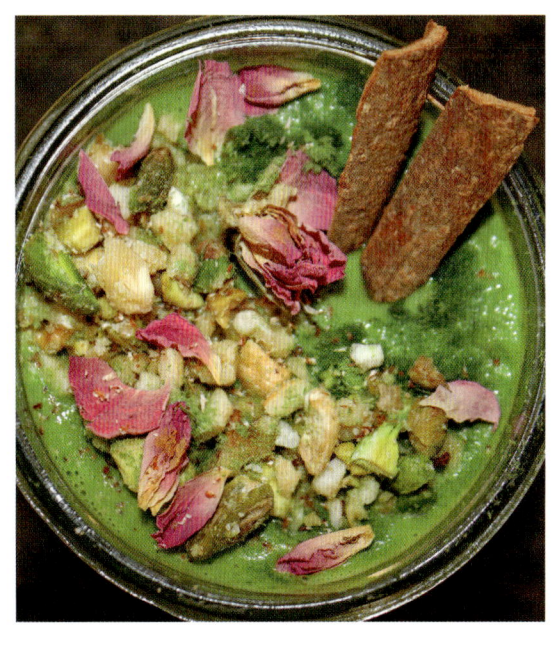

Juices, Lattes, Milks, and Smoothies

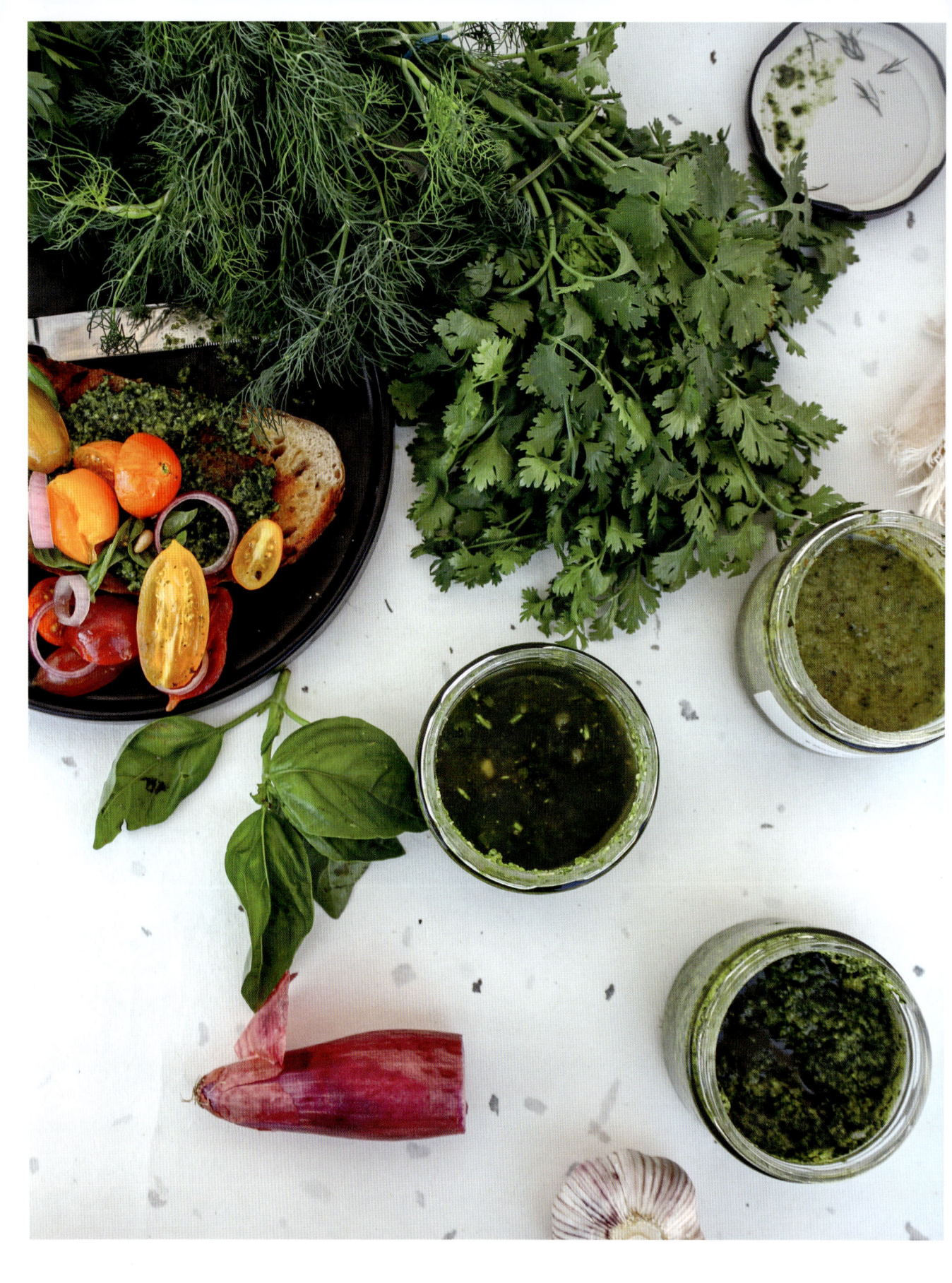

CHAPTER 10

Dressings and Pestos

Homemade, organic, fresh dressings are free of preservatives and other unpronounceable chemicals, and making your own can save you money. Better still, an investment of just 10 minutes of time can yield enough dressing to last you for a month. Having a variety of homemade dressings on hand means you can enjoy a different flavor each day. Once you learn the basic principles for making vinaigrettes and creamy dressings, you can unleash your creative impulses and make your own blends based on your favorite tastes and textures.

Pesto is a traditional Italian sauce made from basil, pine nuts, garlic, parmesan cheese, olive oil, and sometimes lemon juice. It's fresh, aromatic, and savory, and widely used in everyday dishes. The pesto recipes I offer in this chapter will help you become a pesto alchemist, creating your own variations using different oils, herbs, cheeses, nuts, and other ingredients with diverse flavors, textures, colors, and nutritional benefits. To create authentic pesto, a granite mortar and pestle is strongly recommended. This imparts a distinctive and delectable texture that sets the pesto apart from those made using a food processor or blender.

More Great Dressing Recipes

You'll also find some great vinaigrette recipes in chapter 15.

Miso-Ginger Vinaigrette (page 197)
Cherry Vinaigrette (page 212)
Blood Orange–Hazelnut Oil Vinaigrette (page 203)
Green Grape Vinaigrette (page 200)

Vinaigrette 101

MAKES 1 CUP (240 ML)

Whisk some excitement and enjoy the alchemy of dressings made from oil and fruits or vinegar. The basic ratio for a vinaigrette is 3 parts oil to 1 part vinegar. There are so many great choices of vinegars: brown or white rice, apple cider, balsamic, red wine, white wine, plum, yuzu, or ponzu.

The same formula also works well with any type of fresh-squeezed juice in place of vinegar, but keep in mind that their acidity levels vary. A citrusy tea such as hibiscus tea can also fill the role of the vinegar component. Depending on what ingredients you choose, you might increase the proportion of oil to suit the level of acidity you want in the finished vinaigrette. (As a basic comparison, the pH of white vinegar is about 2.5.) Consuming highly acidic foods can have an effect on the body's pH balance. Listening to your body is important to see how it responds to consuming highly acidic foods like vinegars. See "pH Balance and Bone Health" on page 61 for more details about how food can affect the pH balance in the body.

Juice pH Levels

lemon juice: 2.0–2.6
lime juice: 2.0–2.8
blue plum juice: 2.8–3.4
grape juice: 2.9–3.8
pomegranate juice: 2.9–3.2
grapefruit juice: 3.0–3.8
blueberry juice: 3.1–3.3
pineapple juice: 3.2–4.0

1. Add all the ingredients for the vinaigrette to an 8-ounce (240 ml) glass jar, close the lid tightly, and shake it until the ingredients are blended well.
2. Use immediately, or store in the refrigerator for up to 4 weeks.

Amino-Sesame Vinaigrette

¼ cup (60 ml) liquid aminos
3 tablespoons (45 ml) sesame oil
2 tablespoons rice vinegar
2 tablespoons Dr. Laura's Bone Vinegar (page 137)
1 tablespoon black sesame seeds
⅛ teaspoon grated fresh ginger
1 garlic clove, minced
Pinch umami powder

Classic Olive Oil–Lemon Vinaigrette

⅔ cup (160 ml) extra-virgin olive oil
6 tablespoons (90 ml) fresh lemon juice
    or ¼ cup (60 ml) any vinegar
¼ teaspoon Dijon mustard
¼ teaspoon grated lemon zest
½ garlic clove, minced
Pinch salt
Pinch ground black pepper

Hibiscus Passion Vinaigrette

⅔ cup (160 ml) extra-virgin olive oil
¼ cup (60 ml) hot filtered water
1 tablespoon dry hibiscus
⅛ teaspoon lava salt
1 medium garlic clove, minced
Pinch cracked black pepper

Mediterranean Herb and Grape Vinaigrette

⅔ cup (160 ml) flaxseed oil or extra-virgin olive oil
¼ cup (60 ml) grape juice from Concord
    or green grapes
¼ cup (15 g) finely chopped mixed fresh herbs
    such as parsley, basil, thyme, and rosemary
1 garlic clove, minced
⅛ teaspoon fennel seed
⅛ teaspoon sea salt

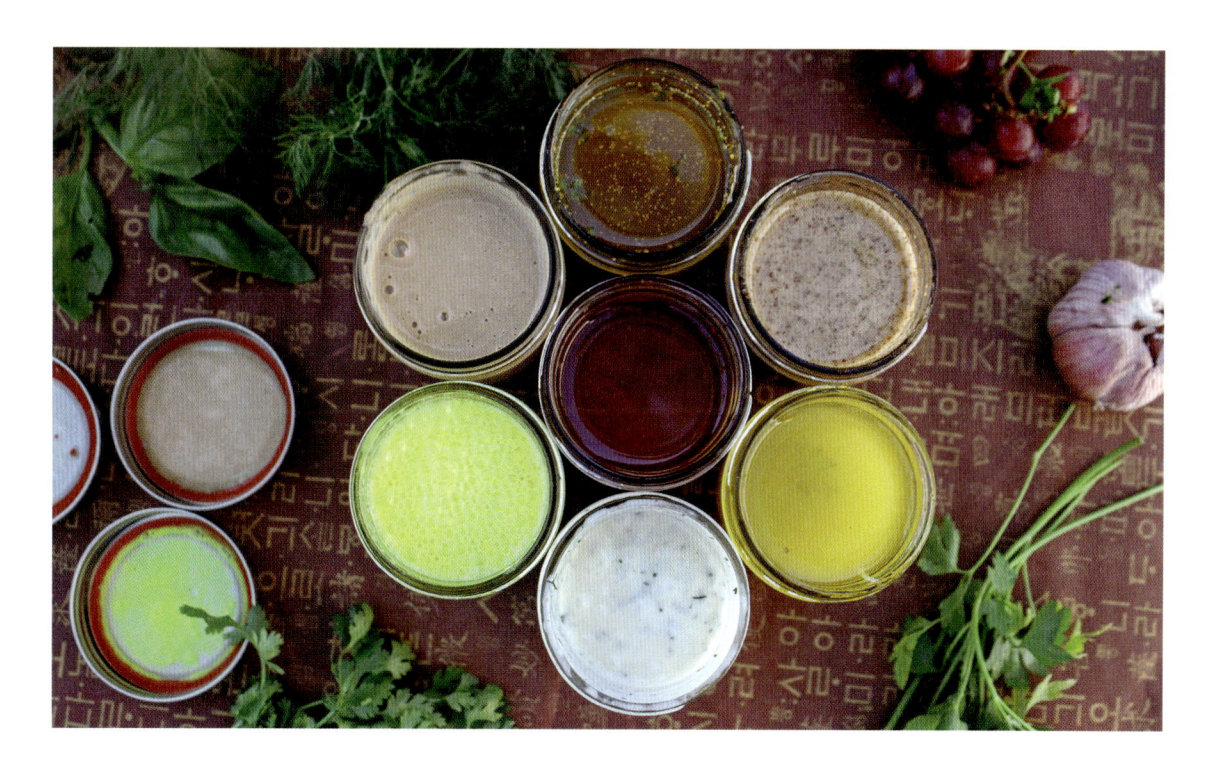

Dressings and Pestos • 121

Dressings 101

MAKES 1 CUP (240 ML)

For making creamy dressings, a blender works well.

1. Add all the ingredients to a mini blender, and blend well, starting on lowest speed and increasing to high, 3 to 5 minutes.
2. Use immediately, or store in a glass jar in the refrigerator for up to 4 weeks.

Creamy Golden Ranch Dressing

This powerhouse ranch dressing pairs healthy good fats in coconut with turmeric, a strong anti-inflammatory remedy. Fresh pineapple adds a tropical twist to the flavor. Triple or quadruple the recipe to have enough dressing to store and use for a month.

⅔ cup (160 ml) coconut milk
3 tablespoons apple cider vinegar
3 tablespoons chopped pineapple
1 tablespoon chopped shallot
1 teaspoon ground turmeric
¼ teaspoon green salt
Ground black pepper to taste

Yogurt-Orange-Dill Dressing

Vegan yogurt is a creamy dairy replacement that can boost gut health, and it provides essential bone-health nutrients. This dressing would make a perfect dairy-free ranchlike dressing for topping a vegan Happy-Go-Lucky Caesar Salad (page 208).

⅓ cup (80 ml) vegan yogurt
¼ cup (60 ml) orange juice
1 tablespoon chopped fresh dill
1 tablespoon extra-virgin olive oil
1 medium garlic clove, minced
⅛ teaspoon ground ginger
⅛ teaspoon sea salt
Ground black pepper to taste

Tahini-Apple-Ginger Dressing

Tahini is a perfect replacement for peanut butter, and it blends well with apple and ginger in this creamy dressing. You'll enjoy the hint of spiciness after the first taste of creamy nutty flavor. Packed with nutrients for bone health, this blend will dress any Asian dishes or salads well.

½ cup (120 ml) tahini
¼ apple, cored and chopped
3 tablespoons brown rice vinegar
2 tablespoons liquid aminos
2 tablespoons chopped shallot
¼ teaspoon grated fresh ginger
Ground black pepper to taste

California Vegan Chipotle Sauce

This staple dressing has an amazing flavor, is incredibly easy to prepare, and doesn't require any cooking.

¾ cup (180 ml) vegan yogurt
½ cup (110 g) canned adobo sauce or 3 tablespoons chipotle powder
¼ cup (60 g) vegan mayonnaise
1 tablespoon fresh lime or lemon juice
1 teaspoon maple syrup
1 teaspoon minced garlic
½ teaspoon smoked paprika
⅛ teaspoon sea salt

More Great Dressing Recipes

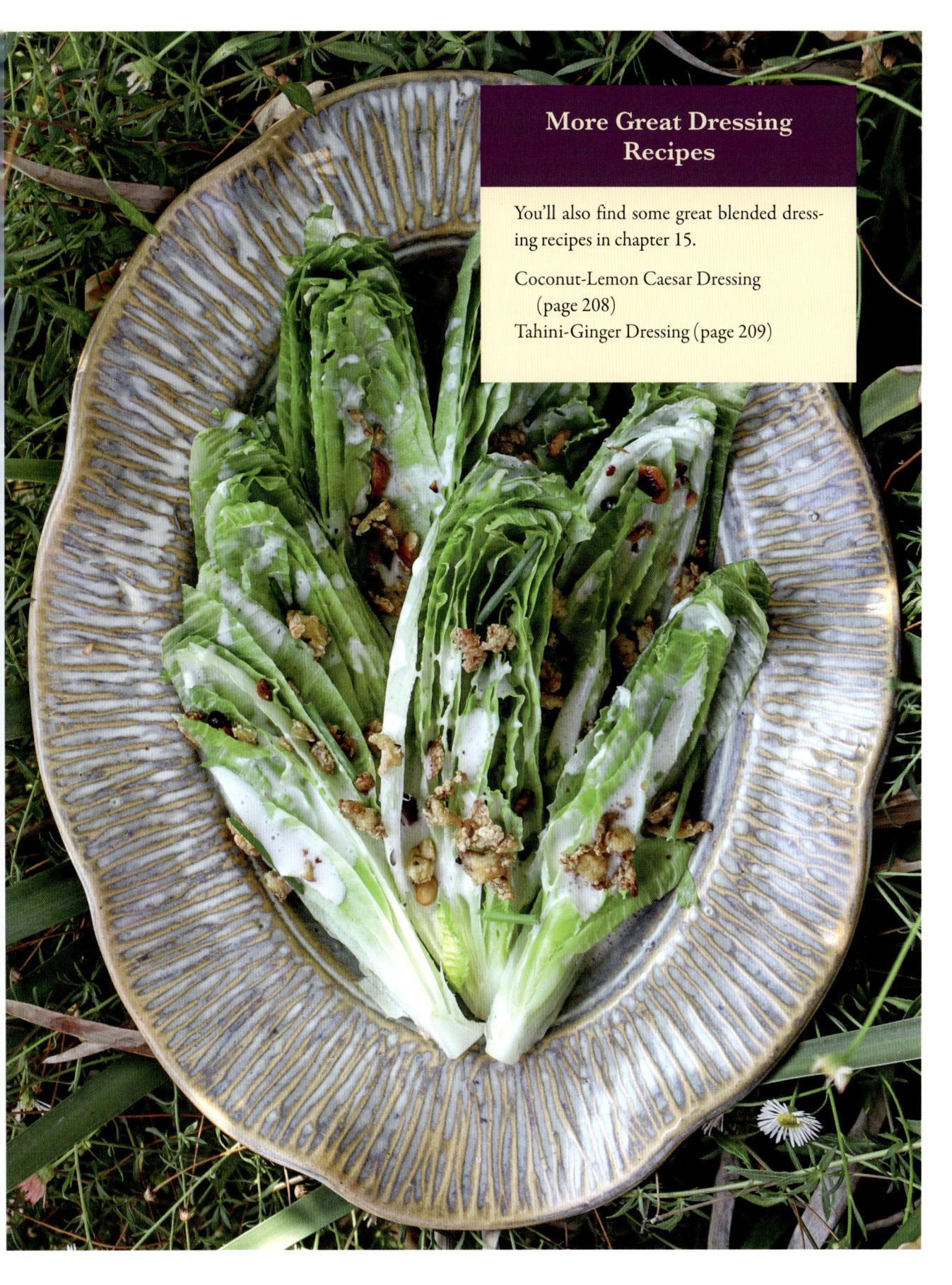

You'll also find some great blended dressing recipes in chapter 15.

Coconut-Lemon Caesar Dressing (page 208)
Tahini-Ginger Dressing (page 209)

Bone Health Classic Pesto 101

A classic pesto is delicious and nutritious. Pestos are helpful for appetite control due to their protein and healthy fats. Basil has anti-inflammatory properties, contains antioxidant-rich compounds, and supports digestive health. Pine nuts contain heart-healthy monounsaturated fats and antioxidants like vitamin E.

When you have mastered the basics of making pesto, branch out to creating your own signature pesto recipe. Set aside time to make a few batches of different pestos at once. They will store well in the refrigerator for several weeks.

Here are the basic components for making a pesto (for quantities of each ingredient, see the variations below):

HERBS AND GREENS

Herbs: basil, chives, cilantro, dill, parsley, sage, thyme

Greens: arugula, broccoli rabe, collard greens, kale, mustard greens, spinach, turnip greens

NUTS AND SEEDS

Nuts: almonds, cashews, walnuts

Seeds: pine nuts, pumpkin seeds, sunflower seeds

CHEESE

Grated parmesan cheese or vegan parmesan

SEASONINGS

Garlic, salt, pepper, lemon juice

OIL

Avocado oil, extra-virgin olive oil, flaxseed oil, hemp seed oil, pistachio oil, pumpkin seed oil, safflower oil, walnut oil

1. Wash the herbs and nuts, then roughly chop and set aside.
2. Grate the cheese and set aside.
3. Using a large mortar and pestle, add the garlic (if using) and gently grind it to a paste. Add the nuts and herbs, and grind until mixed well to an almost pasty texture.
4. Add the oil and continue grinding until the ingredients are well blended.
5. Add the cheese and give it a few gentle mixes. Season with salt, pepper, lemon juice, or other ingredients as desired.
6. Transfer the pesto to a glass jar or container. Use immediately, or refrigerate for up to 4 weeks.

> **TIP**
> If you prefer a quicker method, use a mini blender. You will need to blend in short pulses, turning the machine off and on, for less than 5 seconds at a time. The goal is to maintain a chunky consistency.

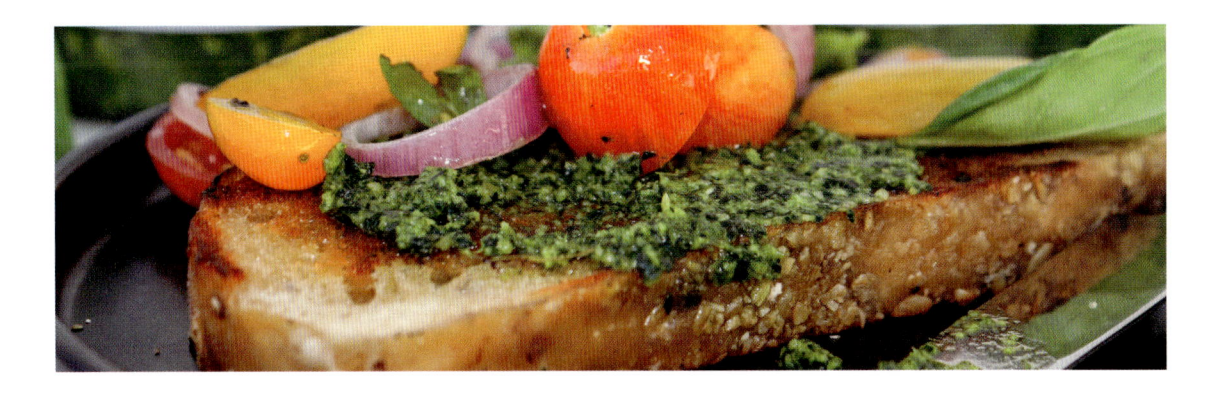

Basil-Walnut Pesto

¼ cup (15 g) chopped fresh basil
¼ cup (60 g) soaked walnuts
½ garlic clove
⅓ cup (80 ml) extra-virgin olive oil
⅛ teaspoon sea salt
Pinch ground black pepper

Kale-Cashew Pesto

3 to 4 kale leaves (see Tip)
¼ cup (60 g) hemp seeds
1 tablespoon nutritional yeast
½ garlic clove
¼ cup (60 ml) sunflower or pumpkin seed oil
1 teaspoon fresh lemon juice
⅛ teaspoon sea salt
Pinch ground black pepper

TIP
Briefly blanch the kale in boiling water, and then place the leaves in an ice bath for 5 minutes, and drain them well.

Hemp Seed Pesto

3 basil sprigs
1 tablespoon hemp seeds
1 teaspoon sesame seeds
1 teaspoon nutritional yeast
½ cup (120 ml) extra-virgin olive oil

Parsley–Pine Nut Chimichurri Pesto

¼ cup (15 g) chopped fresh parsley
¼ cup (35 g) pine nuts
¼ cup (20 g) grated parmesan cheese
1 garlic clove
½ cup (120 ml) hemp seed oil
⅛ teaspoon sea salt
Pinch ground black pepper
Pinch chili powder (optional)

Three Herbs Bone Pesto

3 tablespoons chopped fresh cilantro
3 tablespoons chopped fresh dill
3 tablespoons chopped fresh parsley
¼ cup (35 g) crushed raw cashews
¼ cup (20 g) grated parmesan cheese
½ garlic clove, minced
⅓ cup (80 ml) extra-virgin olive oil
⅛ teaspoon sea salt
Pinch ground black pepper

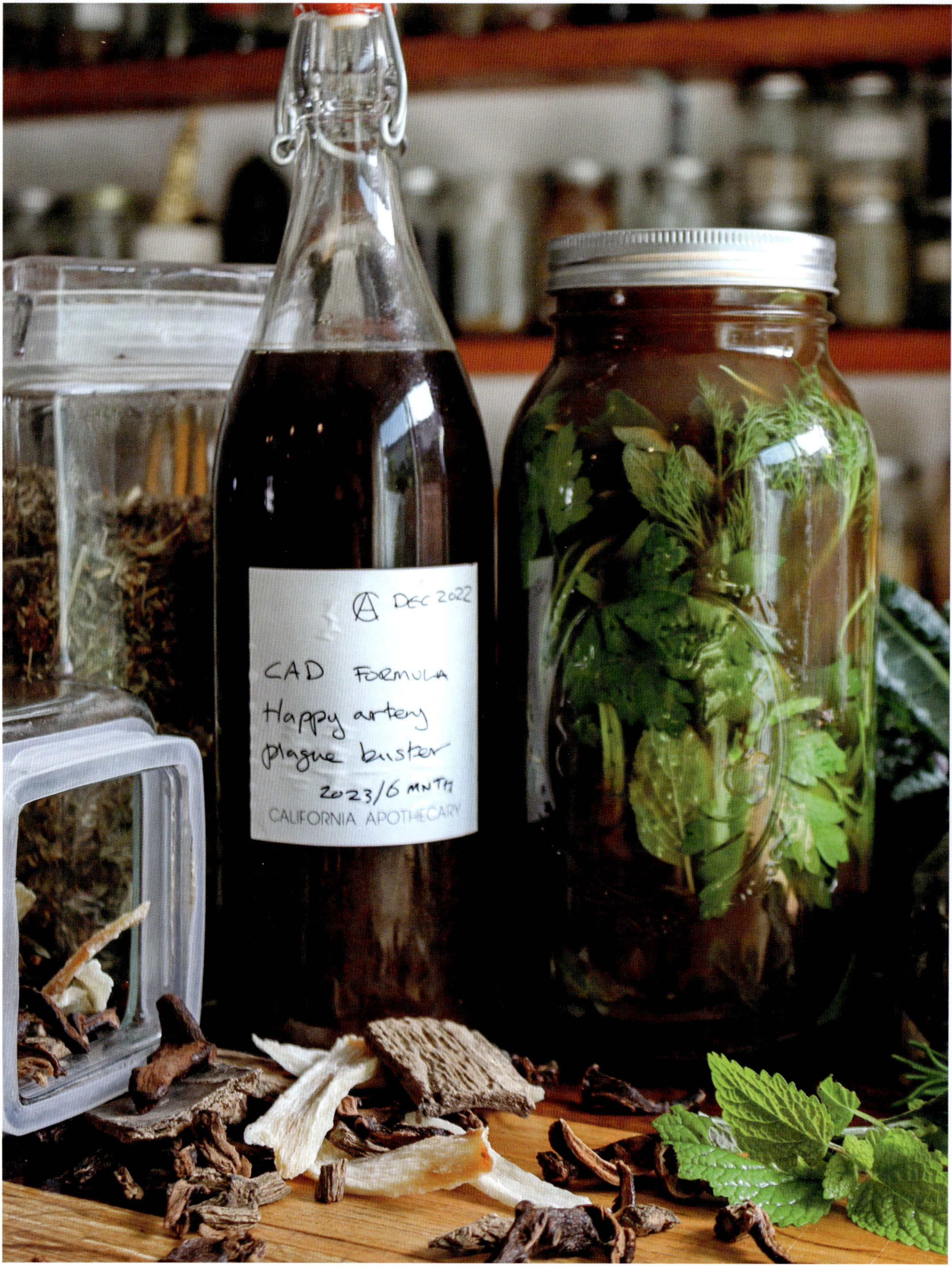
DEC 2022
CAD FORMULA
Happy artery
plague buster
2023/6 MNTH
CALIFORNIA APOTHECARY

CHAPTER 11

Fermented Slow-Aged Pickles and Bone Vinegar

The natural fermentation process involved in pickling is pure magic. The art of slow-aged pickling requires only a few ingredients: air, water, salt, and time. It's a jewel we cannot replicate quickly. Crafting your own pickles is a radical act of self-love, creating food that not only carries rich nutritional value for bone health but also can be stored for many months. The flavor profile of a pickle remains a constant surprise as it evolves with time.

The recipes in this chapter are nested deep in my heart, and I am thrilled to share them with you. In Korea, kimchi is a humble yet vital pickle, essential to surviving harsh winters. We bury it, and nature does the rest. The cold ground is an organic refrigerator, performing its magic. Kimchi holds deep cultural significance, symbolizing our identity. Kimjang, the communal preparation of kimchi during the harvest full moon, unites families and communities to create and share this beloved staple. Each culture has inherited wisdom about how to preserve foods, a testament to their ability to sustain balanced nutrition even during the harshest of winters.

In southern California, where I now live, I can leave jars of kimchi and pickles outdoors year-round to ferment. But if you live in a cold-winter climate and you don't want to bury your kimchi or pickles, you can put them in a shaded, cool spot in your house, ideally where the temperature is between 65° and 72°F (18°–22°C).

It's crucial to use unprocessed, unfiltered sea salt when making pickles, kimchi, and sauerkraut. Unfiltered sea salt is packed with essential minerals, vitamins, and a complex mix of sea microbes that aid in the fermentation process. Refer to page 103 for suggestions on how to season your creations to taste.

Each time I make kimchi I'm grateful to my mother, who instilled in me the importance of cooking fresh, seasonal, nourishing food. I invite you to create this recipe and experience the love that has been passed down from generation to generation in my family. Invite your friends and family and fill your kitchen with laughter and joy as you make kimchi together.

Vinegar also held a special place in my childhood home as a remedy for digestive issues. Our living room displayed jars of vinegar, some of them years old, symbolizing their significance in our family tradition. Back then, I was told that vinegar aids digestion, eliminates harmful bacteria, and acts as a food preservative. In this chapter, we will explore homemade apple cider vinegar to promote bone health. The simplicity of this ancient medicinal food, passed down through generations, is truly astonishing. Incorporating medicinal vinegar into daily life, whether as a dressing, marinade, or simply a spoonful a day, unveils its potential as a medicinal food.

Beet-Cauliflower Pickle

MAKES ABOUT 2 QUARTS (2 L)

In this recipe, I have distilled and simplified the process to encourage you to create your own pickles. The process is straightforward, and the outcome is tangy, crunchy pickles that are as beautiful to behold as they are to consume. I like to chop the vegetables and apple for these pickles into 1-inch (2.5 cm) cubes. And I'm a garlic lover, so I always throw in a few cloves for extra flavor.

A key part of the pickling process is to pour the broth into the jar before the broth begins to cool. The hot broth, when it touches the vegetables, locks in a crunchy texture, which becomes the signature of the pickle making.

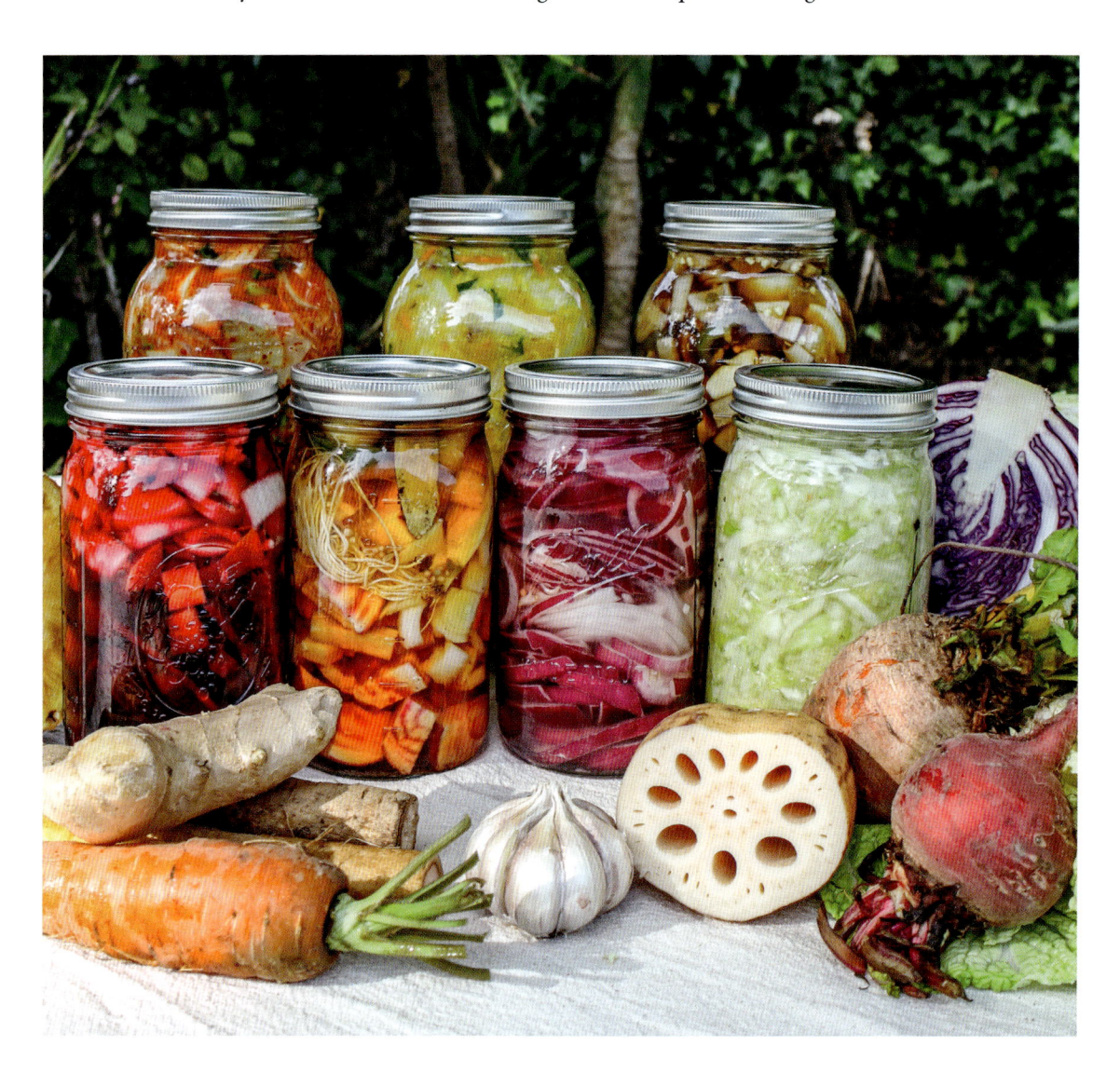

3½ cups (450 g) chopped beets
3½ cups (440 g) chopped cauliflower
½ cup (40 g) chopped yellow or sweet onion
1 medium green apple, cored and chopped
1 scallion
3 or 4 garlic cloves (optional)

FOR THE BROTH

4 cups (1 L) filtered water
5 tablespoons (75 ml) white vinegar or rice vinegar
5 licorice roots, sliced, or ¼ teaspoon licorice powder
1 cinnamon stick
1 tablespoon chopped garlic
1 tablespoon chopped fresh ginger
¼ teaspoon fennel seed
¼ teaspoon mustard seed
¼ teaspoon sea salt

> **TIPS**
>
> For a delightful twist perfect for the summer months, give Persian cucumbers and fresh dill pickles a whirl. They're not only delicious but also incredibly refreshing, helping to keep you hydrated and cool as a cucumber (pun intended), and they are good for your bones. Toss in some naturally sweet veggies like carrots and onions for a burst of flavor.
>
> Feeling adventurous? Try pickling shredded fennel and kale. This combination is one of my favorites. The tasty results will nurture your bones and are a feast for the eyes, too.

1. Place the beets, cauliflower, onion, and apple in a large bowl. Cut the scallion into 1- to 2-inch (2.5–5 cm) lengths and add it to the bowl. Add the whole garlic cloves, if using. Mix all the ingredients well. Set aside.
2. Prepare to can the pickles. Wash and dry a 2-quart (2 L) canning jar. Spread a dry towel on the countertop and place the jar on the towel. Put a canning funnel in the mouth of the jar.
3. Make the broth: Add the water to a pot along with the vinegar, licorice, cinnamon stick, chopped garlic, ginger, fennel seed, mustard seed, and salt. Bring to a boil, then reduce to a gentle simmer and cook for 5 to 10 minutes.
4. Add the vegetables to the jar and pack tightly. Carefully pour in enough of the hot broth to fill the jar, including any whole spices from the remaining broth. Ensure there are no air bubbles.
5. Tightly cover the jar and label with the date and contents.
6. Place the jar on a tray (in case of leakage) and put it in a cool, dark area. Check your pickles after 2 days to see how the vegetables and liquid are settling. The vegetables may settle to the bottom, leading to formation of bubbles, or liquid may leak out of the jar in a few days.
7. Once you start to see bubbles forming in the jar, it's time to open the lid and taste. If the flavor is not tangy or sour enough, put the lid back on, but do not tighten fully, to avoid buildup of too much pressure. Allow fermentation to continue, and check the flavor every 1 or 2 days. When the taste suits your liking, move the jar into the refrigerator. Use immediately or refrigerate for up to 1 year.

Fermented Slow-Aged Pickles and Bone Vinegar

Green and Red Everyday Sauerkraut

MAKES ABOUT 4 QUARTS (4 L)

This simple yet powerful recipe has been passed down for over 2,000 years. Sauerkraut is rich in fiber, vitamins, minerals, and probiotics that ease nutrient absorption.

Making a large batch of sauerkraut is easy to do. Selecting fresh, local, organic cabbages will bring the best result. I encourage you to use both green and red (purple) cabbage to add vibrant colors and nutritional diversity. Beyond aesthetics, this variety can aid in digestion and leave you feeling better after your meal. The taste and texture of homemade sauerkraut is nothing like store-bought brands.

Using fermentation crocks will give you the best results and be the easiest way to make your kraut. Fermentation crocks are airtight, enabling anaerobic bacteria to thrive. However, using glass jars with a tight-fitting lid works well, too.

1 large green cabbage (about 5 pounds [2.25 kg])
1 large red cabbage (about 5 pounds [2.25 kg])
4 tablespoons (90 g) coarse sea salt, plus more if needed
¼ cup (36 g) caraway seed (optional)
¼ teaspoon fennel seed
¼ teaspoon mustard seed
Ground black pepper

1. Shred the cabbage evenly. Place the shredded cabbage in two large bowls, one for green cabbage and another one for red.
2. Sprinkle 3 tablespoons of the salt into each bowl of cabbage. Here's where the magic happens. Use your hands to massage and gently squeeze the cabbage until it turns watery and limp, which typically takes 5 to 10 minutes. Add the caraway seed (if using), fennel seed, mustard seed, and pepper to taste, apportioning about half the total amount of each spice per bowl. Gradually season the mixture in each bowl with more salt, tasting to see if you are satisfied with the results.
3. Wash and dry two 2-quart (2 L) glass jars or fermentation crocks. Place a canning funnel on a jar's mouth. Take handfuls of mixed cabbage and firmly pack them into the jar. Use your fist to tamp down the cabbage, repeating the process until the jar is filled. Repeat with the other jar. Pour any liquid remaining in the bowl into the jars. It is important to press the cabbage firmly and pack it into place so that no air remains in the jar. Air can support aerobic bacteria and mold. For fermentation, we want anaerobic bacteria only. If you are using a fermentation crock, pack in the cabbage in the same manner, pour in remaining liquid, and seal the crock with the lid.

4. If using a jar, insert a smaller jar into the mouth of the filled jar to weigh down the cabbage during fermentation. Put some clean stones or marbles into the smaller jar to provide weight.
5. Cover the mouth of the large jar (including the small jar) with doubled cheesecloth or a dish towel and secure it using a rubber band or twine. This allows for the release of pressure during fermentation while keeping contaminants out.
6. Place the jar on a tray to catch any potential overflow during fermentation. Keep it in a location with a temperature between 65° and 75°F (18°–23°C) and allow to ferment. After 2 to 3 days, begin checking daily and press the cabbage down if any is floating on the surface of the liquid. Taste the sauerkraut and, if desired, continue fermenting, tasting daily for up to 10 days until you achieve your preferred flavor.
7. Once you're satisfied with the taste, remove the cloth, seal the jar tightly with a lid, and transfer it to the refrigerator. You can enjoy the sauerkraut immediately or allow it to slowly ferment further in the fridge for up to 1 year.

> **TIPS**
>
> As the fermentation unfolds, you'll notice fascinating signs of the process. Watch for bubbles rising through the cabbage, a frothy layer forming on top, or even some white scum. Don't be alarmed; these are all indicators of a healthy and active fermentation! If you see that white scum, you can simply skim it off during the fermentation period or just before transferring the cabbage to the fridge.
>
> I like to let sauerkraut mature for at least 2 months, and often even longer when stored in the refrigerator. The cold temperature slows down the fermentation.

Immortal Root Kimchi

MAKES 2 QUARTS (2 L)

I have vivid memories of my mom's perfect herbal home remedies from whenever I was in pain or feeling under the weather. Those memories inspired me to explore infusing the broth of accessible medicinal plants and herbs into pickles and kimchi. It worked, and resulted in significant improvements in my clients' gut health.

In this recipe, the rich, medicinal earthy flavors of the burdock and licorice-infused broth are truly a remedy in pickle form. The broth is mild, tangy, sweet, sour, and bitter. Green jalapeño, radish, and just a hint of maple syrup also make this kimchi irresistible. Licorice adds sweet flavor without sugar. It's a great choice if you have a sugar addiction. At 2 to 3 tablespoons per serving, this recipe will make a 1- to 2-month supply of kimchi.

Kimchi is living proof of one of the healthiest probiotic food medicines to revitalize gut health and support digestion. Remember, your gut is your second brain, so trust your gut and follow your bliss!

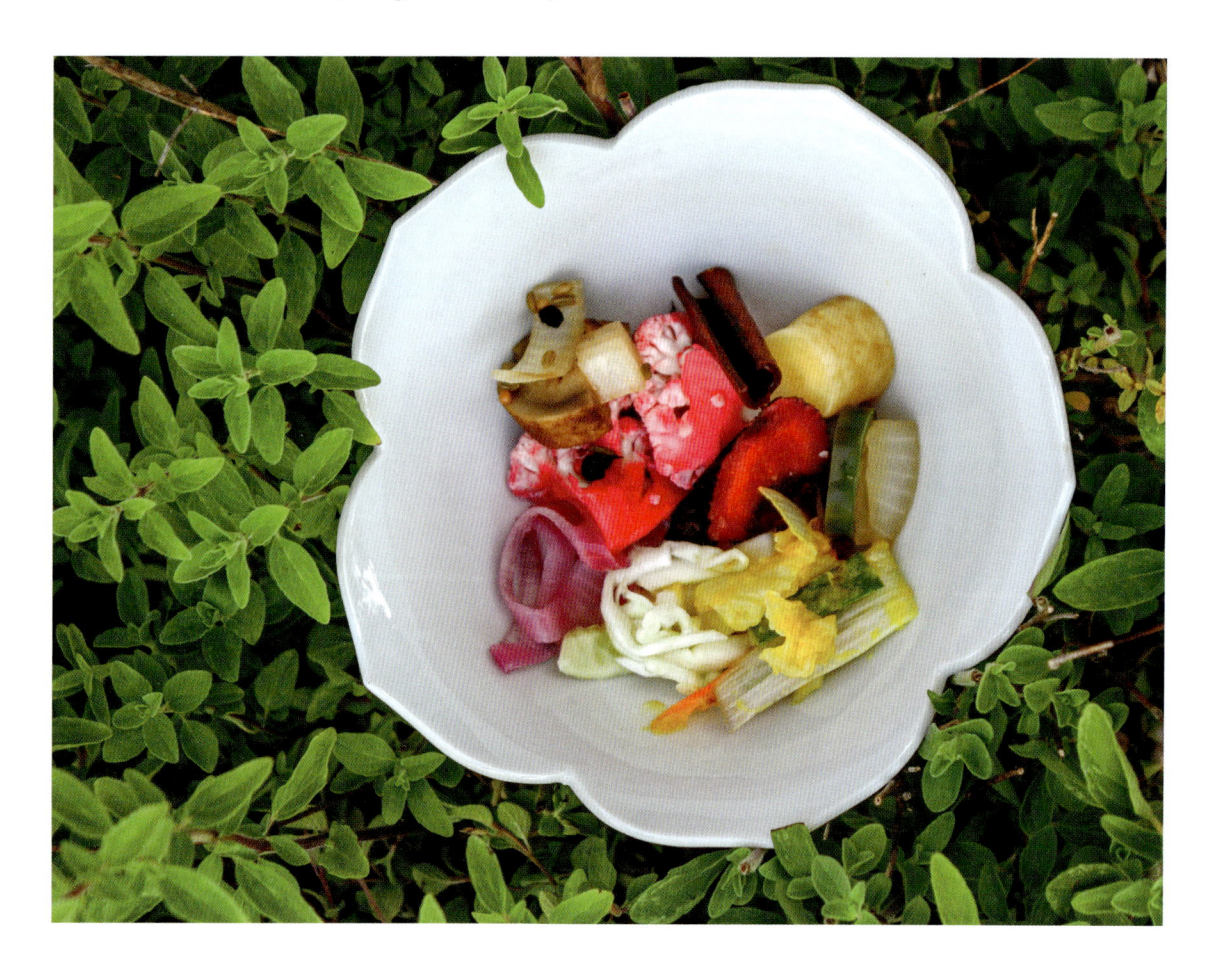

FOR THE BROTH

3 cups (720 ml) filtered water or Root and Leaf Magnesium Broth (page 177)
½ cup (120 ml) liquid aminos or soy sauce
½ cup (120 ml) rice vinegar
2 tablespoons coconut sugar
2 tablespoons maple syrup
1 5-inch (13 cm) cinnamon stick
½ teaspoon ground cardamom
½ teaspoon ground ginger
½ teaspoon licorice powder or 2 or 3 dried licorice roots
½ teaspoon freshly grated nutmeg
½ teaspoon mustard seed
½ teaspoon vanilla extract

FOR THE KIMCHI

2 cups (250 g) chopped onion
2 cups (250 g) chopped radish
1 cup (63 g) chopped burdock root or parsnip
1 cup (125 g) chopped jalapeño, stemmed and seeded (optional)
½ cup (68 g) garlic cloves, peeled
1 tablespoon finely chopped fresh ginger

1. Make the broth: In a large pot, combine the water, liquid aminos, vinegar, coconut sugar, maple syrup, cinnamon stick, cardamom, ginger, licorice, nutmeg, mustard seed, and vanilla and stir well. Bring it to a boil over high heat, then lower the heat to the minimum. Let the broth simmer for 20 to 30 minutes, until you can smell it and it has reduced to one-fifth of its original volume. Remove from the heat and let cool for 5 to 10 minutes.

2. Make the kimchi: Combine the onion, radish, burdock, jalapeño, garlic, and ginger in a large bowl, mix well, and set aside.

3. Wash and dry two 1-quart (1 L) glass jars. Place a canning funnel on a jar's mouth. Add the vegetables to each jar and pack tightly. Carefully pour the hot broth into the jars and seal them immediately. Don't forget to label the jars.

4. To ferment, place the jar in a cool, shaded outdoor area for a few days. When you notice bubbles forming, open the lid briefly to allow any gas to escape. The fermentation time varies with the season. In winter, it may take 3 to 5 days, while in summer, you could have kimchi ready in 1 to 2 days. Taste it periodically, and ferment until the taste is pleasing, then cover the jar and refrigerate for up to 1 year.

> **TIPS**
>
> You can find fresh burdock root in Korean and Japanese grocery stores. If you don't have access to fresh burdock, try parsnip, celery root, carrots, or turnip instead.
>
> Experiment with a combination of green delights like celery, fennel, fresh dill, kale, and green onion to provide a super mix for bone health.

Fermented Slow-Aged Pickles and Bone Vinegar

Jummee's Signature Pineapple-Turmeric Kimchi

MAKES ABOUT 2 QUARTS (2 L)

What's your favorite childhood memory of food? One that's tattooed in my mind is from winter breaks spent with my relatives in the remote countryside where my parents grew up. The kids, including me, would sneak into the neighbor's backyard and uncover a giant buried clay pot filled with kimchi. The kimchi was frozen, with ice crystals glistening on the edges. We grabbed a piece or two, savoring the cold, crunchy, sweet-tangy flavor. Food can evoke such powerful emotions, and my memories of this kimchi have left a lasting imprint.

This recipe is a blend of tradition and contemporary American foodways. I've eliminated the fish sauce and processed sugar, adding sweetness from licorice root instead. Ayurvedic spices are a digestive aid, and the pineapple, apple, onion, and rice powder provide natural sugars. The fermentation process of this nutritional powerhouse creates probiotics, enhancing gut health.

TIPS

If you're short on time, dissolve the salt in warm water for 20 to 30 minutes, then pour it over the cabbage. This trick may cut the pickling time in half, though it may also reduce the crunchiness of the pickles.

If any of the broth spills while you fill the jar, save it to drink during a meal as probiotic shots. It is pure medicine.

If you're making kimchi for the first time, I recommend using napa cabbage as your primary ingredient. It has a satisfyingly crunchy texture and is packed with nutrients beneficial for bone health. As you gain experience, try other types of cabbage, too!

Try these other ingredient combinations for splendid kimchi: kale and fennel; onion and chives; cauliflower and carrots; radish and beets; lotus, burdock, ginseng, and reishi mushroom powder.

1½ large napa cabbages (4 to 5 pounds [1.8–2 kg])
4 cups (1.2 kg) coarse sea salt
¼ cup (45 g) thinly sliced bell pepper
¼ cup (40 g) thinly sliced onion
¼ cup (31 g) shredded carrot
¼ cup (31 g) shredded celery
¼ cup (31 g) shredded radish
¼ cup (6 g) thinly sliced fresh chives or scallions
3 tablespoons shredded red chili pepper

FOR THE NATURAL SUGAR WET MIXER
½ cup (56 g) chopped pineapple
½ cup (31 g) chopped apple
¼ cup (40 g) chopped onion
3 to 5 slices licorice root or ½ teaspoon licorice root powder
3 medium garlic cloves
2 tablespoons ground ginger
1 teaspoon coconut sugar

FOR THE STICKY RICE WARM BROTH
2 cups (480 ml) filtered water
¼ cup (75 g) sweet rice powder
2 tablespoons ground turmeric
⅛ teaspoon ground cinnamon
⅛ teaspoon cumin seed
⅛ teaspoon fennel seed
⅛ teaspoon mustard seed
Ground black pepper

1. Cut the cabbage vertically into quarters, keeping the core intact, and make small slits into the bases. Place the cabbage quarters in a large bowl. Insert handfuls of salt into the slits, place each cabbage in line, and sprinkle it across two or three layers of leaves in each quarter. Be generous with the salt.
2. Add enough water to the bowl to almost cover the cabbage. Place a heavy weight on top of the cabbage to keep it submerged. Let it sit for 4 to 6 hours, flipping the cabbage quarters every 2 hours.
3. When the cabbage leaves become soft and have shrunk to about half their original size, wash the cabbage quarters at least three times or until a leaf tastes slightly salty. The volume of the cabbages will reduce 30 percent during this process. Remove the cabbage from the bowl, squeezing it to remove excess water. Cut the quarters into 2-inch (5 cm) pieces, slicing horizontally. Let the pieces drain in a colander for 30 minutes.
4. Make the natural sugar wet mixer: Place the pineapple, apple, onion, licorice, garlic, ginger, and sugar in a high-speed blender or food processor and blend until smooth.
5. Make the broth: Combine the water and rice powder in a medium saucepan and whisk for 1 to 2 minutes over medium heat. Add the turmeric, cinnamon, cumin, fennel, mustard seed, and pepper to taste. Continue to whisk until the broth thickens and bubbles appear. Remove from the heat and let cool for 10 minutes.
6. Add the bell pepper, onion, carrot, celery, radish, chives, and chili pepper to the pickled cabbage. Add the wet mixer and broth, and mix well.
7. Wash and dry two 1-quart (1 L) glass jars. Place a canning funnel on a jar's mouth. Pack the cabbage mixture into the jars tightly.
8. If you live in a mild climate, allow the jar to sit in a cool, shaded outdoor area for 1 to 2 days in spring to fall, or 3 to 5 days in winter. When the kimchi starts bubbling, move it to the refrigerator. Kimchi can be stored for over a year refrigerated, and the longer it's stored, the more complex its flavors become.

Fermented Slow-Aged Pickles and Bone Vinegar

Apple Cider Vinegar

MAKES ABOUT 1 QUART (1 L)

Apple cider vinegar is a cornerstone of a healthy life, particularly because it enhances mineral absorption from plant-based foods. Including apple cider vinegar in her daily routine has been vital to Helen's success, and I (Jummee) am sure you'll find it valuable as well.

Any type of apple will work for this recipe. Experiment with combinations of sweet and tart apples. The muscovado (unrefined brown) sugar lends a touch of sweetness and accelerates fermentation. You can substitute the sweetener of your choice; I like coconut sugar or maple syrup.

3 organic apples
1 tablespoon muscovado sugar
About 6 cups (1.4 L) filtered water

1. Wash the apples thoroughly and dry with a cotton towel. Peel the apples if desired, and cut them into chunks, removing the stems but keeping the cores. Place the apple pieces in a sterilized 2-quart (2 L) jar with a wide neck.
2. Mix the sugar with 1 cup (240 ml) of the water. Pour the sugar water over the apples. Add enough additional water to cover the apples completely.
3. Cover the jar with cheesecloth or a paper towel and secure it with a rubber band. Place it in a location where it won't be disturbed. You'll notice bubbling as the apples and water start turning into cider.
4. After 1 to 2 weeks, when you start to see small bubbles, strain the liquid. Press on the apple chunks in the strainer to extract as much liquid as possible. Return the liquid to the same jar.
5. Cover the jar again and leave it for 3 to 6 weeks. Occasionally check for the development of the mother of vinegar. Taste it after 3 weeks to check its strength. Once the vinegar is as strong as you like, transfer it to a sterilized bottle or jar with a tight-fitting lid. Stored in a cupboard at room temperature, homemade apple cider vinegar will stay good for up to 5 years but will taste best within 2 years.

TIPS

You can also make vinegar using the scraps after preparing an apple dish. Use the peels and cores from six to eight apples.

If you make a larger batch, be sure to adjust the sugar quantity. More sugar accelerates the conversion of water to alcohol and reduces fermentation time.

Dr. Laura's Bone Vinegar

MAKES 3 QUARTS (3 L)

This homemade vinegar helps support bone health with fresh and medicinal herbs and plants that are easy to find. The bone-building herbs are infused into organic raw apple cider vinegar to release their nutrients. Using raw apple cider vinegar is important because it is full of good bacteria to help the digestive system. See the sidebar for choices of herbs. You can use this vinegar to make salad dressing or serve it on any vegetables. This recipe is for a 6-month to 1-year supply.

A selection of dried or freshly snipped herbs (see Dr. Laura's Vinegar Herbs below)

6 to 7 cups (1.4 to 1.7 L) raw apple cider vinegar (page 136)

1. Thoroughly wash three 1-quart (1 L) glass jars in boiling water to sanitize. (You can use smaller jars if you prefer.)
2. Fill the jars about one-third full with dried herbs or two-thirds full with freshly snipped herbs.
3. Fill the jars to the brim with vinegar, then seal tightly.
4. Label the jars with the date and ingredients and store in a cool, dark cupboard for a minimum of 6 weeks.
5. Strain the vinegar and return the strained liquid to the jars. Store it in a cupboard at room temperature for up to 3 years.

Dr. Laura's Vinegar Herbs

Dandelion (*Taraxacum officinale*)
Horsetail (*Equisetum arvense*)
Mugwort (*Artemisia vulgaris*)
Oatstraw (*Avena sativa*)
Red clover (*Trifolium pratense*)
Stinging nettle (*Urtica* spp.)

Alternatively, you can use many other herbs and greens that grow in the United States, such as motherwort, mint, wild arugula, chickweed, shepherd's purse, alfalfa, parsley, comfrey, raspberry leaves, blackberry leaves, thimbleberry leaves, sage, amaranth leaves, lamb's-quarter, kale, or cabbage.

Molasses-Kale-Herb Vinegar

MAKES 2 QUARTS (2 L)

Here is an herb-infused vinegar that only gets better as time goes by, both in flavor and health benefits. It becomes a powerful elixir with incredible medicinal purposes. So, don't hesitate to make a large batch and let it age gracefully. The taste will only improve.

6 kale leaves
3 to 5 dill sprigs
5 parsley sprigs
Handful fresh sage
Handful fresh oregano
Handful fresh mint
5 tablespoons (75 ml) blackstrap molasses
About 7 cups (1.7 L) raw apple cider vinegar (page 136)

1. Place a 2-quart (2 L) glass jar on the countertop and gently add the kale and herbs. Put a canning funnel in the mouth of the jar. Carefully pour in the molasses and then the apple cider vinegar until it reaches the top.
2. Seal the jar with a lid, label it with the ingredients and date, and store it in a cool, shaded area for at least 6 weeks. During this time, the vinegar will develop its unique taste and become ready for use.
3. Strain, and return the strained liquid to the jar. Store it in a cupboard at room temperature. It will keep for up to 6 months.

CHAPTER 12

Dips and Breads

When you're in the mood for some seriously tasty dips, how about serving up a selection of dips in a funky set of mismatched bowls of different shapes and colors? I love to bring folks together for informal, delicious eats and conversation in this way.

Making your own bread to pair with your meal is a very rewarding experience, as breadmaking holds deep historical roots. As Helen and Laura note on page 54, there are concerns about the quality and potential health effects of the wheat produced on an industrial scale in North America. Because of that, and because of my personal interest in developing gluten-free recipes, the bread recipes I offer in this chapter use gluten-free flours and grains. You may also want to seek out local bakers who make healthy, nutritious breads with organically grown wheat flour and fermented dough.

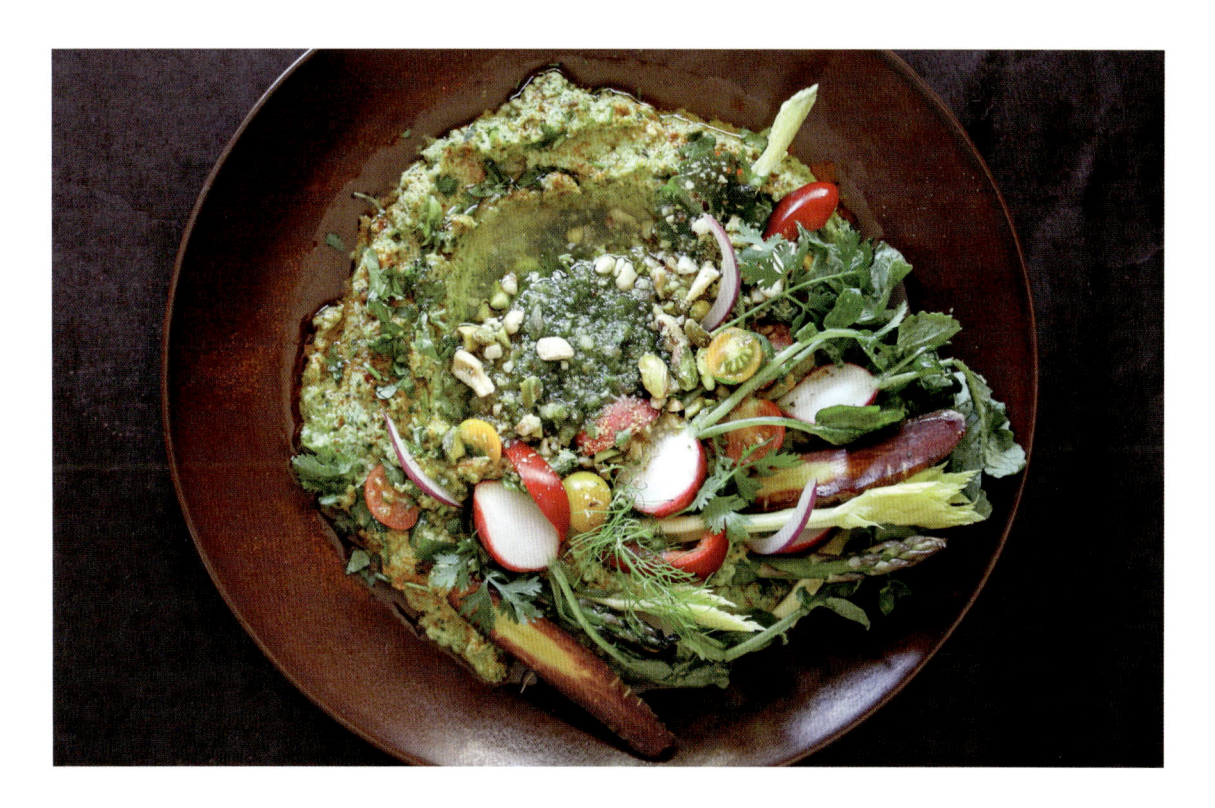

Edamame Dip

MAKES 2 SERVINGS

Edamame's story goes back over 2,000 years to South Asia, but this protein-packed legume has only recently become a beloved snack and ingredient in Western cuisine. Dip some celery, baby carrots, radishes, or even fruits in this tasty, easy-to-make edamame dip, and you're good to go.

DIP

- 2 cups (320 g) frozen precooked peeled edamame
- 5 tablespoons (16 g) roughly chopped fresh cilantro
- 1 small shallot, chopped
- 1 garlic clove, minced
- ⅛ teaspoon ground cumin
- ⅛ teaspoon fennel seed
- 2 tablespoons coconut milk
- 2 tablespoons walnut oil
- 1 tablespoon white miso paste
- ½ teaspoon fresh lemon juice
- Sea salt
- Ground black pepper

TO SERVE

- 2 or 3 baby red radishes, with leaves
- 2 asparagus spears
- 1 or 2 celery ribs, with leaves
- 3 golden cherry tomatoes (optional)
- 1 tablespoon chopped fresh dill
- ¼ teaspoon fresh orange juice or lemon juice
- 1 tablespoon crushed macadamias

1. Make the dip: Thaw the edamame by placing it in water in a large bowl for 10 minutes. Rinse in cold water and drain. Bring a large pot of water to a boil, and cook the edamame for 5 minutes. Drain and allow to cool for 10 minutes.
2. Combine the edamame, cilantro, shallot, garlic, cumin, and fennel seed in a food processor and pulse the ingredients for 2 to 3 minutes to form a mash. Add the coconut milk, walnut oil, and miso and pulse again for 1 to 2 minutes until all the ingredients combine into a smooth, silky, hummuslike texture. Add the lemon juice and season to taste with salt and pepper.
3. Prepare the vegetables for serving: Cut the radishes, asparagus, celery, and cherry tomatoes (if using) into creative shapes of your choice.
4. To serve, spread the edamame mash in a large circle on a plate. Place the cut vegetables on top. Place the dill around the edges of the plate. Drizzle with the orange or lemon juice and sprinkle with crushed macadamias.

> **TIP**
> Try pumpkin or Japanese yam as a substitute for edamame in the fall for a dip of a different color and different nutritional boost. Adzuki beans or black beans are also good choices for their high-protein content and similar texture..

Silky Tofu–Spinach Dip

MAKES 4 SERVINGS

This rich, tangy, oil-free spinach dip is a nutritional powerhouse, unlike traditional spinach dips, which are loaded with heavy sour cream. It incorporates coconut yogurt, water chestnuts, and dill to promote digestion, boost immunity, and provide fiber and protein to nourish your body.

Serve with your favorite tortilla chips, Red Lentil–Saffron Tortillas (page 150), Triple Kale Chips (page 258), fresh seasonal veggies, or Broccoli and Mushroom Buffalo "Wings" (page 156).

½ cup (75 g) thawed frozen spinach or about 2 cups (60 g) fresh spinach, cooked
½ cup (65 g) water chestnuts
1 cup (275 g) soft silken tofu
¼ cup (60 ml) coconut yogurt or vegan mayonnaise
1 tablespoon apple cider vinegar
1 garlic clove, minced
2 tablespoons chopped fresh dill
1 teaspoon fresh lemon juice
⅛ teaspoon grated lemon zest
Sea salt
Ground black pepper

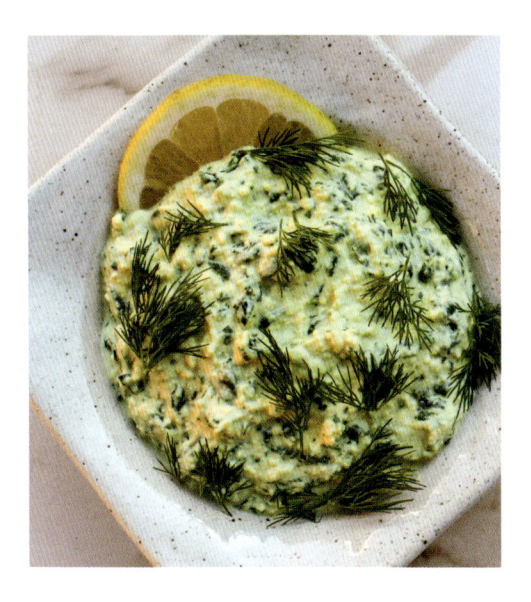

1. If using frozen spinach, rinse it, strain, and squeeze well to remove excess water. If using fresh spinach, simmer in water for 2 to 3 minutes, rinse under cold water, and squeeze out the excess. Rinse the water chestnuts thoroughly with water, then drain.
2. In a food processor, combine the spinach, water chestnuts, tofu, yogurt, vinegar, and garlic. Blend everything into a creamy paste. If you prefer a crunchy texture, pulse the ingredients until you achieve the desired texture.
3. Transfer the mixture to a bowl and add the dill, along with the lemon juice and lemon zest. Gently stir to combine, then season to taste with salt and pepper. Mix again to ensure even seasoning. If possible, refrigerate the dip for 30 minutes to 1 hour before serving.
4. Store any leftovers in an airtight container in the refrigerator for up to a week.

TIP
Be careful not to overblend this dip to avoid formation of excess liquid.

Deep Purple Hummus

MAKES 2 SERVINGS

Beautiful beets are one of my favorite roots. Beets are not grown or available at markets in Korea, so I was mesmerized by their striking color and flavor when I met them for the first time in the United States. There are so many ways to prepare beets: a dip or mash like this hummus, roasted beets sliced and served with arugula and sprouts, pickled beets, and more.

Beets are a perfect fall-to-winter root based on the Five Elements of Traditional Chinese Medicine (see page 98). You will feel more energy flow through your body when you eat beets!

This recipe incorporates hibiscus and cinnamon sticks to increase vitamin C and iron, and the lemon juice reduces the effects of the oxalates in the beets. This hummus is an excellent dip for your favorite crudités. Or, if you are tired of heavy servings of mashed potatoes, substitute this magical deep purple mashed beet recipe instead. It will leave you feeling light but well satisfied.

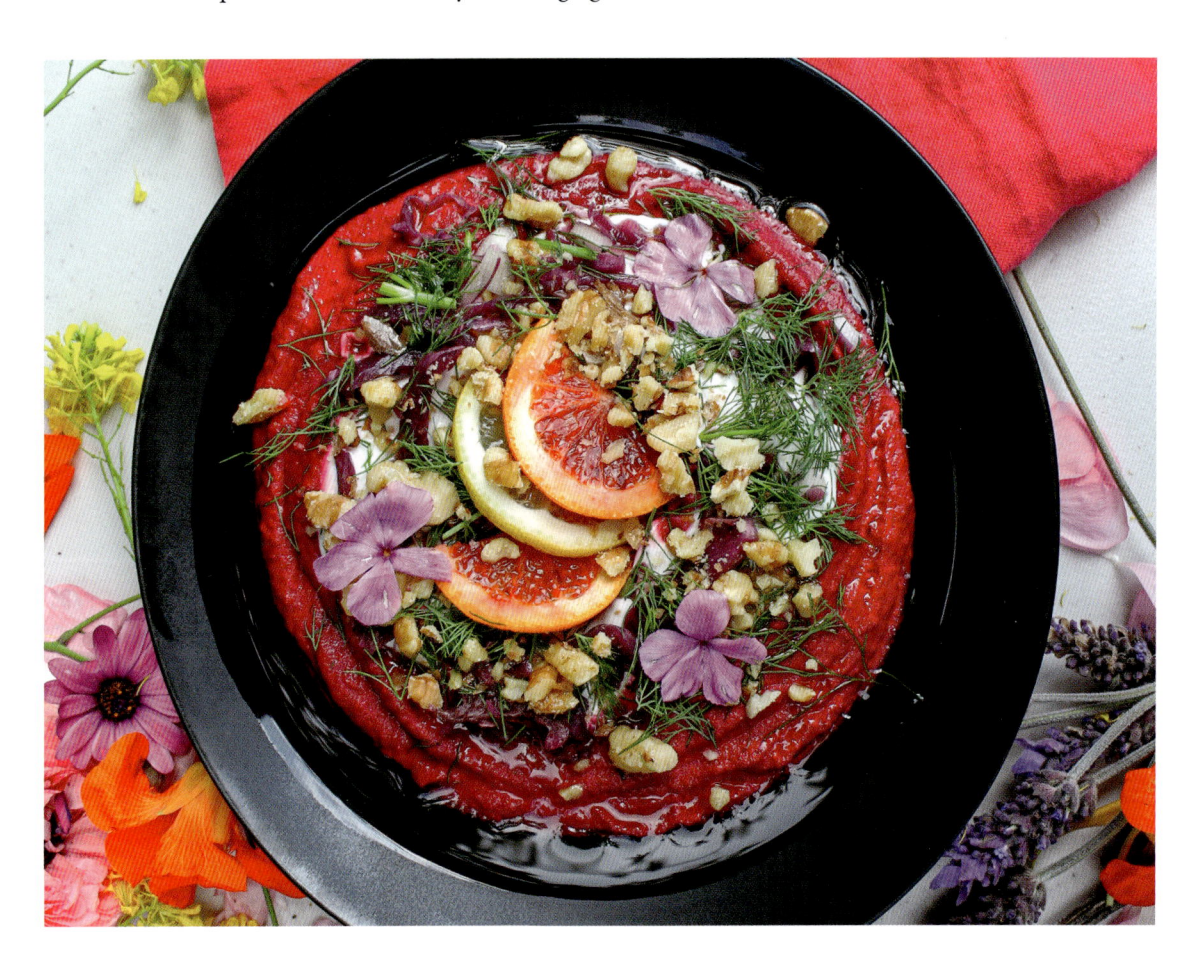

2 small beets, quartered
2 tablespoons dry hibiscus tea
1 rosemary sprig or 1 teaspoon dried rosemary
1 cinnamon stick (about 3 inches [8 cm])
1/8 teaspoon fennel seed
1/8 teaspoon ground cumin
1/8 teaspoon mustard seed
Sea salt
Ground black pepper
1 tablespoon raw cashews, soaked
1 tablespoon coconut milk
2 to 3 tablespoons walnut oil
1/4 teaspoon fresh lemon juice

FOR THE GREEN OIL

2 tablespoons walnut oil
2 or 3 parsley sprigs
Sea salt
Cracked black pepper

FOR GARNISH

2 tablespoons crushed walnuts
1/2 orange, thinly sliced
1/4 teaspoon fresh orange or lemon juice
Chopped fresh dill or dried dill

> **TIPS**
>
> If you like, you can add diced baby red radishes or carrots to the serving plate as well.
>
> Green oil is a fantastic topping for a variety of dishes. A drizzle of it adds brightness and a professional-chef touch, enhancing the overall presentation. If you wish, try substituting basil or mint for the parsley to customize the flavor profile of the oil.
>
> Making colorful garnish oil is a great culinary technique. You can mix this oil with leftover cooked beet broth for a striking purple salad dressing.

1. Fill a 2-quart (2 L) saucepan about two-thirds full of water and set it over high heat. Add the beets, hibiscus, rosemary, cinnamon stick, fennel seed, cumin, mustard seed, and a pinch of salt and ground pepper. Bring to a simmer, then reduce the heat to medium-low.
2. Check the beets at the 15- to 20-minute mark by inserting a small sharp knife into a piece of beet; when the beets are done it should pierce the flesh smoothly. If they are not done, add more water if needed and continue cooking up to 10 minutes longer.
3. When the beets are cooked through, drain them well (reserve the cooking liquid for adding to a vegetable stock or salad dressing). Set the beets aside to cool for 15 to 20 minutes. Remove the cinnamon stick and hibiscus and set aside for use in garnishing the hummus.
4. Place the cooled beets in a food processor with the cashews. Pulse for 2 to 3 minutes, until the beets are uniformly mashed. Add the coconut milk; the color will change to a bright pink-purple. Gradually add the walnut oil, finishing with the lemon juice and seasoning with salt and ground pepper. Give it a final pulse for a few seconds.
5. Make the green oil: In a mini blender, combine the walnut oil and parsley, a pinch of salt, and cracked pepper. Blend for 1 to 2 minutes until the oil turns a vibrant green; pour it into a small sauce bowl.
6. To serve, spread the beet mash in a large circle on a serving plate. Work artistically, using bold brush strokes. Sprinkle the crushed walnuts over the dish and top with the orange slices. Garnish with the reserved hibiscus and cinnamon stick. Randomly drizzle over the green oil and orange juice, creating a beautiful contrast of purple and green. Sprinkle the dill over all.

Dips and Breads

Mushroom Cashew Pâté

MAKES 2 CUPS (100 G)

Pâté is a beloved French staple—a rich, savory spread or paste traditionally made from finely ground duck liver. This recipe breaks away from the original and reinvents pâté as a richly flavored plant-based paste. This simple yet luxurious dish is designed for easy preparation. Enjoy it as an everyday spread or a perfect appetizer for a special occasion. Take note that the cashews should be set to soak while you prepare the rest of the ingredients.

Serve with toasted Flourless Mung Bean Olive Loaf (page 148) or spread the pâté on your lunch sandwich.

1 cup (150 g) raw cashews
½ leek or 1 small shallot, chopped
4 tablespoons (60 ml) extra-virgin olive oil
5 garlic cloves, roughly crushed
½ cup (30 g) chopped fresh parsley
2 tablespoons chopped fresh rosemary, sage, or thyme
1 tablespoon herbes de Provence
1 celery rib, chopped
8 ounces (250 g) button or cremini mushrooms, sliced (about 2 cups)
6 tablespoons (90 ml) filtered water
⅛ teaspoon saffron
Sea salt
Ground black pepper

1. Put the cashews in a medium bowl and cover with clean water. Let them soak for 30 minutes to 1 hour, and then rinse them under running water, drain well, and set aside.
2. Put the leek pieces in a bowl with water to soak for 10 to 15 minutes to remove trapped soil or sand particles. (If using shallot, you can skip this step.) Drain them well, and set aside.
3. Heat a large, dry skillet over medium heat. Toast the soaked cashews in the skillet for 1 to 3 minutes until they turn golden brown, enhancing their flavor. Remove them from the skillet and set aside in a small bowl.
4. In the same pan, add 3 tablespoons of the olive oil, the garlic, parsley, rosemary, and herbes de Provence and sauté for 2 to 3 minutes. Add the leeks and celery; sauté for an additional 1 to 2 minutes.
5. Add the mushrooms and sauté until they turn golden brown, about 5 minutes. Add the water and saffron, cover the skillet with a lid, reduce the heat to a minimum, and cook until liquid barely covers the mushrooms, about 10 minutes, stirring occasionally to distribute the flavor evenly. Season with salt and pepper. Remove from the heat and allow the mixture to cool for 10 to 20 minutes.
6. When the mushroom-leek mixture has cooled, put it in a food processor with the toasted cashews and the remaining tablespoon of oil. Pulse, pausing to scrape the sides as needed, until you achieve a pâté texture.

7. Press the mixture into a serving container, using a spatula to smooth the surface. Cover tightly. Chill in the refrigerator until completely set before serving. The pâté will keep, refrigerated, in an airtight container for 2 to 3 days.

> **TIPS**
>
> Collect garlic skins in a cotton bag and store in the freezer for use in making broth (see page 175). Collect onion roots and skins in the same way. Embrace a "no waste" mindset to save money and stay healthy.
>
> Before you slice and cook the mushrooms, set them in the sun for 30 minutes to encourage production of vitamin D, as described on page 94.
>
> Try this pâté recipe substituting walnuts for the cashews. Walnuts are a great bone-health, high-protein, brain-boosting food.

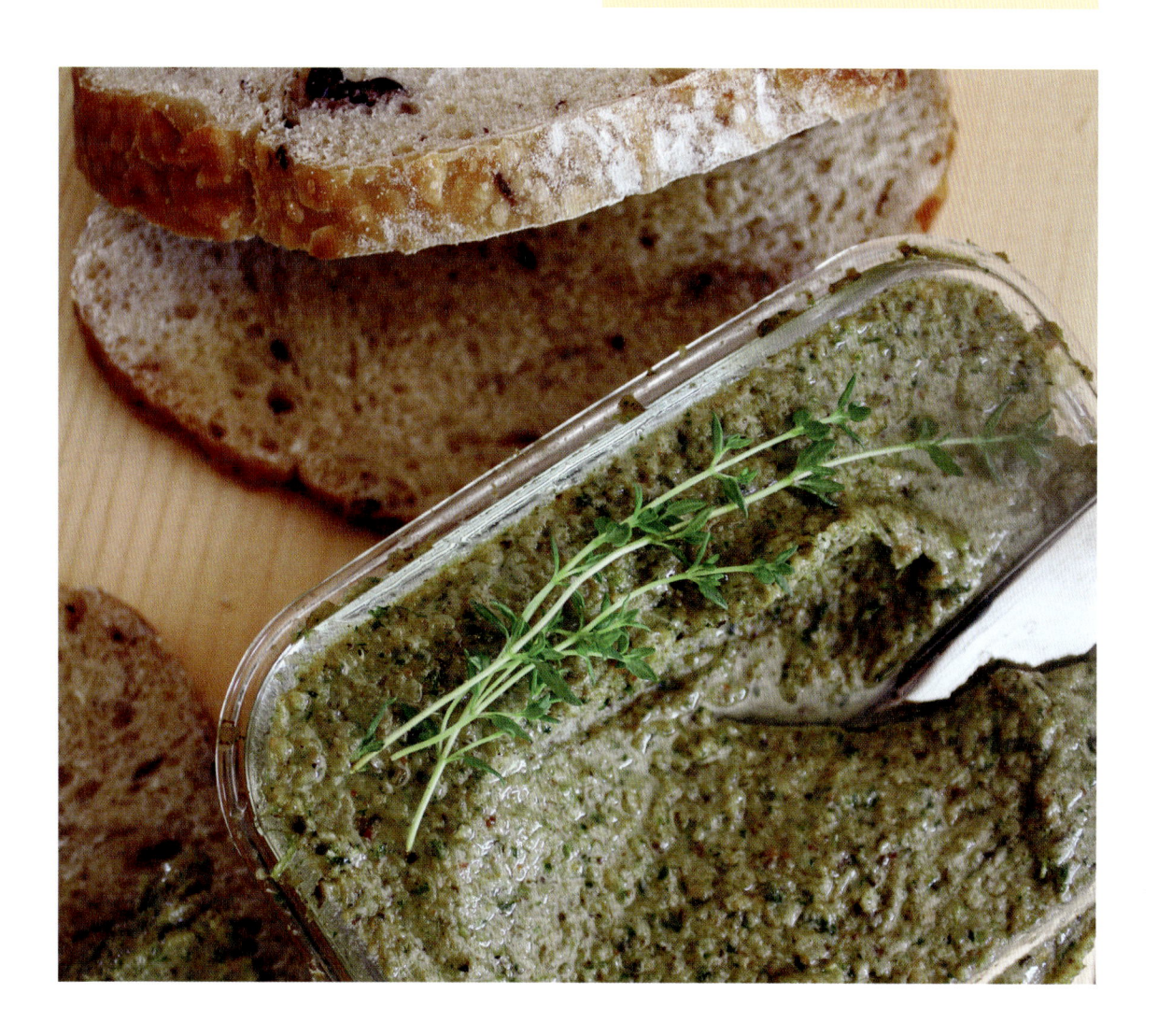

Dips and Breads

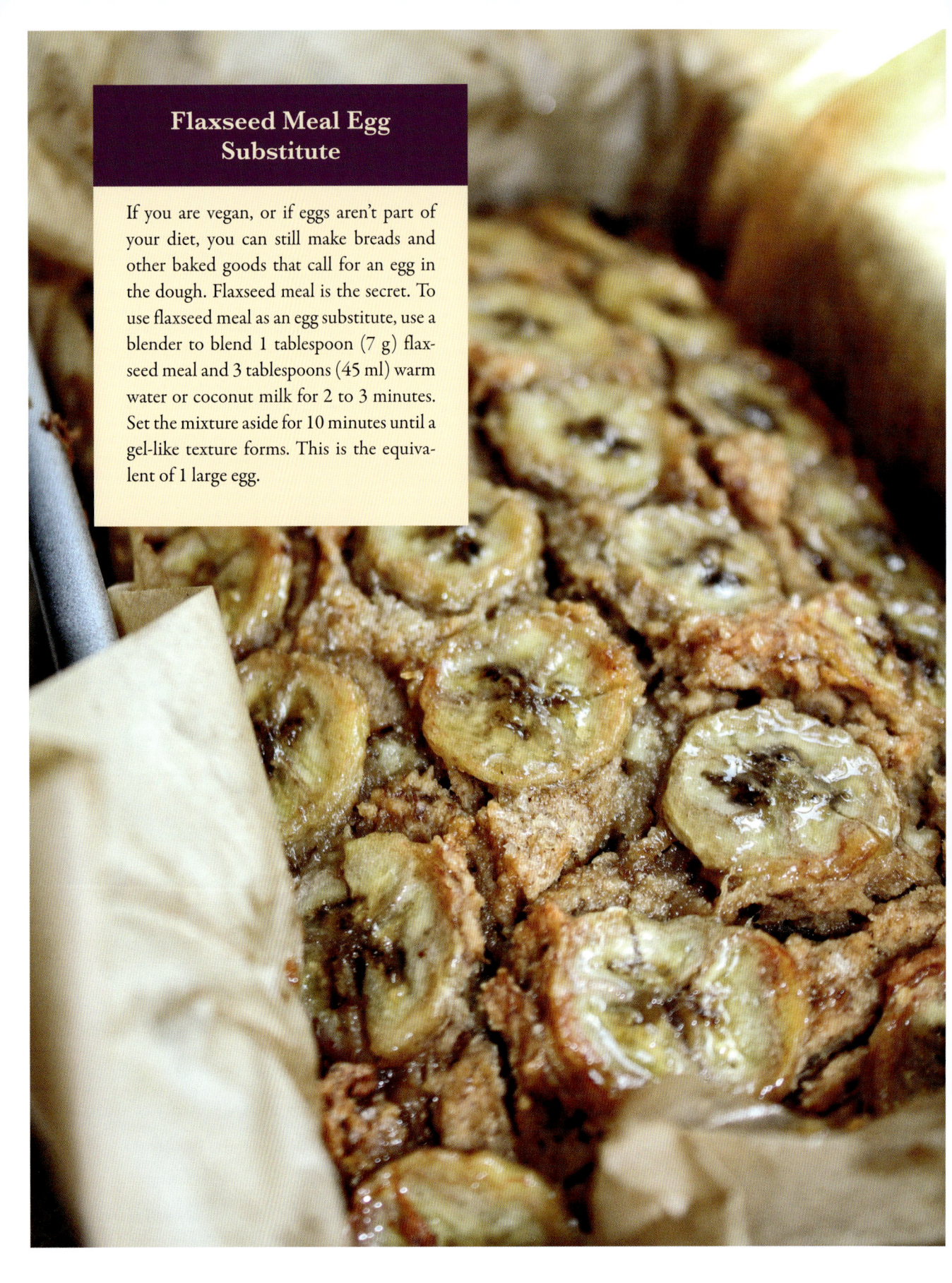

Flaxseed Meal Egg Substitute

If you are vegan, or if eggs aren't part of your diet, you can still make breads and other baked goods that call for an egg in the dough. Flaxseed meal is the secret. To use flaxseed meal as an egg substitute, use a blender to blend 1 tablespoon (7 g) flaxseed meal and 3 tablespoons (45 ml) warm water or coconut milk for 2 to 3 minutes. Set the mixture aside for 10 minutes until a gel-like texture forms. This is the equivalent of 1 large egg.

Feel-Good Banana Bread

MAKES 1 LOAF

My banana bread is a clean, lean, gluten-free, vegan treat made with a blend of hearty, nutty oat and almond flours. Bananas are superstars when it comes to bone health, thanks to their potassium content, which helps maintain calcium levels in bones. They also provide vitamin K and magnesium for bone strength. Plus, their prebiotic fiber aids the nutrient absorption that is essential for overall bone health.

This bread is a smart alternative to a typical sugar-rush snack. One slice of this afternoon delight might make you go bananas! Oh, don't forget to *smell* the bread as you slice the loaf. There is nothing like the aroma of fresh-baked banana bread.

4 large, ripe bananas
Flaxseed meal egg substitute (page 146), or 1 egg
6 tablespoons (90 ml) extra-virgin olive oil
¼ cup (60 ml) melted coconut oil
¼ cup (50 g) coconut sugar
1 teaspoon vanilla extract
1½ cups (144 g) oat flour
1 cup (100 g) almond flour
1½ teaspoons baking powder
1 teaspoon baking soda
⅛ teaspoon ground cinnamon
¼ cup (30 g) chopped walnuts
6 pitted dates, minced
Olive oil or coconut oil, for brushing

TIPS

Black dots on the skin are an indicator that bananas have reached the perfect stage of ripeness for this recipe.

You can substitute sprouted spelt flour for the almond flour, but keep in mind that spelt is not gluten-free.

There are many alternatives to conventional white sugar. This recipe uses coconut sugar. For more options, see the "sweet liquids" list on page 106.

1. Preheat the oven to 350°F (180°C). Line a standard loaf pan with parchment paper.
2. Peel three of the bananas, place them in a medium bowl, and mash thoroughly using a potato masher or a fork.
3. In a larger bowl, prepare the flaxseed egg substitute or beat the egg.
4. Add the mashed bananas to the flaxseed mixture or beaten egg. Add the olive oil, coconut oil, sugar, and vanilla and gently stir until well mixed. Then, stir in the oat flour, almond flour, baking powder, baking soda, and cinnamon. Add the walnuts and dates, giving the batter a final good mix.
5. Pour the batter into the prepared loaf pan. Peel the fourth banana, cut it in round slices, and decorate the top of the loaf. To keep the loaf moist, brush the top with a bit of olive oil or coconut oil. Tap the sides of the pan with your fingers a few times to get rid of air bubbles in the batter.
6. Bake for 55 to 65 minutes, or until the surface of the loaf is golden brown. To check doneness, insert a skewer or toothpick into the center of the loaf; it should come out clean or with just a few crumbs. If the top is browning too quickly but the inside needs more time, cover the pan with a piece of foil to prevent overbrowning.
7. Let the finished bread cool on a rack for about 3 hours, or until it reaches room temperature, before removing from the pan and slicing. Store in a sealed container in the refrigerator for up to 4 days or freeze for up to a few weeks.

Flourless Mung Bean Olive Loaf

MAKES 1 LOAF

Eating bread has been a daily ritual since ancient times, and this must-have staple is fermented with hardships, gratitude, comfort, and survival. In this recipe you are keeping up the tradition and updating it to our modern times for a gluten-free, bloating-free, healthy, yummy, and bone-strong nutritious loaf. The olive and rosemary aroma of this focaccia-inspired bread reminds me of small-town Italian bakeries.

Mung beans are nutrient-dense legumes rich in protein, fiber, vitamins, and minerals. Eating mung beans promotes digestion and may help stabilize blood sugar levels. Mung beans contain antioxidants, and incorporating them into your diet can enhance overall well-being. The more you eat mung beans, the better you feel. The heart-healthy fats from olives, combined with rosemary's antioxidants, also offer a boost to your health.

In order to remove toxins from the skins of the mung beans, they first need to soak as described on page 102.

- 2 cups (910 g) dried mung beans, soaked
- 1 cup (240 ml) warm filtered water
- 5 tablespoons (80 ml) extra-virgin olive oil, plus more for brushing
- ¼ cup (37 g) flaxseed meal or 1 egg
- 1 small garlic clove, minced
- 1 teaspoon baking soda
- 1 teaspoon fresh thyme leaves
- 1 teaspoon salt
- 3 tablespoons chopped pitted olives of your choice
- 3 tablespoons fresh orange juice or lemon juice
- 2 tablespoons chopped fresh rosemary, plus 1 sprig for garnish

1. Preheat the oven to 350°F (180°C) and line a standard loaf pan with parchment paper.
2. Drain the mung beans, rinse under running water, and place them in a large bowl. Add the warm water, olive oil, flaxseed meal, garlic, baking soda, thyme, and salt, and stir well. Transfer to a food processor and process until it forms a thick paste. Add the olives, orange juice, and chopped rosemary, and pulse to incorporate.
3. Place the dough in the prepared pan, brush with olive oil, and put a rosemary sprig on top for decoration.
4. Bake for 30 to 40 minutes. Poke a thin knife into the bread to test for doneness. If the blade comes out clean and the top is golden, it's cooked properly.

> **TIPS**
>
> Explore different flavors by adding chopped, drained sundried tomatoes to this bread. Vegan parmesan cheese or aged parmesan cheese would make this bread pleasantly cheesy.
>
> Experiment with sweet and savory options by adding sprouted pumpkin seeds, walnuts, and soaked raisins, goji berries, or currants.

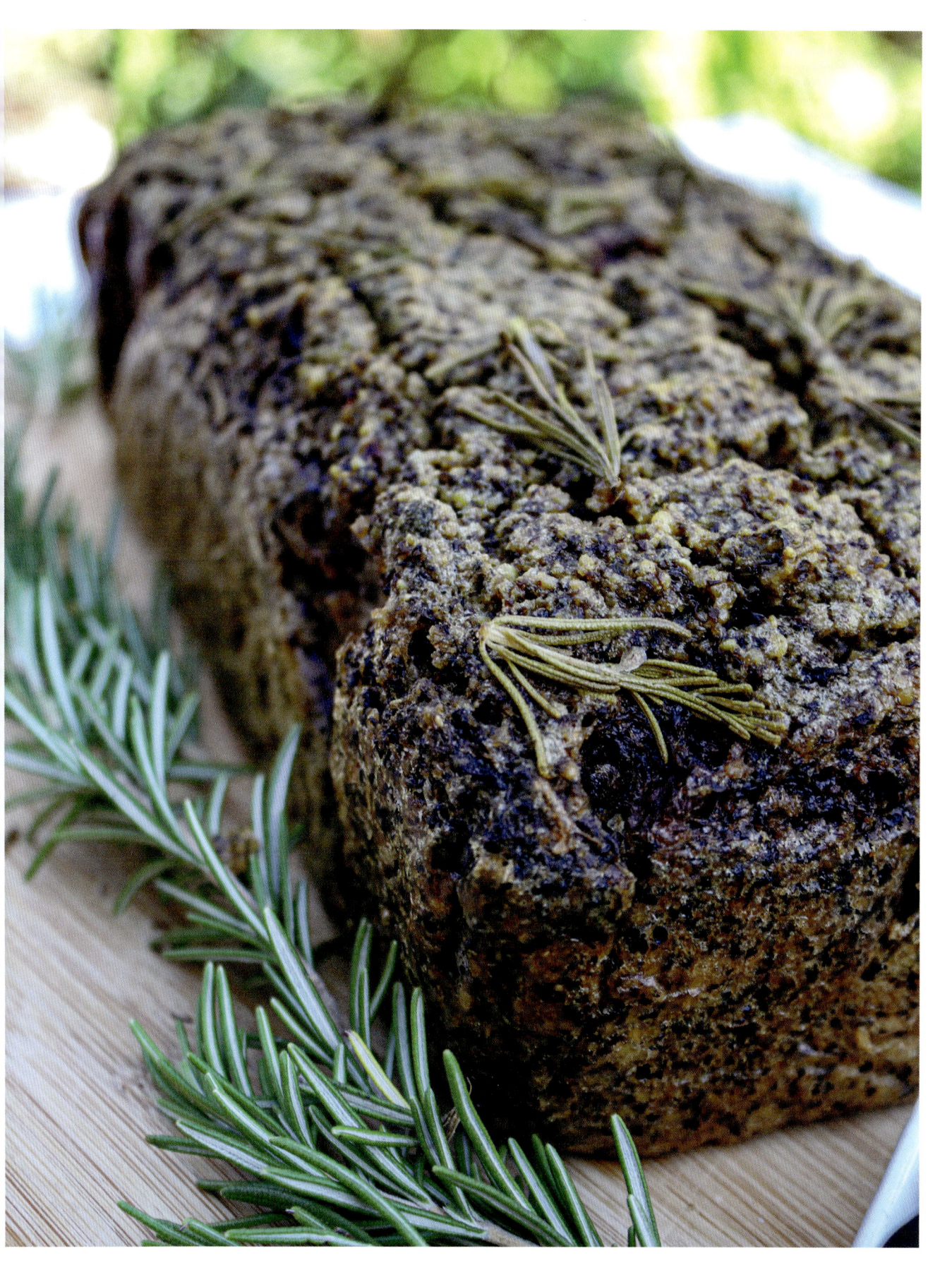

Red Lentil–Saffron Tortillas

MAKES SIX 6-INCH (15 CM) TORTILLAS

This recipe combines a delicious Mexican tortilla with Indian flavors of saffron and turmeric. The nutty, tender red lentil tortillas are nutritious and high in protein to promote bone and heart health, aid digestion, and stabilize blood sugar. And with only seven ingredients, they are ridiculously easy to make.

The pliable nature of these tortillas makes them perfect for roll-ups, tacos, dipping, or serving on the side of your favorite Indian curry. They work equally well for savory or sweet fancy sides.

Using a powerful high-speed blender or food processor for this recipe will ensure success in creating a silky-textured, smooth batter. Use a tortilla pan or tortilla maker for a round tortilla shape.

1 cup (250 g) red lentils
1½ cups (480 ml) warm hemp milk or warm filtered water
4 to 6 saffron threads
2 tablespoons flaxseed meal
½ teaspoon ground turmeric
¼ teaspoon apple cider vinegar (optional)
¼ teaspoon sea salt

1. Soak the lentils in water for at least 30 minutes or up to 2 hours. Drain and set aside.
2. Pour the hemp milk into a medium bowl. Add the saffron and allow it to melt into the liquid for 30 minutes; the liquid will turn golden yellow.
3. In a high-speed blender or food processor, combine the soaked lentils and saffron-infused hemp milk, along with the flaxseed meal, turmeric, apple cider vinegar (if using), and salt. Blend well for 3 to 5 minutes, until the texture resembles pancake batter.
4. Heat a dry nonstick pan over medium heat and scoop some lentil batter into the pan using a large spoon or a measuring cup. Use the back of the spoon or underside of the cup to spread the batter evenly, moving the spoon or cup with a circular motion.
5. Cook the tortilla for 4 to 5 minutes, until it has set and can be easily flipped. Flip and cook the second side for 4 to 5 minutes. Then move the tortilla to a plate and cover with a cloth to keep warm. Repeat until you are out of batter. Serve immediately.

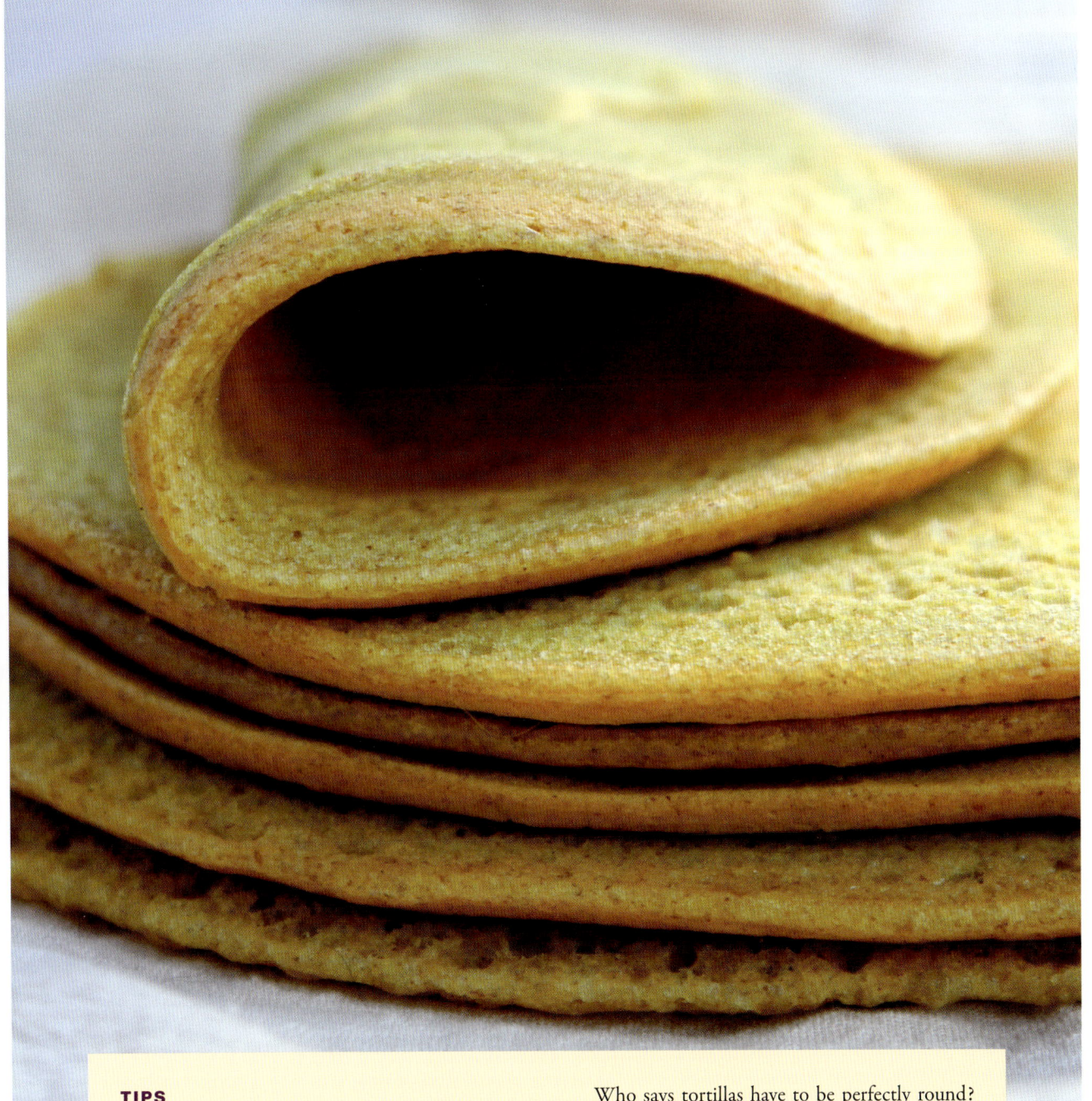

TIPS

If you don't have a high-speed blender or food processor, combine the batter ingredients in a large bowl and blend them with an immersion blender.

If you wish, you can add a little bit of ghee to the pan before pouring in the tortilla batter. This will give the tortillas a rich flavor, but oil is not essential for this recipe.

Who says tortillas have to be perfectly round? An irregular shape would give your dish a more rustic touch. Have fun, and invite your children to make the tortillas with you!

For a change of flavor, try substituting green lentils. You could also use black beans or quinoa (keep in mind that these would require presoaking for 2 days as described on page 102).

Savory Mung Bean Flatbread

MAKES 2 FLATBREADS

When I first tried avocado toast, spread with creamy avocado and sprinkled with sprouts and red onion pickles, I couldn't believe how delicious it was. But because I am gluten sensitive, I've always wanted to remake this tasty new-age dish that emerged from the California conscious-health movement *without* any gluten. So, I decided to create a gluten-free, high-protein mung bean flatbread using simple ingredients.

This classic nutty, earthy mung bean dough allows you to get creative with shapes, textures, and thicknesses. You could also use it to make pizza, savory pancakes, and crunchy chips. Let's make it and have fun!

Be sure to plan in advance, because the mung beans need to be presoaked for 2 days.

1 cup (202 g) dried mung beans, soaked (see page 102)
¼ cup (15 g) chopped fresh basil (20 to 25 leaves)
3 tablespoons brown rice flour
3 tablespoons extra-virgin olive oil, plus more for brushing
1 tablespoon flaxseed meal
1 tablespoon kelp powder
⅛ teaspoon ground cinnamon
⅛ teaspoon ground cumin
⅛ teaspoon fennel seed

1. Preheat the oven to 400°F (200°C).
2. Drain the mung beans and place them in a large bowl. Add the basil, brown rice flour, olive oil, flaxseed meal, kelp powder, cinnamon, cumin, and fennel seed and mix to combine.
3. Transfer the mixture to a food processor and blend by pulsing on and off. When the ingredients are well-blended and develop a thick consistency similar to hummus (this should take 5 to 7 minutes) stop the processor. If the dough seems watery, add more rice flour to reach the consistency of a thick dough.
4. Line two baking sheets with parchment paper and brush olive oil over the paper. Divide the dough into two equal portions. Spread each portion evenly on the parchment, as thinly as possibly. Place another piece of parchment on top of each sheet of dough, and use a rolling pin to even out the dough to a consistent thickness. Remove the top pieces of parchment from the dough.
5. Put the pans into the oven and bake for 5 to 10 minutes, until the top surface becomes golden, yet still moist.
6. Remove from the oven and let cool for 30 minutes. Cut your flatbread any size you like, and stack flatbread pieces in plastic bags. Stored in the freezer, they will keep well for months.

TIPS

Soak three to five times more mung beans than needed for this recipe, and store the extra soaked mung beans in zip-top plastic bags in the freezer. This is a giant time saver. Thaw by soaking a bag in water for 30 minutes.

Instead of oven baking, you can cook this flatbread in a medium sauté pan over medium-high heat. Use a fresh rosemary sprig to brush oil in the pan and then spread the dough in the pan as thinly as possible. Cook it until golden brown, 2 to 3 minutes each side.

To thaw frozen flatbread, warm it in the oven for 20 minutes at 300°F (150°C).

Try flatbreads with guacamole or Mushroom Cashew Pâté (page 144). Sprinkle on some sprouts, pickled red onion, and chopped olives, and drizzle with extra-virgin olive oil.

You can use this dough to make crunchy, yummy, nutty mung bean chips too. Spread the dough very thinly on dry baking sheets and broil it at 450°F (230°C) for 5 to 10 minutes. Monitor it closely while it's under the broiler and remove it when it starts to look crunchy. When it is cool enough to handle, break into chips.

Sprouted Seeds Bread

MAKES 1 LOAF

Digestion, nutrition, deliciousness! According to Traditional Chinese Medicine principles, digestion is ruled by earth elements, and digestion is the source of energy. In this recipe, the sprouted seeds are high in protein and healthy fats. Psyllium is great medicine for a leaky gut. The brown rice and almond milk provide balanced protein for bone health.

Get ready for a slice of yumminess that fuels your body and activates your taste buds. Enjoy with almond butter, honey, or pesto sauce, or use this great bread to make avocado toast for your lunch, with radish or broccoli sprouts sprinkled on top.

½ cup (100 g) amaranth seeds
½ cup (95 g) brown rice
½ cup (40 g) rolled oats
½ cup (65 g) pumpkin seeds
½ cup (95 g) quinoa
½ cup (70 g) sesame seeds, plus 3 tablespoons to top the loaf
¼ cup (30 g) flaxseed meal
1 tablespoon hemp seeds
1¼ cups (300 ml) almond milk (see page 111)
⅔ cup (160 ml) warm filtered water
2 tablespoons coconut oil
1 tablespoon psyllium powder
1 tablespoon baking powder
1 teaspoon baking soda

1. Place the amaranth seeds, brown rice, rolled oats, pumpkin seeds, quinoa, ½ cup (70 g) sesame seeds, flaxseed meal, and hemp seeds in a large bowl. Rinse well under running water, drain, and then add three times more water to let it hydrate. The whole seeds will begin to sprout. Soak in the refrigerator for at least 10 hours.
2. Preheat the oven to 350°F (180°C). Line a standard loaf pan with parchment paper.
3. Remove the sprouted mixture from the refrigerator. Transfer it to a colander to drain. Let sit (not refrigerated) for 30 minutes, until the water is completely drained.
4. Add the mixture back to the bowl, then incorporate the almond milk, warm water, coconut oil, psyllium powder, baking powder, and baking soda. Mix well. Pour the mixture into the prepared loaf pan. Sprinkle the remaining 3 tablespoons sesame seeds over the top of the loaf.
5. Bake for 1 hour. If the top begins to brown too much, cover the pan with foil. After about 40 minutes, begin checking whether the loaf is fully baked by inserting a knife into the bread. When the blade comes out clean, remove the loaf from the oven. Let it cool for 20 to 30 minutes before serving.

TIPS

This bread tastes best after it has completely cooled down. After cutting one or two slices, store the remaining bread by wrapping it in a damp cloth and keeping it in the refrigerator for a week or two.

In place of the seed mixture in this recipe, you can combine 1½ cups sprouted quinoa and 1½ cups sprouted amaranth, yielding a nutty and delicious fully protein-based bread.

CHAPTER 13

Small Meals

I love to start a meal with an intriguing appetizer that ignites my senses and satisfies my cravings, creating an intimate experience that brings a smile to my face. Appetizers and other small meals are the gateway to an extraordinary dining adventure, with their enticing aromas, unique composition, delightful colors and textures, and bold flavors that leave us yearning for more. In this chapter, I dive into a dish as sensory awareness, exploring small meals that are both simple to prepare and bursting with flavor. These recipes are versatile, perfect as stand-alone delights or as flavorful additions to your main courses.

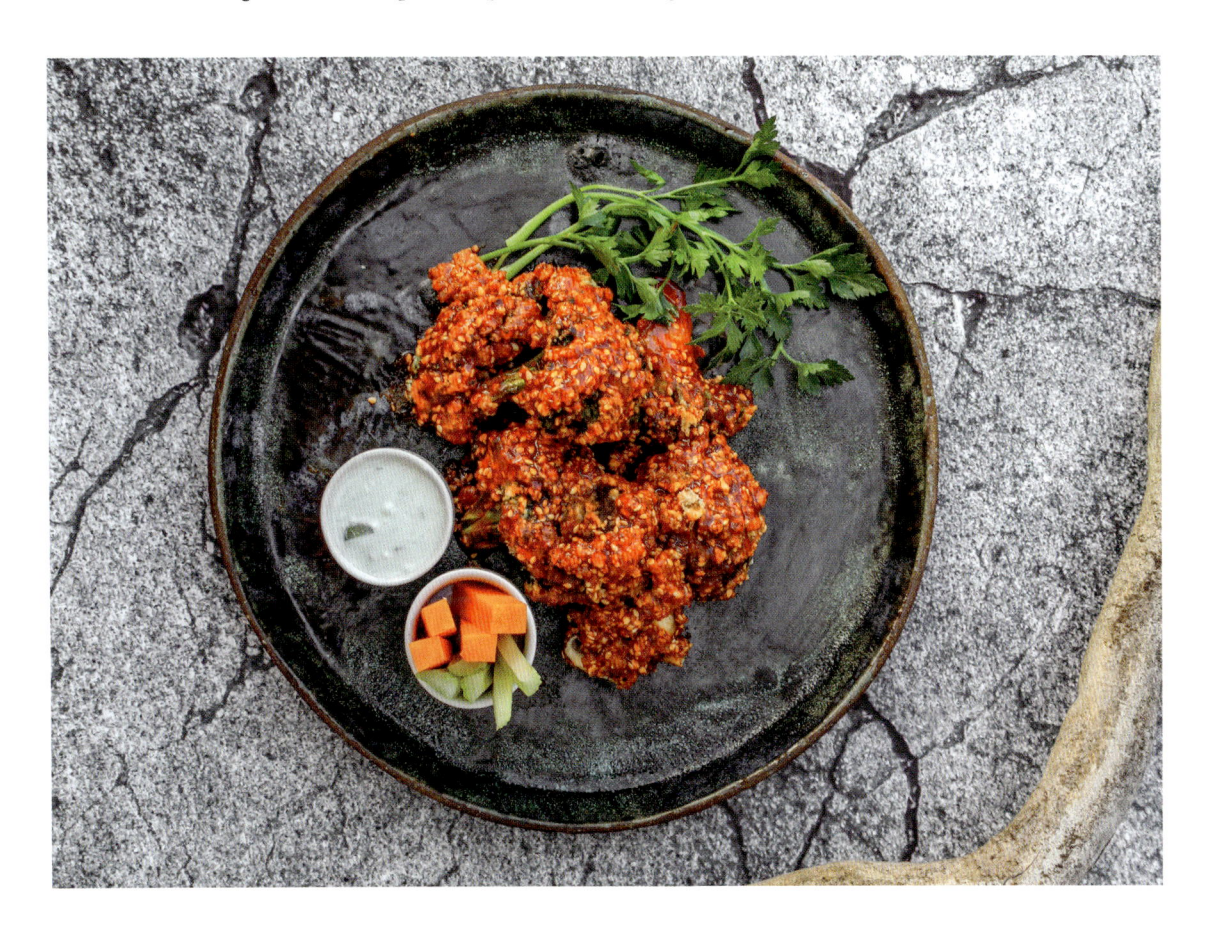

Broccoli and Mushroom Buffalo "Wings"

MAKES 2 SERVINGS

Wings are an American staple, and this recipe takes the legacy of those spicy, crunchy, savory flavors to the next level in a fantastic broccoli and mushroom version. I couldn't resist the temptation to merge American and Korean flavors, dressing the wings in irresistible Korean spicy sauce and pairing them with classic blue cheese.

Broccoli has gotten a bad reputation because it's often served overcooked and soggy, with the message "It's good for you—eat it." Unfortunately, this stereotype has led to the misconception that healthy food is unappetizing, lacking in taste, and entirely unappealing.

Let's give broccoli a whole new perspective. This dish will have you saying, "Wow, I love broccoli now!"

1 celery rib
2 small carrots
½ large broccoli head
6 medium button mushrooms

FOR THE WET BATTER

6 tablespoons (60 g) brown rice flour or any gluten-free flour
1½ teaspoons baking powder
1 teaspoon garlic powder
Sea salt
Cracked black pepper
¼ cup (60 ml) filtered water, plus more as needed

FOR THE DRY COATING

½ cup (100 g) brown rice flour or gluten-free flour
½ cup (60 g) raw cashews or unsalted peanuts, finely ground
1 tablespoon flaxseed meal
⅛ teaspoon paprika

FOR THE BUFFALO SAUCE

2 tablespoons Korean sweet chili paste (gochujang) or any hot sauce
2 tablespoons extra-virgin olive oil
1 tablespoon black sesame seeds
1 tablespoon maple syrup
1 tablespoon rice vinegar
1 tablespoon sesame oil

FOR THE BLUE CHEESE DRESSING

¼ cup (35 g) crumbled blue cheese
1 tablespoon coconut yogurt
1 tablespoon vegan mayonnaise
1 teaspoon cornichons, finely chopped
1 medium garlic clove, minced
½ teaspoon fresh lemon juice
Sea salt
Cracked black pepper

TO SERVE

Fresh lemon juice
¼ cup (32 g) crushed raw cashews
1 tablespoon black sesame seeds
1 tablespoon hemp seeds
Fresh parsley sprigs

1. Preheat the oven to 400°F (200°C).
2. Cut the celery and carrots into thin, 3-inch (8 cm) sticks. Place them in a container with water and refrigerate them for at least 30 minutes (this helps keep them crunchy). Cut the broccoli into bite-sized "wings," retaining some stem. Clean the mushrooms with a wet cloth or kitchen towel.
3. Make the wet batter: In a large bowl, combine the brown rice flour, baking powder, garlic powder, and a pinch of salt and pepper. Add the water and mix thoroughly. If the batter is too thick, add a little more water. Set the batter aside.
4. Make the dry coating: Mix the brown rice flour, ground cashews, flaxseed meal, and paprika together on a large plate.
5. Arrange the batter bowl and the coating plate side by side. Place a wire rack over a baking sheet and position the pan next to the coating plate. Hold each broccoli floret by the stem, dip it into the batter, coat it with the dry coating, and place it on the wire rack. Repeat this process with the mushrooms, holding them by the stem or edge.
6. Transfer the pan and wire rack of broccoli and mushrooms to the oven to roast for 15 minutes. Use tongs to flip the vegetables, and roast for an additional 15 minutes. Set aside and allow them to cool for at least 15 minutes.
7. Make the buffalo sauce: In a medium bowl, combine the gochujang, olive oil, sesame seeds, maple syrup, rice vinegar, and sesame oil and whisk well. Add the mixture to a mini blender and blend for 1 to 2 minutes until well blended. Transfer the sauce back to the bowl. Dip the broccoli and mushrooms into the sauce and coat them evenly. Set aside.
8. Make the blue cheese dressing: Combine the blue cheese, yogurt, mayonnaise, cornichons, and garlic, whisking them thoroughly. Stir in the lemon juice and season to taste with salt and pepper.
9. Remove the carrot and celery from the refrigerator, drain them, and place them in a small bowl. Sprinkle them with lemon juice. On a serving plate, arrange the wings in a mountainlike pile. Garnish with the nuts, seeds, and parsley.

TIPS

Try this recipe with cauliflower instead of broccoli. It's an equally exciting, low-carbohydrate superfood.

If you love Asian flavors, try dipping the wings in Tahini-Apple-Ginger Dressing (page 122).

Small Meals • 157

TIPS

Roasting beets (at 375°F [190°C] for 1 hour) is another popular way to cook them. Roasting tends to bring out more flavor, while boiling beets results in a softer, more tender consistency.

This recipe dresses up a plain lemon and olive oil vinaigrette with acai powder. You can use other superfood powders, such as pomegranate or beetroot powder, instead, to create colorful, visually appealing dressings. The bold, vibrant colors can stimulate your appetite and add a sense of excitement to a meal.

Beets, spinach, and collard greens are high in oxalates, which can impair nutrient absorption in the digestive tract (see page 43). One way to solve this problem is by pairing beets with lemon juice.

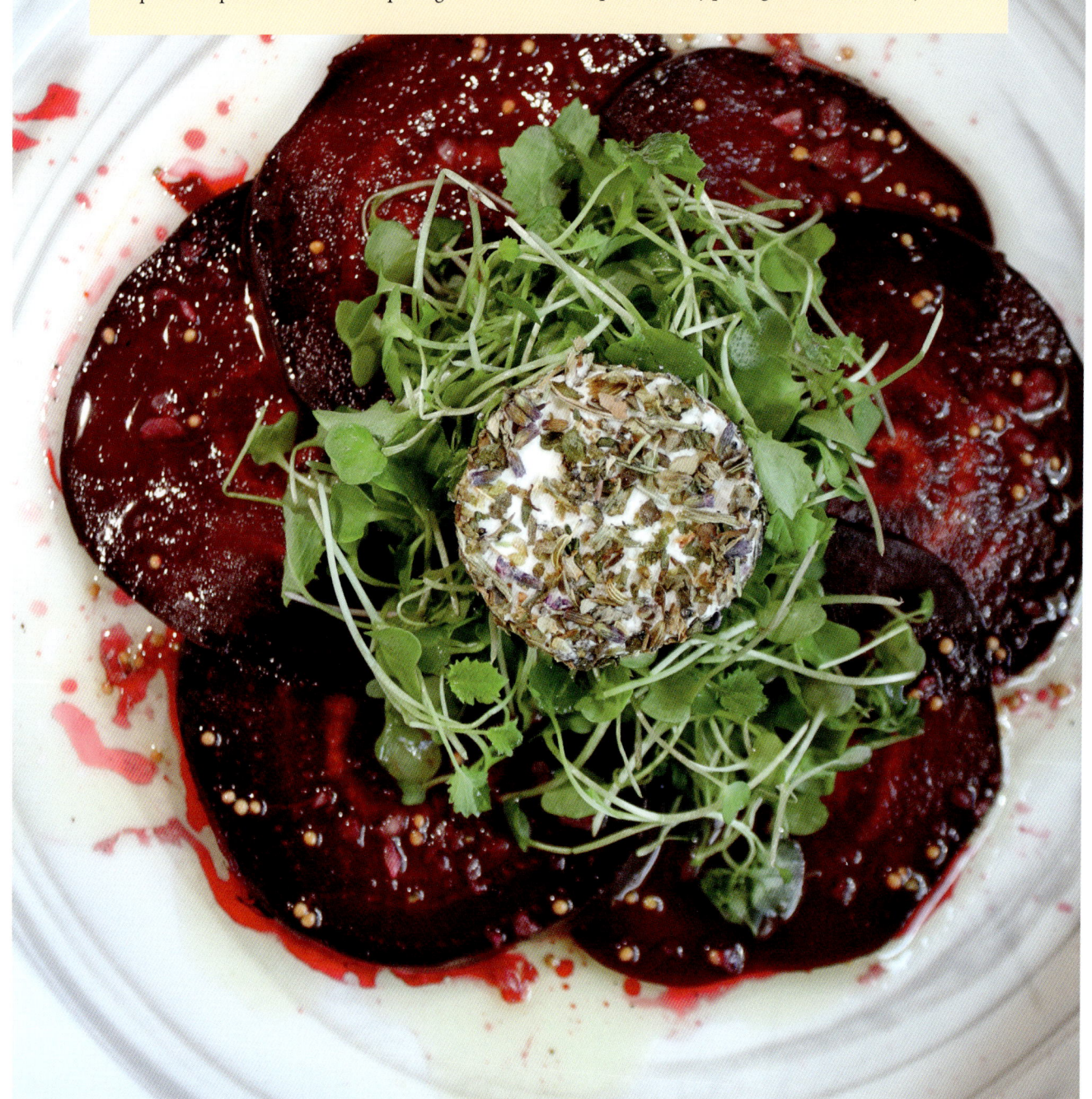

Beets with Herbed Goat Cheese

MAKES 2 SERVINGS

The vibrant red-purple hue and tender texture of boiled beets is a perfect pairing with creamy goat cheese. Beets are high in nitrates, which can help lower blood pressure and potentially reduce the risk of heart disease and stroke. They are also an excellent source of folate, manganese, and copper—bone-health essentials. The more beets you consume, the healthier your heart can become. By preparing this dish, you may find an added touch of love in your heart.

2 large beets, 4- to 5-inch (10 to 13 cm) diameter
6 cups (1.4 L) filtered water
4 ounces (110 g) goat cheese
1 teaspoon herbes de Provence
⅛ teaspoon lava salt
¼ cup (10 g) microgreens
¼ cup (10 g) baby kale

FOR THE ACAI-LEMON VINAIGRETTE

3 tablespoons extra-virgin olive oil
1 tablespoon acai powder
½ garlic clove, minced
½ teaspoon fresh lemon juice
⅛ teaspoon mustard seed
Sea salt
Cracked black pepper

1. Place the beets in a medium-sized pot and cover with water. Bring the water to a boil, then reduce the heat and let the beets simmer for about 10 minutes. Lower the heat to medium-low and continue cooking the beets for 40 to 50 minutes. Check for doneness by poking one of the beets with a knife. If it pierces easily through to the middle, the beets are ready. Remove the beets from the pot and set them aside to cool.
2. Cut the goat cheese into neat 3-inch (8 cm) medallions. On a small, flat plate, combine the herbes de Provence and lava salt. Roll the goat cheese medallions in this mixture until thoroughly coated, then set aside.
3. Make the vinaigrette: In a mini blender, combine the olive oil, acai powder, garlic, lemon juice, mustard seed, and a pinch of salt and pepper, and mix thoroughly for 1 to 2 minutes. Set aside.
4. After the beets have cooled, remove the skin. Slice the first beet horizontally into thin rounds, and arrange the rounds on a serving plate. Place the other beet in a container and refrigerate it for another use. Top the beet slices with a layer of microgreens and baby kale and place the herbed goat cheese on top in the center. Drizzle the vinaigrette over the top and serve.

California Rainbow Spring Rolls

MAKES 2 ROLLS

California rolls are a refreshing option for a quick and easy small meal, and crafting a roll is fun and artistic. This playful recipe uses lots of vegetables instead of the usual sea greens, and you can experiment with other fillings. I like to include avocado because of its nourishing fats and heart- and bone-health benefits.

1 Persian cucumber, trimmed
½ medium bell pepper, stemmed and seeded
½ avocado, pitted and peeled
2 sticks (4 inches [10 cm] long) feta cheese or vegan feta cheese
3 or 4 cilantro sprigs
1 small carrot, shredded
¼ cup (10 g) alfalfa sprouts
1 teaspoon fresh lemon juice
Sea salt
2 rice paper wrappers, 8½ inches (22 cm) diameter
Sesame oil

FOR THE DIPPING SAUCE
½ cup (130 g) almond butter
¼ cup (60 ml) filtered water
¼ cup (30 g) shredded apple
1 tablespoon maple syrup
2 teaspoons rice vinegar
½ garlic clove
⅛ teaspoon ground ginger
Crushed almonds
Sliced scallion

1. Cut the cucumber, bell pepper, and avocado into slices about 4 inches long and ½ inch wide (10 × 1 cm). Cut two slices of feta of similar size. Chop the cilantro. Arrange these ingredients on a large plate with the shredded carrot and alfalfa sprouts. Sprinkle the fillings with the lemon juice and a pinch of salt to season lightly.

2. Pour some warm water onto a large plate. Submerge the rice paper in the water to moisten it on both sides. As soon as the paper is softened, transfer it to a plate or cutting board. Place two or three slices of avocado in the center, about two-thirds of the way down the rice paper. Layer half of the alfalfa sprouts, shredded carrots, cucumber, bell pepper, feta cheese sticks, and cilantro on top. Wrap the ingredients quickly, firmly pressing down as you roll up the rice paper halfway. Then fold in the edges and continue rolling, applying light pressure to create a well-formed cylinder. To maintain the moisture of the roll, coat the surface of the roll with a small amount of sesame oil.

3. Repeat the process with the second piece of rice paper and other half of the fillings. Cut each roll in half to create four pieces. Arrange the rolls on a serving plate.

4. Make the dipping sauce: In a mini blender, combine the almond butter, water, apple, maple syrup, vinegar, garlic, and ginger and blend thoroughly. Transfer the sauce to a serving bowl and sprinkle crushed almonds and scallions over the sauce.

5. Serve the rolls with the dipping sauce. Any leftover sauce can be refrigerated for a few days.

TIPS

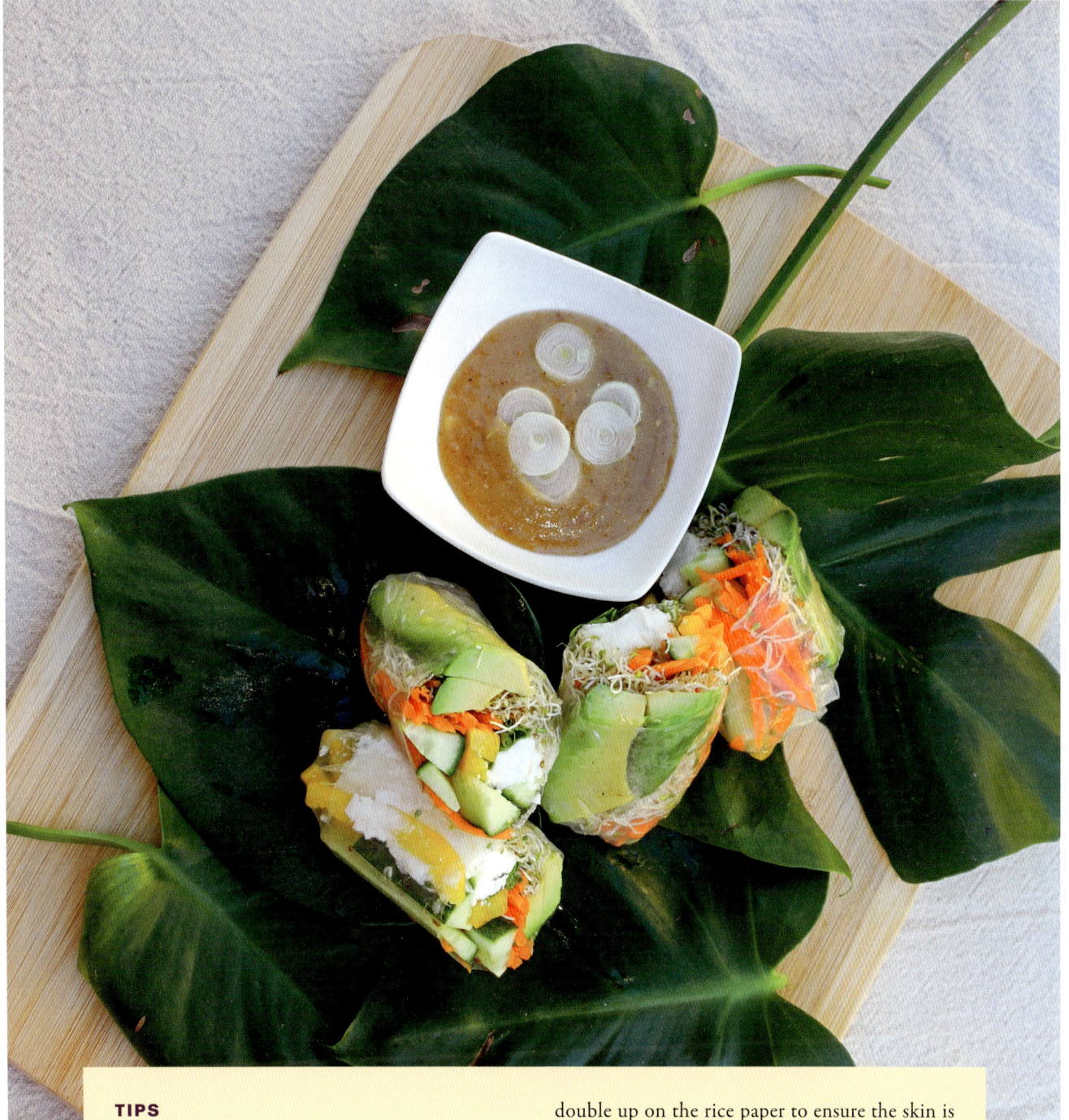

Keep the feta in the refrigerator so it stays firm until you are ready to slice it.

When moistening the rice paper, act swiftly to make the rolls. As soon as the paper is softened, promptly stuff it with vegetables and roll it up. If you're new to working with rice paper, you can double up on the rice paper to ensure the skin is strong enough to securely hold the shape of the rolls.

Add BBQ Tempeh (page 230) to make this as a main dish. This option is a quick and easy solution when you're feeling extremely hungry and not in the mood for an extensive cooking session.

Golden Triangle Indian Mash

MAKES 2 SERVINGS

This humble side dish made of mashed potato and cauliflower mixed with Indian spices became a favorite of mine during my travels in India's Golden Triangle. Think of it as a more flavorful version of boring old mashed potatoes.

This recipe is easy to make, with nutritious cauliflower and chickpea protein, as well as India's most popular medicinal root, turmeric. Turmeric is used every day by many in India, traditionally for supporting the skin, upper respiratory tract, joints, digestive system, and more. This spice not only gives the dish a beautiful yellow color, it assists your body in staying strong and healthy.

3½ ounces (100 g) cauliflower, roughly chopped
2 medium Yukon Gold potatoes
1 small onion
½ celery rib
1 tablespoon coconut oil
1 garlic clove, minced
¼ teaspoon ground turmeric
⅛ teaspoon ground cumin
⅛ teaspoon paprika
½ cup (120 g) canned chickpeas, drained and rinsed
1 bay leaf
Saffron
¾ cup (180 ml) filtered water
2 tablespoons coconut milk
Salt
Cracked black pepper
Chopped fresh parsley

1. Cut the cauliflower, potatoes, and onion into 1-inch (2.5 cm) cubes. Cut the celery into ½-inch (1 cm) pieces.
2. In a medium-sized sauté pan over medium heat, add the coconut oil, garlic, turmeric, cumin, and paprika and cook for 1 to 2 minutes, until fragrant. Add the cauliflower, potato, onion, celery, chickpeas, bay leaf, a pinch of saffron, and the water. Cook for 5 to 10 minutes over medium-high heat until all the ingredients are tender enough to mash. Mash them gently with a masher. Add the coconut milk just before serving, stirring it into the mash. Season with salt and pepper and garnish with parsley.

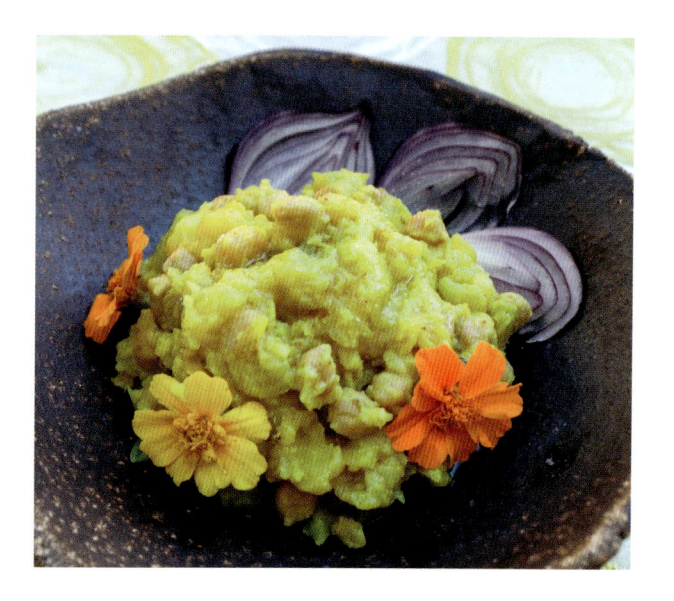

TIP
Try adding your favorite cooked vegetables to this dish. I love combinations with fresh asparagus and broccoli. Or okra and carrots!

Steamed Eggplant with Apple-Tahini Sauce

MAKES 2 SERVINGS

Eggplant is one of the stars of low-calorie, nutrient-packed recipes. This shiny purple veggie is loaded with fiber, vitamins, and minerals. Eggplant can help boost heart health, lower high cholesterol, and even keep blood sugar in check.

This recipe calls for steaming the eggplant rather than sautéing. This cooking trick makes eggplant an even healthier food because it reduces the need for oil, which eggplant flesh readily absorbs when sautéed.

So go ahead, load up on eggplant. Each bite, with its silky, tender texture, might just put a smile on your face.

1 7-inch (18 cm) eggplant

FOR THE CREAMY APPLE-TAHINI SAUCE

¼ cup (60 ml) tahini
1 small apple, cored and roughly chopped
2 tablespoons filtered water
1 tablespoon apple cider vinegar
1 garlic clove, minced
⅛ teaspoon ground ginger
Salt
Cracked black pepper

FOR GARNISH

1 scallion, diced

1. Add 1½ cups (350 ml) water to a large steamer pot and bring it to a boil over high heat.
2. Cut the eggplant in half vertically, then cut each piece in half lengthwise, to end up with four long wedges. Transfer the eggplant wedges into bamboo steamer baskets, ensuring they are evenly spaced. Place the steamer baskets on the steamer pot above the boiling water and steam the eggplant for 20 to 30 minutes. The eggplant should reduce in size by about half and become translucent.
3. Make the tahini sauce: Place the tahini, apple, water, vinegar, garlic, ginger, and a pinch of salt and pepper into a blender. Blend all the ingredients together until they form a smooth sauce.
4. On a serving plate, use a spoon to pour and spread the creamy tahini sauce, creating a large circle. Arrange the steamed eggplant on top of the sauce, forming an appealing spiral shape. Garnish with the scallions for added freshness and flavor.

> **TIP**
>
> Adding a tangy Granny Smith or a sweet yet tart Pink Lady apple (including the skin) to any sauce or dressing can bring a delightful brightness to the flavor, providing a complete taste profile without relying on lemon juice or citrus flavors. It's like having a secret ingredient that brings magic to your cooking! In addition, the skin and flesh of tangy apples contain compounds that may help prevent cancer.

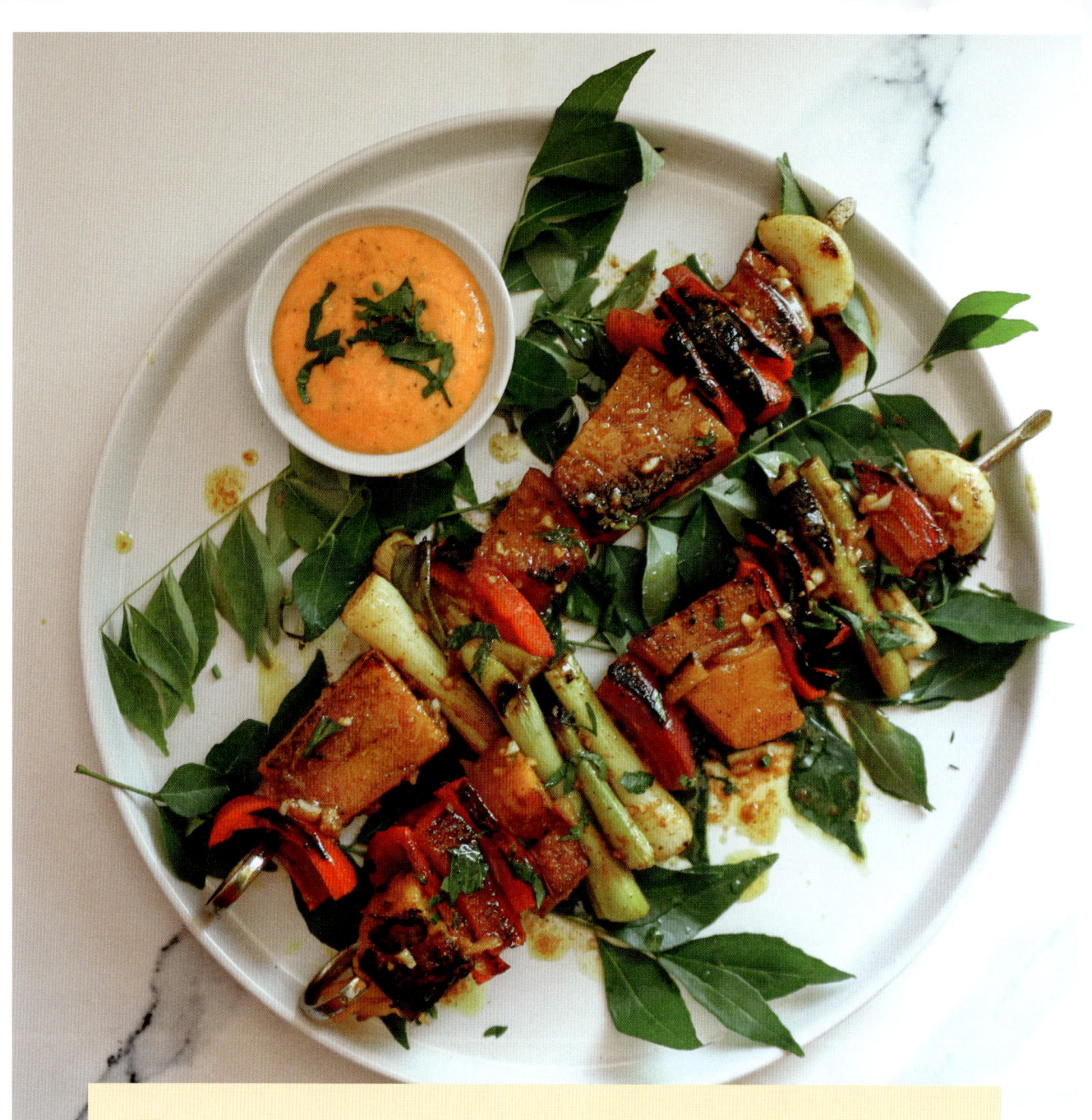

TIPS

Don't discard the pumpkin seeds; they're a good source of protein, healthy fats, and magnesium. Roast them at 425°F (220°C) for 10 minutes for a crunchy snack or as a garnish for the kebabs.

If you're using wooden skewers, soak them in water for 2 hours before preparing the kebabs to prevent the skewers from burning.

If you want to make this dish a main course, you can skewer cubes of barbecue tofu and grill them along with the vegetables. Experiment with mushrooms and other hearty vegetables like potatoes, sweet potatoes, or zucchini.

For a special presentation, place the kebabs on a bed of arugula, lettuce, or your favorite greens.

Curry Lemon-Pumpkin Kebabs

MAKES 2 SERVINGS

In a lively Turkish market, I met a street vendor named Hasan, a master of crafting mouthwatering kebabs. His secret? A time-honored recipe and an unshakable sense of humor. People flocked to his stall, not just for the scrumptious food but also for his contagious laughter.

While kebabs often emphasize meat, this delightful vegan recipe features pumpkin, scallion, and red bell pepper. What sets this dish apart is not only its striking visual appeal but also the delectable sauce that complements the hearty vegetables.

Marinating the vegetables with refreshing lemon juice and curry powder results in a grill-worthy dish bursting with fall-inspired flavors. It's an uncomplicated recipe that your family will undoubtedly savor and devour.

1 small pumpkin, about 6-inch (15 cm) diameter
½ red bell pepper
3 scallions

FOR THE KEBAB SAUCE

¼ cup (60 ml) extra-virgin olive oil
1 tablespoon fresh lemon juice
½ garlic clove, minced
1 teaspoon curry powder
½ teaspoon sea salt
¼ teaspoon paprika

FOR THE PAPAYA–HEMP SEED RANCH DRESSING

½ cup finely chopped papaya
3 tablespoons hemp seed oil
2 tablespoons hemp seeds
2 tablespoons white wine vinegar
¼ teaspoon Dijon mustard
Sea salt
Cracked black pepper

FOR GARNISH

1 teaspoon minced fresh sage or parsley
½ teaspoon grated lemon zest

1. Preheat a grill for direct, high-heat cooking.
2. Slice off the top and bottom of the pumpkin, cut it in half, scoop out the seeds, and peel if desired. Slice the flesh into strips and cut the strips into 2-inch (5 cm) cubes. Cut the bell pepper to match the size of the pumpkin cubes. Remove the green tops from the scallions and cut each of the white stems into three pieces. Set the vegetables aside.
3. Make the kebab sauce: In a large bowl, combine the olive oil, lemon juice, garlic, curry powder, salt, and paprika, stirring them well. Set aside.
4. Make the ranch dressing: In a mini blender, combine the papaya, hemp seed oil, hemp seeds, vinegar, Dijon mustard, and a pinch of salt and black pepper. Blend for about 2 minutes. Set aside.
5. Skewer the pumpkin, pepper, and onion chunks on two metal or wooden skewers and brush them evenly a few times with the kebab sauce. Let them sit for about 10 minutes.
6. Grill the kebabs over high heat for 4 to 5 minutes, turning and basting with the sauce until they are cooked through. Brush on more sauce during the last minute of grilling.
7. Place the kebabs on a serving plate and drizzle them with the ranch dressing or serve the dressing on the side. Garnish with the minced sage and lemon zest.

Small Meals

Sweet and Savory Grilled Peaches and Zucchini

MAKES 2 SERVINGS

Experience the delightful union of sweet and savory by grilling fresh, local, and seasonal peaches. Peaches? Oh, yes, peaches.

Tangy, sweet peaches perfectly complement the smoky flavor of grilled zucchini. Not only do peaches provide a delicious addition to the dish, but they also offer health benefits. They aid in preventing constipation, support gut health, and contain prebiotics that nourish the beneficial bacteria in the gut. Despite their sweet flavor, peaches have a lower impact on blood sugar levels than some other fruits, making this dish a perfect way to satisfy your sweet tooth.

---

2 medium-sized, firm yellow peaches

1 small yellow or green zucchini

Toppings: sprouts (any type), crumbled goat cheese or vegan feta cheese, extra-virgin olive oil, lemon juice, aged balsamic glaze, fresh oregano, edible flowers

Himalayan salt

Cracked black pepper

---

1. Preheat a grill for direct, high-heat grilling (or see Tips for an indoor variation).
2. Halve the peaches and remove the pits. Slice the zucchini horizontally into 1-inch-thick (2.5 cm) rounds.
3. Place the peach halves and zucchini slices on the grill. To achieve grill marks, place a heavy pot on the food to apply pressure. Cook for 2 to 5 minutes, checking the progress of grilling occasionally. When you see the distinctive brown marks, rotate the peaches and zucchini 90 degrees and cook for another 2 to 5 minutes. Flip them over and repeat the process to obtain even grill marks on both sides.
4. Transfer the peaches and zucchini to a wooden carving board. Allow excess moisture to drain to prevent the food from becoming soggy.
5. On a long rectangular plate, arrange the grilled peach and zucchini pieces, alternating them to create an appealing stack. Sprinkle with the toppings of your choice. Season with salt and pepper, and serve immediately.

TIPS

You can also cook this dish indoors in a cast-iron grill pan. First, brush the pan with olive oil or peanut oil and preheat the pan over medium-high heat. Once the pan is heated, increase the heat to high and add the peaches and zucchini and cook as directed. For added flavor, use a sprig of fresh rosemary to brush the oil around the grill pan while it heats up.

Try this dish with grilled watermelon or apple instead of peach. Garnish grilled watermelon with freshly chopped basil and mint, and add a sprinkle of cinnamon and nutmeg to grilled apples. These juicy and delicious variations may even surpass the original!

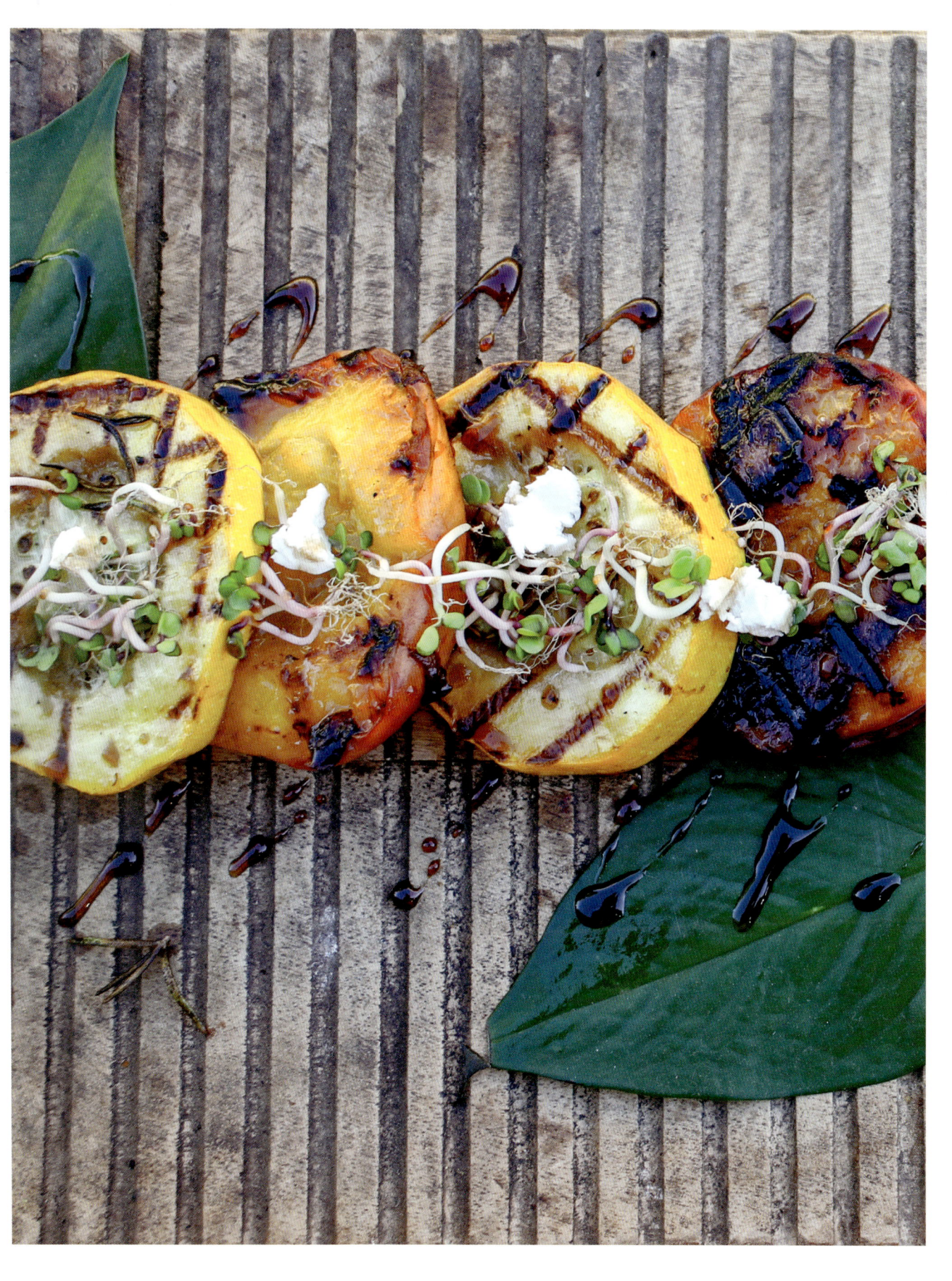

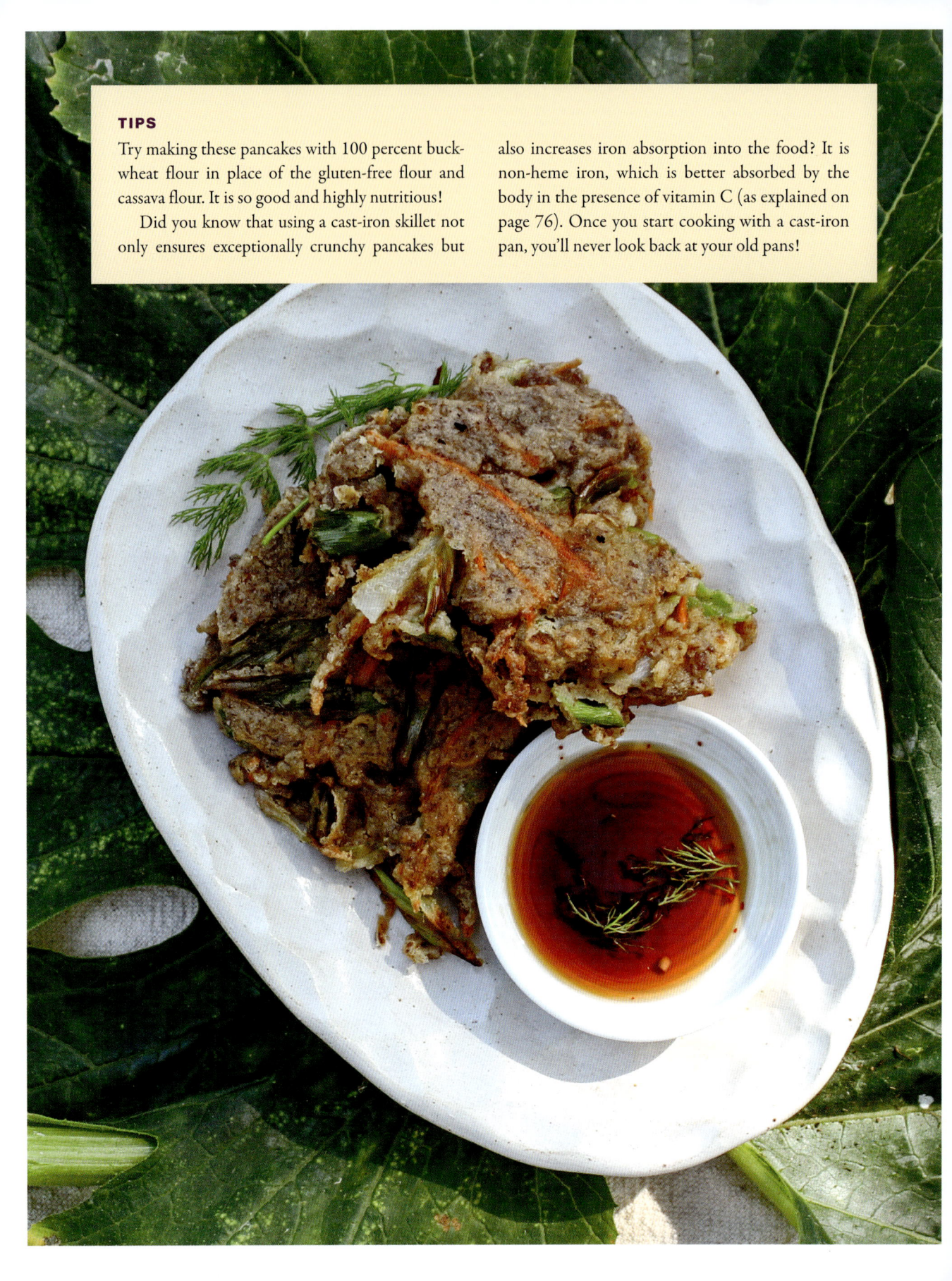

TIPS

Try making these pancakes with 100 percent buckwheat flour in place of the gluten-free flour and cassava flour. It is so good and highly nutritious!

Did you know that using a cast-iron skillet not only ensures exceptionally crunchy pancakes but also increases iron absorption into the food? It is non-heme iron, which is better absorbed by the body in the presence of vitamin C (as explained on page 76). Once you start cooking with a cast-iron pan, you'll never look back at your old pans!

Sweet Potato–Scallion Pancakes

MAKES FOUR 3-INCH (8 CM) PANCAKES

Did you know that eating two or three scallions can provide 30 percent of your daily value (bone RDA) for vitamins A and C? Scallion is more than just a garnish—it can be the star ingredient in your dish. It also contains vitamin K, which helps with blood clotting and strengthens bones. Additionally, scallions are rich in antioxidants. Impressive, right?

Recipes for different kinds of pancakes abound, and people from cultures around the world have been enjoying the versatility of pancakes for centuries. You can customize this recipe to suit your preferences, such as by trying other types of flour.

FOR THE BATTER

½ cup (45 g) gluten-free flour blend or oat flour
¼ cup (35 g) cassava flour
¼ cup (37 g) flaxseed meal
¾ cup (180 ml) filtered water
¼ cup (60 ml) coconut oil
Salt
1 cup (100 g) diagonal sliced scallions
¼ cup (30 g) shredded sweet potato
2 tablespoons minced fresh dill or any fresh herbs

FOR THE DIPPING SAUCE

3 tablespoons liquid aminos
2 tablespoons minced fresh dill or any fresh herbs
1 tablespoon brown rice vinegar
1 teaspoon sesame oil
¼ teaspoon salt
⅛ teaspoon ground ginger
Ground black pepper
Red chili flakes

FOR GARNISH

Chopped fresh dill

1. Make the batter: In a medium bowl, combine the gluten-free flour, cassava flour, and flaxseed meal. Gradually whisk in the water until the batter is smooth. Add 2 tablespoons of the coconut oil and a pinch of salt. When the batter is well mixed and has a thick, liquid consistency, gently fold in the scallions, sweet potato, and dill, and mix well. Set the batter aside.
2. Make the dipping sauce: In a medium bowl, combine the liquid aminos, dill, brown rice vinegar, sesame oil, salt, ginger, a pinch of pepper, and a pinch of chili flakes, and mix well. Transfer to a small sauce bowl and set aside.
3. Heat 1 to 2 tablespoons of the remaining coconut oil in a skillet over medium heat for 1 to 2 minutes. Scoop out pancake-sized portions of the batter into the heated pan (in batches if necessary) and cook for 2 to 3 minutes on each side. Only flip them once; the goal is to achieve a crunchy texture, so allow each side to cook until halfway, and flip when the bottom turns brown.
4. Transfer the cooked pancakes to a cooling rack or wooden board to maintain their crunchiness and prevent them from becoming soggy.
5. To serve, transfer the pancakes to a plate, stacking them alongside the small dish of sauce, then delicately sprinkle dill over the top.

Umami Soy-Glazed Portobello Steak

MAKES 2 SERVINGS

Eating steak can be a primal experience, but if you want to explore meatless options and expand your horizons, try portobello steak instead. You'll be amazed at how closely the texture and flavor of these meaty mushrooms evoke that of traditional beef steak. Portobello mushrooms are easy to digest and offer a rich array of minerals, including potassium, phosphorus, calcium, magnesium, iron, and zinc. If possible, expose the mushrooms to sunlight for 30 minutes before cooking to stimulate them to produce vitamin D.

Using a stone mortar and pestle to grind the ingredients for the chimichurri sauce will give you the best flavors and texture. If you don't have a mortar and pestle, simply chop and mix the ingredients.

2 portobello mushrooms

FOR THE UMAMI GLAZE

¼ cup (60 ml) filtered water
2 teaspoons mild miso paste, plus more as needed
1 tablespoon extra-virgin olive oil
1 tablespoon maple syrup
¼ teaspoon umami powder
1 rosemary sprig, for brushing on the glaze

FOR THE CHIMICHURRI SAUCE

2 tablespoons chopped fresh cilantro
4 walnuts, soaked
1 garlic clove
Sea salt
Ground black pepper
2 tablespoons extra-virgin olive oil

TIP

Umami mushroom powder is a seasoning that can be found in Asian markets. It has a rich, meaty, and woody flavor profile that adds depth and complexity to your dishes. Life is short—why not add umami to drop a flavor bomb!

1. Scrape the gills of the mushrooms using a spoon or a gentle scraping tool. This helps to create a smoother surface. Next, clean the mushrooms by gently wiping them with a damp towel to remove any dirt or debris. Remove the stem by gently twisting or cutting it off.
2. Make the umami glaze: In a small bowl, combine the water, miso, olive oil, maple syrup, and umami powder. Whisk the ingredients together until well combined, then taste for seasoning. If needed, add a little more miso. Set aside.
3. Make the chimichurri sauce: Place the cilantro, walnuts, garlic, and a pinch of salt and pepper in a stone mortar. Use the pestle to grind the ingredients together until you achieve a chunky texture. Slowly pour in the olive oil while continuing to grind, until all the ingredients are well combined.
4. Use the sprig of rosemary to brush all surfaces of the mushrooms with umami glaze, ensuring that the glaze is evenly distributed.
5. Preheat a cast-iron skillet, then cook the mushrooms over high heat for approximately 5 minutes. Flip the mushrooms, brush them again with the glaze, and continue cooking for an additional 5 minutes or until the mushrooms are tender.
6. Serve the mushrooms, drizzled with the chimichurri sauce.

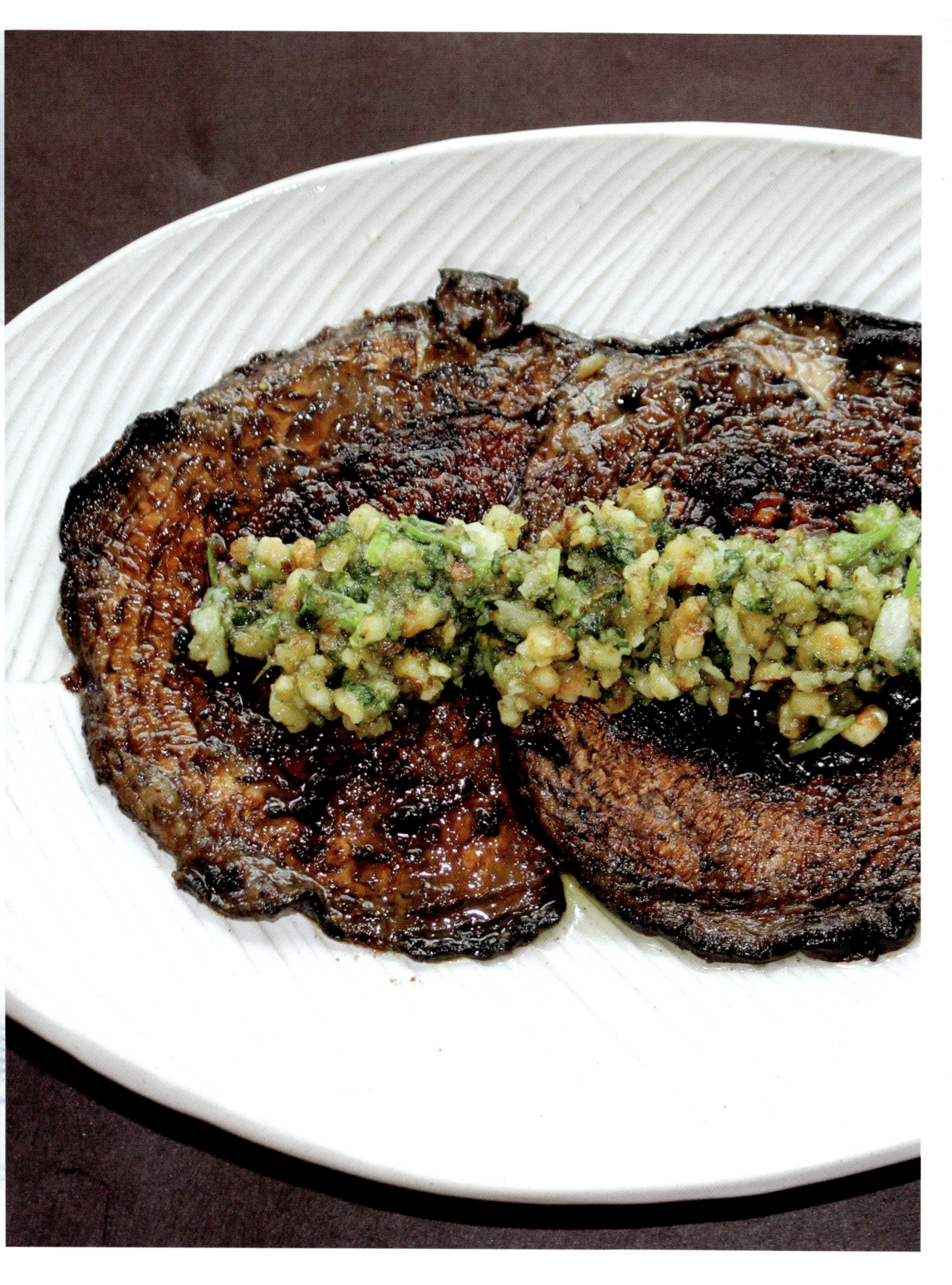

Snap Peas with Tempeh Dust

MAKES 2 SERVINGS

Sugar snap peas are famous for their crunchiness and vibrant texture. They are highly nutritious and very good for your digestive system.

Instead of a typical sauté, this recipe takes a detour to make snap peas super crunchy and incredibly fun—all with minimal nutrient loss. How, you ask? By turning up the heat with a quick broil. After broiling, you make them even more delicious with a coating of fermented tempeh, gluten-free panko breadcrumbs, and vegan parmesan.

12 ounces (300 g) sugar snap peas, trimmed
½ cup (60 g) gluten-free or regular panko
¼ cup (40 g) crushed tempeh
¼ cup (20 g) grated vegan parmesan or parmesan cheese
1 tablespoon nutritional yeast
1 teaspoon chopped fresh parsley
2 tablespoons extra-virgin olive oil
4 basil leaves, chopped

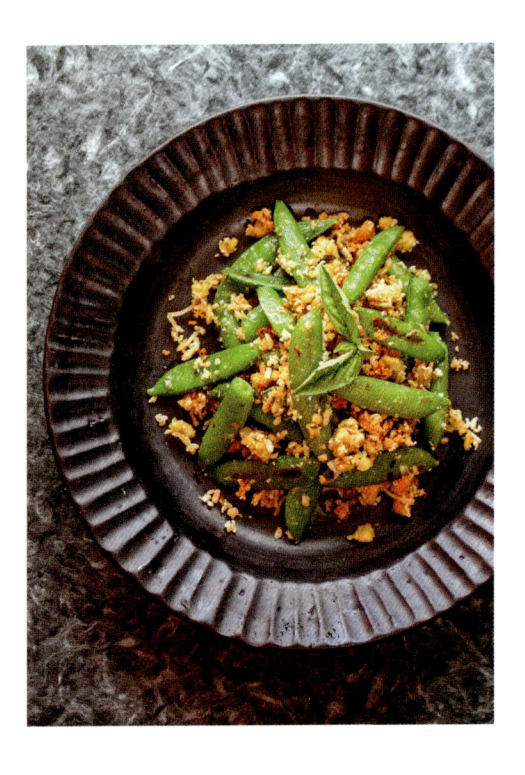

1. Place the snap peas in a small bowl. Add the panko, crushed tempeh, parmesan, nutritional yeast, and parsley. Drizzle the olive oil over the ingredients and toss them well.
2. Set the oven to the broil setting. Pour the peas onto a baking sheet and transfer to the oven. Stay close by the stove while the peas are broiling and check them frequently; it will only take 2 or 3 minutes for them to cook. If the peas are overcooked, their texture will be chewy and soggy. When the peas have reduced 50 percent in volume, remove them from the oven and let sit for 2 to 3 minutes.
3. Transfer the peas to a serving plate and garnish with the basil.

TIP
If your oven doesn't have a broiler setting, you can get similar results by roasting the peas at 425°F (220°C). Check them after 5 minutes, and don't let them overcook. Total cooking time will be 8 to 12 minutes.

CHAPTER 14

Broths, Porridge, and Soups

I remember the cold, brisk winters of my childhood. My mom always made delicious soups, and when I arrived home with a frozen chin, sipping the warm soup would melt my heart and warm my body immediately.

I design broths and soups with diverse seasonal ingredients and different nutritional balances. As you explore this chapter, you may begin creating your own signature soups that will curb your hunger and become good medicine for your body and spirit.

Let's toss out the outmoded idea that healthy food has to be plain and dull. Medicinal healing foods can be delicious, nutritious, easy to make, and affordable, so they are accessible for everyone.

Soup is soulful slow food to feed your body, one delightful spoonful at a time.

Most of my recipes make just two servings, considering the modern trend toward smaller families. However, in this soup section, you can double or triple the recipes so you'll have extra portions saved in the freezer for a quick meal in the future. The flavors become even richer with longer storage.

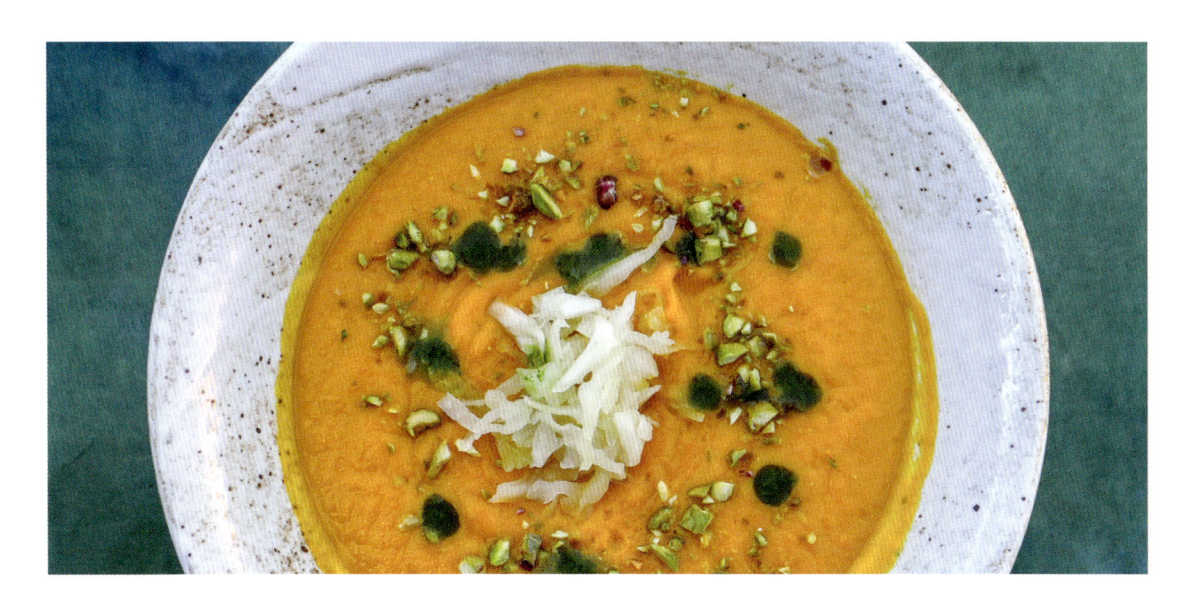

Miso Soup with Dashi Broth

MAKES 4 SERVINGS

Have you tried Japanese miso or noodle soup? You will fall in love with the hearty flavor and feeling of comfort it provides. Miso soup is often served as a starter, preparing the digestive system for a meal with warmth and healthy bacteria.

Miso is a fermented soybean paste widely consumed in Korea and Japan. It comes in many forms, colors, and different taste profiles. The slow-aged fermentation process is the key to the beneficial bacteria. Miso is a complete source of protein and rich in a variety of nutrients and beneficial plant compounds. For this recipe I chose white miso, a mild, low-sodium option. This recipe also contains miyeok, which is a Korean sea green that is called wakame in Japanese.

Make this dashi broth on a lazy Sunday after sourcing all the ingredients from your farmers market, and let it simmer for a couple of hours while you read the paper.

FOR THE DASHI BROTH

2 medium shiitake mushrooms
¼ cup (25 g) bean sprouts or mung bean sprouts
5 cups (1.2 L) filtered water
1 garlic clove
½ cup (60 g) sliced white radish
2 (3-inch [8 cm] square) pieces dried kelp

FOR THE MISO SOUP

¼ cup (60 g) cubed semi-firm tofu
¼ cup (30 g) shredded white radish
2 tablespoons (10 g) small pieces dried miyeok (wakame)
2 tablespoons thinly sliced scallions
4 teaspoons low-sodium white miso paste
⅛ teaspoon ground ginger

1. Make the dashi broth: Clean the mushrooms and rinse the sprouts. In a large cast-iron pot, add the water, mushrooms, sprouts, radish slices, garlic, and kelp and bring to a boil. Then lower the heat and simmer until the broth reduces by 20 percent, which will take 40 minutes to 1 hour. Turn off the heat, and let it sit for another 30 minutes so all the flavors will be incorporated into the broth. Strain the broth and discard the solids. Reserve 3 cups (720 ml) of the broth for the soup; any leftover broth can be stored in the freezer for another day.

2. Make the soup: Divide the tofu, shredded radish, miyeok, and scallions equally between two serving bowls.

3. Add 3 cups (720 ml) of the dashi broth to a medium pot and turn the heat to high. Add the miso and ginger, then reduce the heat to a simmer. Break up the miso paste by whisking it into the broth. After 2 to 3 minutes, remove from the heat. Gently pour the hot broth over the ingredients in the serving bowls. Serve immediately.

TIPS

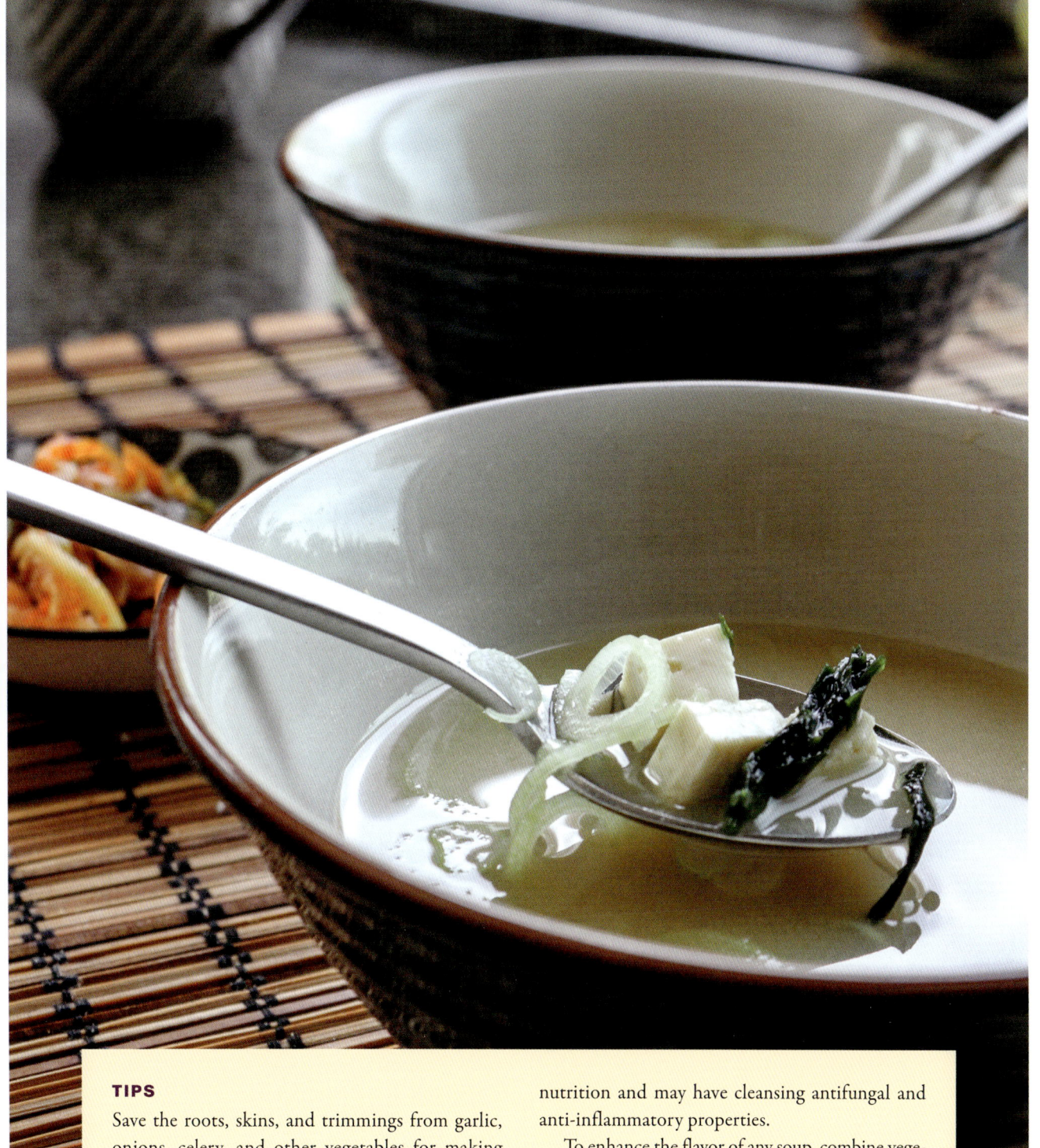

Save the roots, skins, and trimmings from garlic, onions, celery, and other vegetables for making your next vegetable broth or medicinal Root and Leaf Magnesium Broth (page 177). The outer skins and roots provide an excellent source of nutrition and may have cleansing antifungal and anti-inflammatory properties.

To enhance the flavor of any soup, combine vegetable broth and rice water (see "How to Make Rice Water," page 191) in a ratio of 1:1, and boil them to make rice broth. Rice broth is nutty, creamy, and rich.

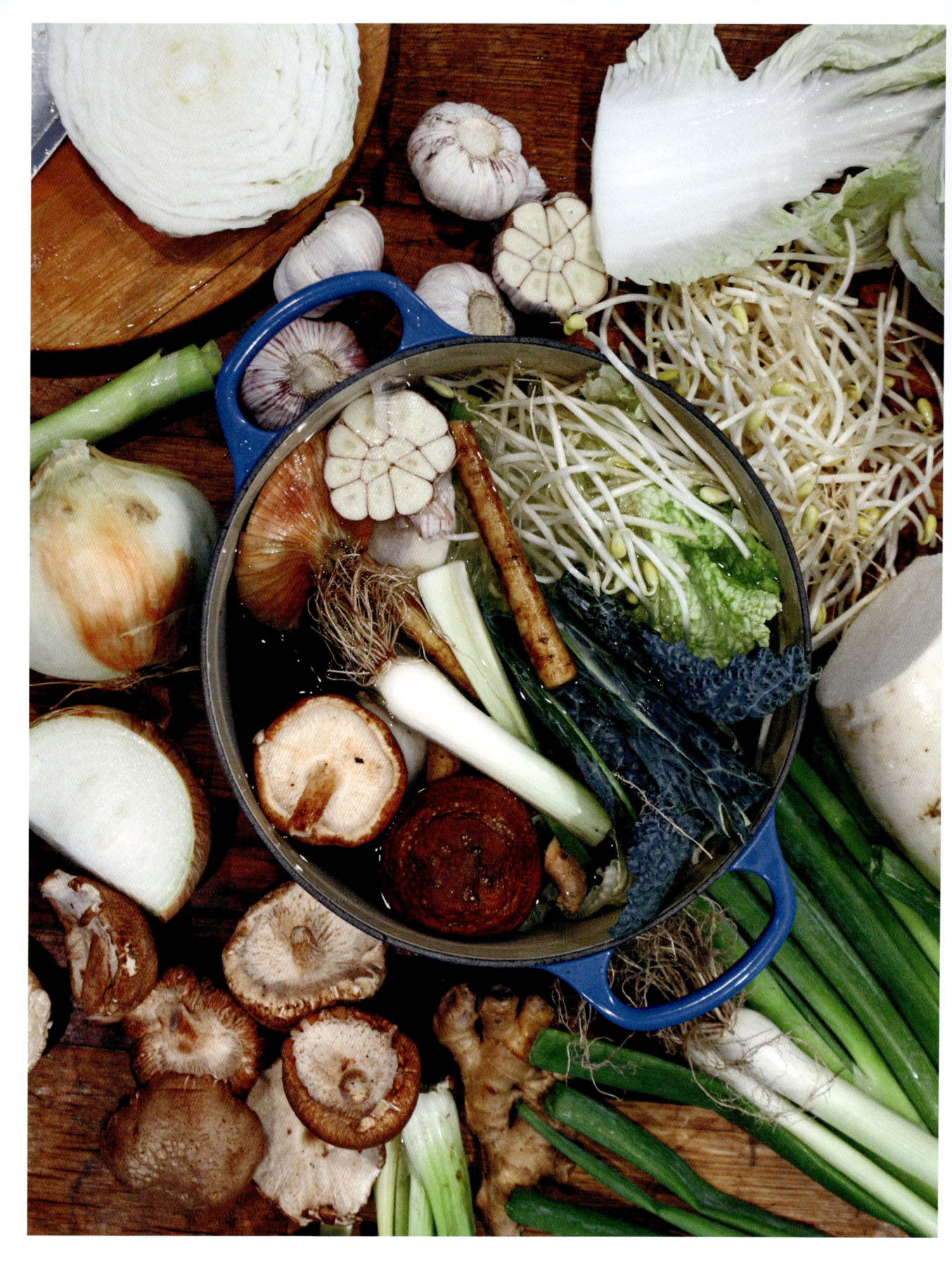

Root and Leaf Magnesium Broth

MAKES 12 QUARTS (11.4 L)

This mineral broth is a key recipe for keeping bones healthy while also providing a good source of potassium and supporting digestion. Slow-cooking roots, mushrooms, and leaves results in a nutrient-dense liquid. When you consume the broth, it delivers high-density minerals directly to your body without needing a long digestive process, conserving the energy that would otherwise be spent on digestion. This makes it a medicinal option that can help with leaky gut conditions and a host of other ailments.

This broth can be a base for any soup, adding flavor and nutrition. You can also use it to break a fast or as a simple liquid diet to rest and reset your gut system. This recipe makes a very large batch, which works well for me because I use this broth in many dishes. I always like to have some in my freezer. You can cut the recipe in half if you don't have the equipment or the wish to make 12 quarts (11.4 L) at one time.

13 quarts (13 L) filtered water
¼ cup (25 g) bean sprouts
4 (3-inch [8 cm] square) pieces dried kelp
4 medium shiitake mushrooms
2 kale stalks with the stem
2 whole scallions or ½ leek
1 small carrot
1 leaf napa cabbage or green cabbage
1 2-inch (5 cm) piece fresh ginger
1 Korean radish (about 3 inches [8 cm] long), sliced into 1-inch (2.5 cm) rounds
½ celery rib
½ medium onion
½ garlic head
¼ fresh burdock root, cut into 3-inch (8 cm) pieces

1. In a large pot, add the water and all of the ingredients. Bring to a boil over high heat, then reduce the heat to a minimum and simmer until the broth reduces by 20 percent, about 2 hours. Remove the broth from the heat and let it sit for an additional 30 minutes to allow the flavors to incorporate.
2. Strain the broth and transfer into freezer-safe containers for storage. Reserve the mushrooms, kelp, sprouts, carrots, radishes, and cabbage for use in another soup, such as a variation on Miso Soup with Dashi Broth (page 174).

> **TIP**
> We highly recommend this broth for a monthly or seasonal cleansing liquid fast. It provides abundant nutrition, curbing hunger while giving your body a break and reset from heavy daily digestion. This practice helps maintain good shape, sharpens brain health, and serves as an ageless rejuvenation and prevention tool. See "Spring Fasting" on page 51.

Broths, Porridge, and Soups

Borscht with Cashew Cream

MAKES 4 SERVINGS

This soulful, vividly red soup became my staple winter meal when I entered the Russian Banya (sauna) community in Brooklyn. I asked one of the spa kitchen staff what the soup was called. The answer, delivered with a strong Russian accent: "Borscht." I asked him to tell the recipe, and I carefully transcribed his description. Since then, I have played with the soup to create my own lean and twisted version. Here's my recipe featuring cashew cream, a wonderful alternative to sour cream for those who don't eat dairy products.

TIPS

Adding a small quantity of water or broth to sautéed vegetables and bringing it to a boil early in the soup-making process intensifies the flavors in a short period of time. I start most of my soups this way, and then add the rest of the broth or water to continue the cooking process.

Making croutons from leftover bread to use as a topping for the soup will add crunchy texture. Alternatively, sauerkraut can provide a tangy and complementary flavor to enhance the silky texture of the dish.

Try parsnip, pumpkin, or sweet potato as a substitute for beets. These variations have a silkier texture than the original recipe.

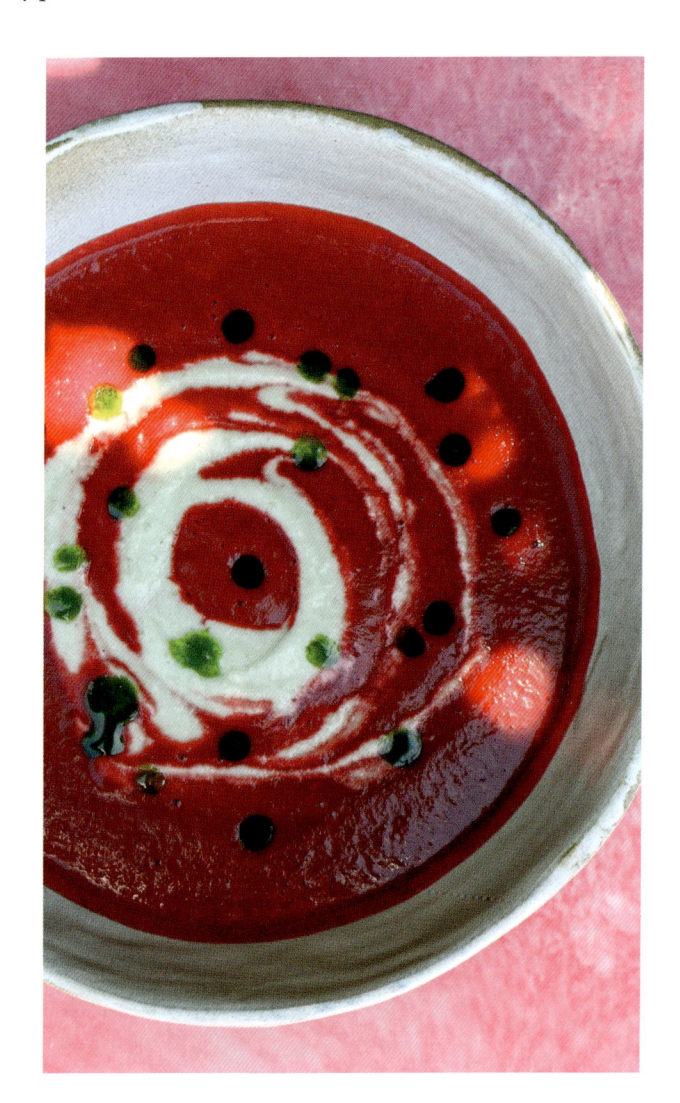

1 medium onion
1 celery rib
1 medium Yukon Gold potato
2 garlic cloves
1 tablespoon extra-virgin olive oil or ghee
1 tablespoon dried dill
6 cups (1.4 L) filtered water or Root and Leaf Magnesium Broth (page 177)
4 cups (580 g) coarsely chopped beets
1 bay leaf
¼ teaspoon ground cinnamon
¼ teaspoon freshly grated nutmeg
¼ teaspoon fennel seed
¼ cup (60 ml) coconut milk or vegan cream
Sea salt
Cracked black pepper

FOR THE CASHEW CREAM
½ cup (120 ml) filtered water
¼ cup (40 g) raw cashews, soaked
2 tablespoons ghee or extra-virgin olive oil
Sea salt
Cracked black pepper

FOR GARNISH
1 tablespoon Green Oil (page 143)

1. Roughly chop the onion, celery, and potato into large pieces. Roughly chop the garlic.
2. In a cast-iron pot over medium-high heat, heat the oil and dill for 1 minute. Add a few tablespoons of the water or magnesium broth, the garlic, onion, celery, and potato, and sauté for 2 to 3 minutes until the vegetables soften. Add the beets and sauté for 5 minutes.
3. Add 3 cups (720 ml) of the water or broth and increase the heat to bring it to a simmer. Add the rest of the water or broth, along with the bay leaf, cinnamon, nutmeg, and fennel seed. Bring the mixture to a boil and then reduce the heat to medium-low. Let it simmer for another 10 to 15 minutes.
4. Once the beets have become translucent, add the coconut milk and continue cooking for 1 to 3 minutes. There should be just enough broth to barely cover the beet chunks. This will result in the perfect texture after blending. Allow the soup to cook at low heat for another 10 to 20 minutes to let the flavors meld together. Remove from the heat and let it cool down at least 5 minutes before blending.
5. Meanwhile, make the cashew cream: In a mini blender, combine the water, cashews, and ghee, and blend well for 3 to 5 minutes, or until the mixture reaches a creamy consistency resembling sour cream. Season with salt and pepper.
6. Pour the contents of the pot into a large blender. Do not fill the blender too full; work in batches if necessary. Blend the soup well, starting at a low speed and gradually increasing to high. Blend for 4 to 5 minutes, or until the soup has a silky texture. Season with salt and pepper.
7. Transfer the soup to individual soup bowls. Place a portion of the creamy cashew mixture on top of each soup bowl, and swirl it in. To add a burst of flavor and visual appeal, drizzle a few drops of green oil over the soup. Enjoy the vibrant and delicious presentation of the dish. Freeze any leftover soup in plastic or silicone containers.

Broccoli-Potato-Leek Soup

MAKES 2 SERVINGS

This silky, super-green soup will make your dinner smooth and sound.

Leeks are related to onions, garlic, and scallions, but have a mild, soft, yet sweet flavor that is not overpowering. Leek is one of my favorite vegetables. If you are not fond of onion or garlic, leek will be your savior.

The tenderness of sweet leeks and green superhero broccoli are a perfect combo in this recipe. Leeks are highly nutritious and contain vitamin K, which may reduce the risk of osteoporosis. Leeks also contain lutein and zeaxanthin, which help support better vision.

½ head broccoli
1 small Yukon Gold potato
½ celery rib
½ small onion
1 medium leek
1 garlic clove
1 tablespoon ghee or extra-virgin olive oil, plus more for serving
2 or 3 oregano sprigs
2 or 3 fresh sage leaves or ⅛ teaspoon dried sage
⅛ teaspoon ground cardamom
3½ cups (840 ml) Root and Leaf Magnesium Broth (page 177) or filtered water
¼ teaspoon moringa powder
1 bay leaf
Salt
Ground black pepper

TO SERVE

Fresh lemon juice
1 teaspoon crushed natto, fresh or dry
1 teaspoon minced fresh parsley
1 teaspoon chopped olives
Green Oil (page 143) or Red Oil (see Tip) (optional)

1. Roughly chop the broccoli, potato, celery, onion, and leek into large pieces. Roughly chop the garlic.
2. Warm the ghee in a medium pot over medium heat. Add the oregano, sage, and cardamom and allow the flavors to infuse into the oil for 1 to 2 minutes. Add the celery, onion, leek, and garlic, and sauté them lightly for 1 to 2 minutes, then add the broccoli and potato and cook for another 2 to 3 minutes. Add 2 cups (480 ml) of the broth and increase the heat to high until it comes to a simmer. Once the broth is simmering, add the remaining 1½ cups (350 ml) broth, the moringa powder, and the bay leaf. Bring the mixture to a boil, then reduce the heat to medium-low and simmer for another 10 to 15 minutes. Look for all the ingredients to become transparent. Keep an eye on the broth and continue to reduce it until it barely covers the vegetable chunks. Remove from the heat and let it cool for 5 minutes.
3. Pour the soup into a blender and blend for 3 to 5 minutes. Season with salt and pepper.
4. Ladle the soup into two soup bowls. Add a squeeze of lemon to each. Place a half teaspoon each of natto, parsley, and olives at the center of each bowl of soup. To add a decorative touch, drizzle with green or red oil.

TIP

You can make Red Oil by following the instructions for Green Oil (page 143) and replacing the parsley with hibiscus extract or beet extract powder and the walnut oil with extra-virgin olive oil.

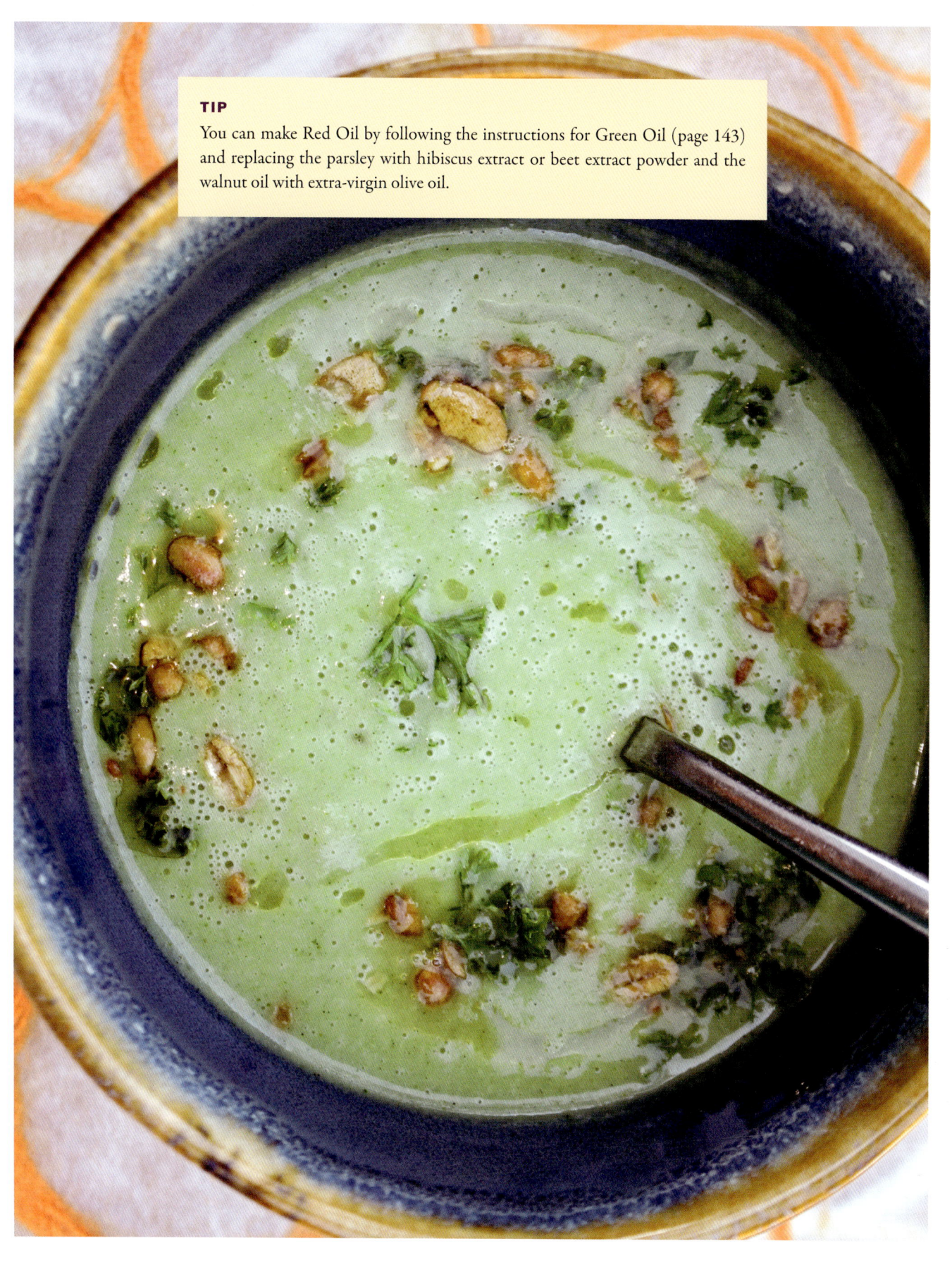

California Creamy Corn Chowder

MAKES 2 SERVINGS

According to the *Dongui Bogam*, an ancient Korean medicinal healing guidebook, there are three simple secrets to longevity: eating local, eating fresh, and eating in season. This recipe uses fresh plant-based ingredients to recreate the taste of clams. That sounds impossible, but it's simpler than you think! The oyster mushrooms, umami-packed dashi broth with kelp and green salt, and a touch of rice flour will do the work.

I love the vibrant colors, fresh textures, and distinct flavors of creamy potatoes, crunchy corn, and carrots in this chowder. Say goodbye to New England clam chowder and say hello to California Creamy Corn Chowder with open arms. This is not your average clam chowder! It's a taste of tradition and a gift to your health, all in one bowl.

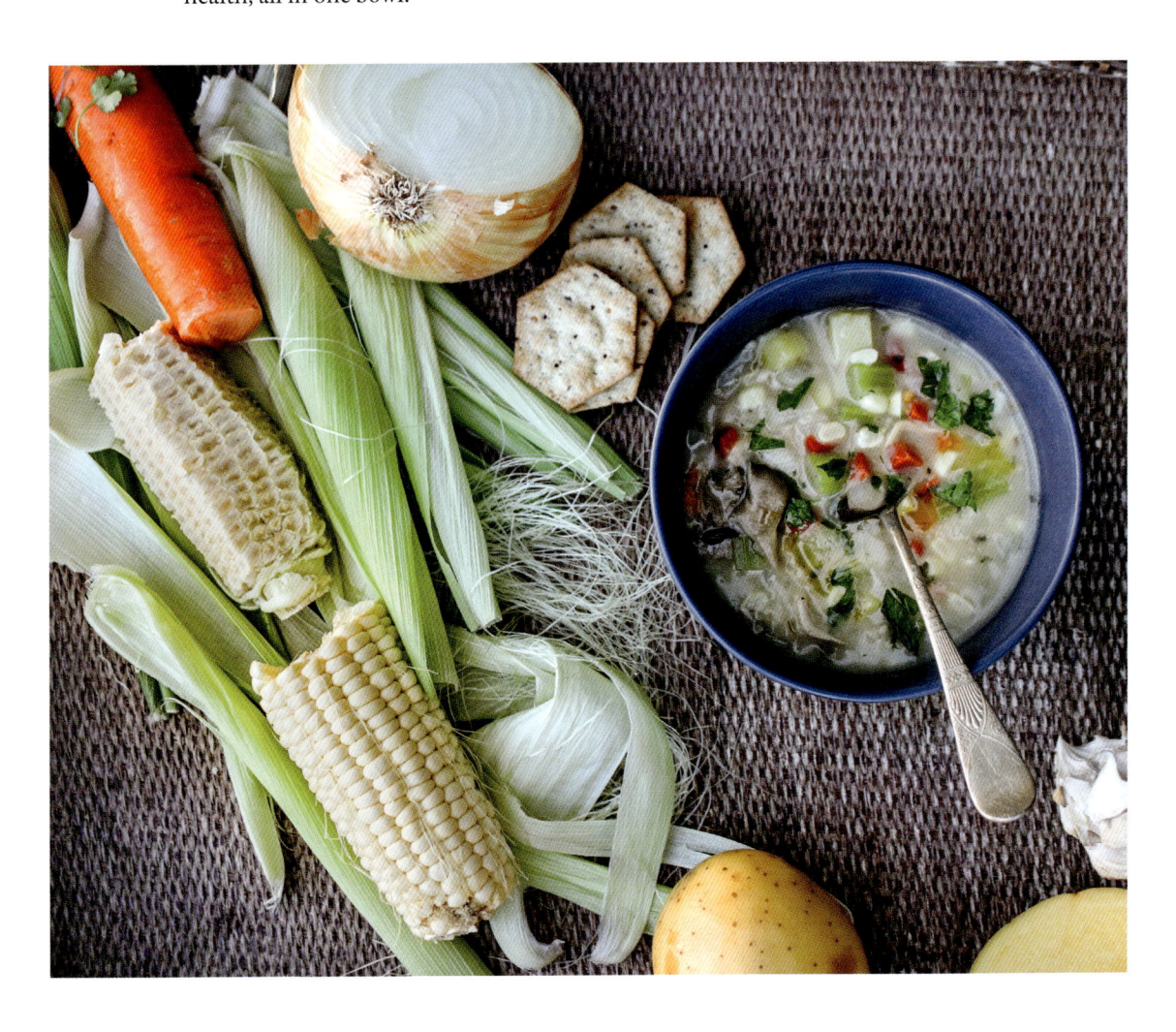

3 medium sun-soaked oyster mushrooms
   (see page 94)
1 medium Yukon Gold potato
1 medium onion
½ celery rib
½ small carrot
1 ear non-GMO sweet corn
   (locally grown if possible)
3 to 4 tablespoons jarred roasted red peppers
1 tablespoon ghee or extra-virgin olive oil
1 garlic clove, minced
Handful chopped fresh parsley
2 cups (480 ml) rice water (page 191)
1 bay leaf
3 cups (720 ml) dashi broth (page 174)
   or filtered water
3 tablespoons rice flour
3 tablespoons coconut milk or vegan cream
3 tablespoons rice flour

TO SERVE
Minced fresh parsley
Cracked black pepper
Umami mushroom powder or nutritional yeast

1. Use a damp cotton cloth to gently wipe the mushrooms clean. Tear the mushrooms into small pieces. Cut the potato, onion, celery, and carrot into ½-inch (1 cm) cubes. Place all the prepared vegetables and mushrooms on a large plate and set them aside.
2. Husk the corn. Hold the ear steady in a vertical position and gently cut off the kernels from top to bottom, rotating the cob little by little until all the kernels are removed. Place the kernels in a small bowl and set them aside.
3. Drain the roasted red peppers and cut them into ½-inch (1 cm) pieces.
4. Set a cast-iron pot over medium-low heat and add the ghee, garlic, and parsley. Sauté for 1 minute so the aromatic flavors release into the oil. Add the onion and celery and sauté for an additional 1 minute. Add the corn, potato, carrot, and mushrooms and sauté for 2 to 3 minutes. Add 1 cup (240 ml) of the rice water and the bay leaf. Bring the mixture to a simmer and cook for 2 to 3 minutes. Slowly stir in the remaining 1 cup (240 ml) rice water and the dashi broth.
5. In a small bowl, combine the rice flour with 5 tablespoons water and whisk well. Gently pour the flour water into the soup and stir to blend well. Reduce the heat to medium-low and stir in the coconut milk. Let the soup simmer gently for approximately 5 minutes, stirring occasionally, until the vegetables are fully cooked and the flavors have melded together. Add the roasted red pepper during the last minute of cooking. It's important not to overcook the soup, as you want to preserve the distinct flavors and textures.
6. Ladle the chowder into two soup bowls and top it with a sprinkle of parsley and black pepper and a dusting of umami powder.

> **TIP**
> Try making this chowder with asparagus and lion's mane mushrooms, which offer a wealth of bone-health nutrition and beneficial properties for brain cells.

Broths, Porridge, and Soups

Golden Dal Moringa Khichuri

MAKES 2 SERVINGS

One of the major healing dishes of India is khichuri—a staple in everyday Indian cuisine and a key element of the panchakarma cleansing and rejuvenating program. Panchakarma follows Ayurvedic principles, seeking to balance the five elements of Ether, Air, Fire, Water, and Earth.

This recipe will guide you to create a simple yet powerful and nutritious healing meal and teach you how to apply the same method to make other versatile soups. Moringa, a drought-resistant native Indian superfood, enhances the flavor and nutritional value.

With a blend of basic Indian spices and simple cooking techniques, this recipe will help you gain confidence in Indian cooking.

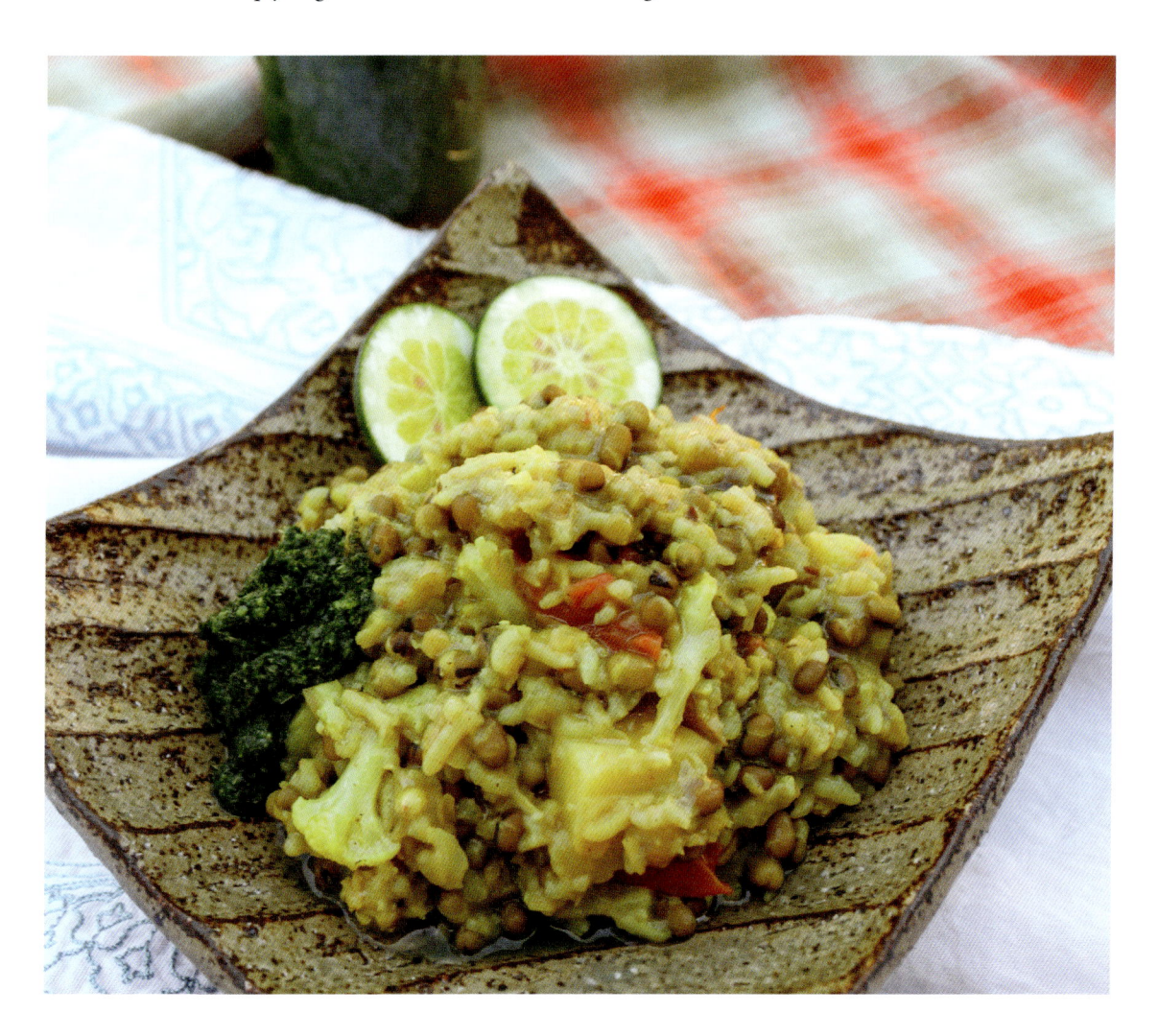

½ cup (95 g) mung beans

½ cup (95 g) basmati rice, soaked

1 small to medium potato, any kind

1 small tomato

¼ cup (30 g) cauliflower florets

1 tablespoon ghee

1 whole cardamom pod or
    ⅛ teaspoon ground cardamom

⅛ teaspoon ground coriander

⅛ teaspoon ground cumin

⅛ teaspoon ground ginger

⅛ teaspoon red chili flakes

⅛ teaspoon ground turmeric

Ground cinnamon

1 whole clove

1 garlic clove, minced

1 teaspoon moringa powder

1 bay leaf

5 cups (1.2 L) filtered water or Root and Leaf Magnesium Broth (page 177)

FOR THE SWEET AND TANGY MINT CHUTNEY

1 cup (30 g) fresh mint

¼ cup (15 g) fresh cilantro

3 tablespoons filtered water or yogurt (vegan or whole-milk)

1 fresh green chile, stemmed and chopped

1 small garlic clove, minced

2 teaspoons honey, maple syrup, or date syrup

1 tablespoon lime juice or pineapple juice

⅛ teaspoon ground ginger

Salt

1. One day in advance, soak the mung beans as described on page 102. Drain.
2. Cut the potato into ½-inch (1 cm) cubes. Cut the tomato into four wedges, remove the seeds, and then cut the wedges into ½-inch (1 cm) cubes. Set these vegetables aside with the cauliflower florets.
3. Melt the ghee in a large pot over low heat. Add the cardamom, coriander, cumin, ginger, chili flakes, turmeric, a pinch of cinnamon, and the clove. Sauté for 1 to 2 minutes, then add the garlic and sauté for 1 to 2 minutes more. Add the mung beans and sauté for 3 minutes; add the rice, potato, tomato, and cauliflower and sauté for an additional 2 to 3 minutes; then add the moringa powder and bay leaf and sauté for 2 to 3 minutes.
4. Add 2 cups (480 ml) of the water; bring to a boil, then reduce to a simmer. Add the remaining 3 cups (720 ml) water, raise the heat again to a boil, and again reduce to a simmer. Continue cooking for 20 minutes. Remove from the heat and let the pot sit, covered, for 20 to 30 minutes, until the rice and mung beans are completely cooked.
5. Make the chutney: In a mini blender, add the mint, cilantro, water, chile, garlic, honey, lime juice, and ginger. Blend well for 2 to 3 minutes, pulsing the blender on and off (too much blending will make the mint bitter). Season gradually with salt to taste.
6. Serve the dal with the chutney.

TIPS

You can substitute parsnip or broccoli for the potato to create a lower-carb version of this dish.

To make the mint chutney creamier and health-friendly, use yogurt instead of water—it's delicious!

To add color and texture to the dish, add ¼ cup (25 g) green peas 5 minutes before you serve the dal to preserve the bright green color of the peas.

Broths, Porridge, and Soups

Hearty Quinoa Minestrone

MAKES 2 SERVINGS

This is the ultimate winter soup that never fails to amaze dinner guests. Every time I whip up this richly flavored recipe, it elicits exclamations like, "Oh, that hits the spot!" (Remember to double or triple this recipe if you're planning on inviting guests over.)

This soup is also just right for a chilly winter day when you're home alone with leftover veggies in the fridge, and you have the craving for something warm to eat. Instead of pasta or rice, my minestrone features black quinoa, a treasure of nutrients. The vegetables are the core of this soup, and I have chosen mushrooms, root veggies, zucchini, cabbage, and a delightful tomato sauce. You can substitute other vegetables of your choice—even pumpkin for a twist! Minestrone is versatile enough to enjoy during the summer, too. Be careful, though—this soup can be quite addictive.

1 small zucchini
2 portobello mushrooms
1 small parsnip
1 wedge cabbage
½ small onion
½ celery rib
½ small carrot
2 fingerling potatoes
3 tablespoons extra-virgin olive oil or ghee
1 garlic clove, minced
¼ teaspoon dried basil
4½ to 5 cups (1 to 1.2 L) filtered water or Root and Leaf Magnesium Broth (page 177)
1 cup (240 ml) canned tomato sauce
¼ cup (45 g) black quinoa
1 tablespoon tomato paste
1 tablespoon maple syrup
1 bay leaf
¼ cup (15 g) chopped collard greens or kale
Salt
Ground black pepper
Fresh basil leaves, for garnish

1. Chop the zucchini, mushrooms, parsnip, cabbage, onion, celery, carrot, and potatoes into small cubes (about ½ inch [1 cm]). Set aside.
2. In a soup pot, heat the oil over medium heat. Add the garlic and dried basil and cook for 1 minute. Then add the parsnip, onion, celery, and carrot and cook for 2 to 3 minutes. Add the zucchini, mushrooms, cabbage, and potatoes and sauté for 5 minutes.
3. Pour in 1½ cups (350 ml) of the water or broth and increase the heat to high. Once it's simmering, add 3 cups (720 ml) water or broth and the tomato sauce, quinoa, tomato paste, maple syrup, and bay leaf. Bring the mixture to a boil and then reduce the heat to medium-low and simmer for 10 to 12 minutes. Watch for the quinoa to expand and increase in volume and for the broth to reduce to the point where it barely covers the ingredients. Add an additional ½ cup (120 ml) water or broth only if needed to fully cook the quinoa.
4. Add the collard greens and cook for 1 to 2 minutes. The greens add a touch of beautiful green color in the rich red broth. Season with salt and pepper to taste.
5. Serve the soup immediately, garnishing each bowl with the fresh basil.

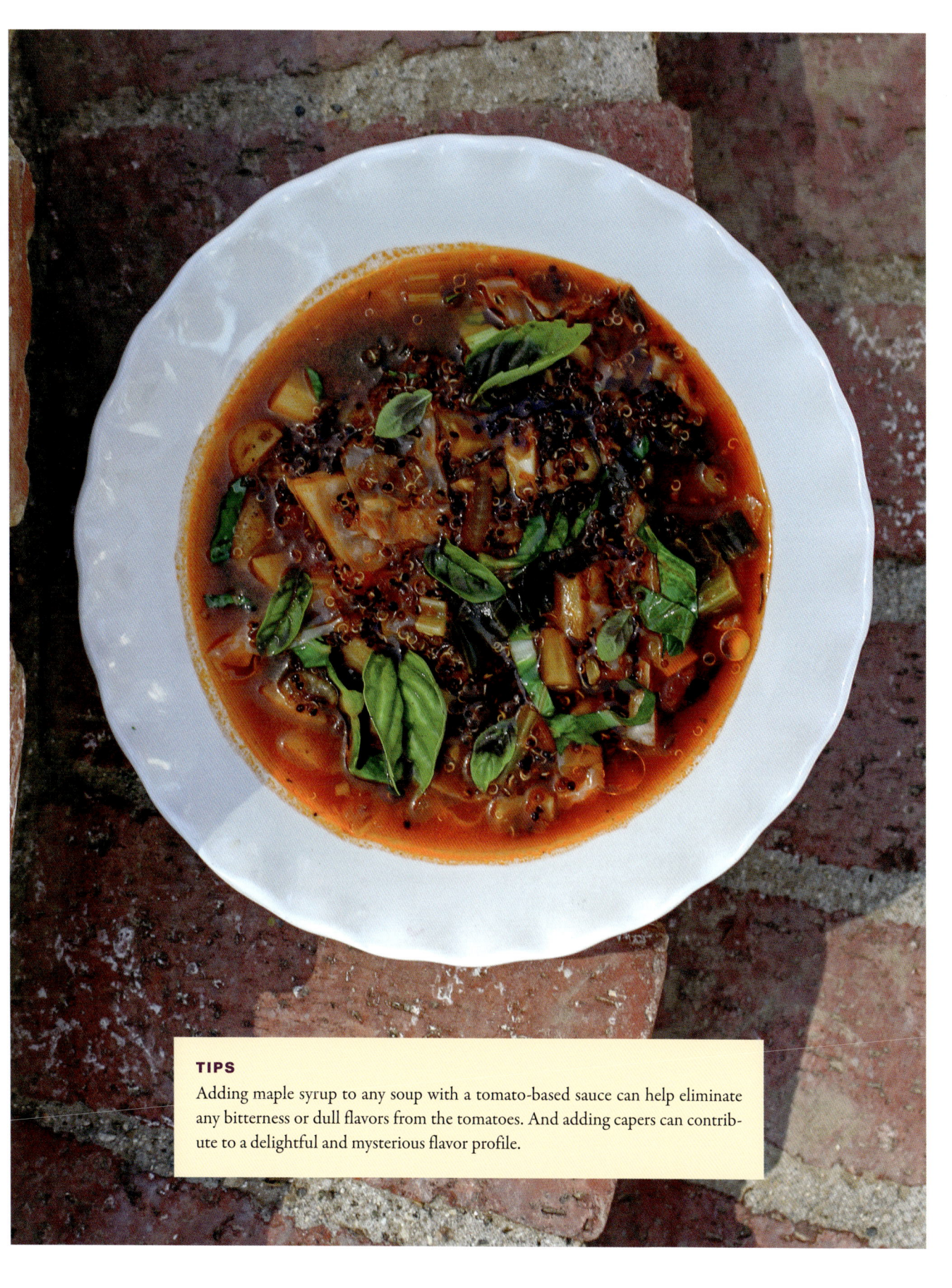

TIPS

Adding maple syrup to any soup with a tomato-based sauce can help eliminate any bitterness or dull flavors from the tomatoes. And adding capers can contribute to a delightful and mysterious flavor profile.

Recover-Restore-Reboot Porridge

MAKES 2 SERVINGS

Porridge holds a special place in my heart and kitchen. It's my go-to, nourishing food remedy when I'm cooking for my private clients, especially for those on the path to healing and restoring their digestive health. This humble dish takes me back to the warm, comforting meals my mother lovingly prepared when I was a little kid, and it remains a cherished option for a soft and tender breakfast.

Porridge, also known as congee, is a dish with deep ancestral roots that is commonly enjoyed in East Asian and Southeast Asian cultures. Traditionally consumed as a breakfast food, this dish has been cherished by our ancestors as a source of comfort and healing. The rice is cooked until it reaches a soft and tender consistency, requiring less digestive work for the body. In this vegan alternative to chicken soup for the soul, I use brown rice instead of white rice.

According to the principles of Five Elements in Traditional Chinese Medicine, brown rice, cabbage, and shiitake mushrooms are considered natural center core foods, playing a vital role in stabilizing both the body and mind, especially when confronted with extreme heat or cold in other food ingredients. By incorporating these natural center core ingredients, we can ground ourselves and find balance. This dish is an essential aid for recovering, reenergizing, and healing the body and soul. Often enjoyed as a meal before—or after—fasting, this porridge serves as a timeless reminder of our ancestral connections.

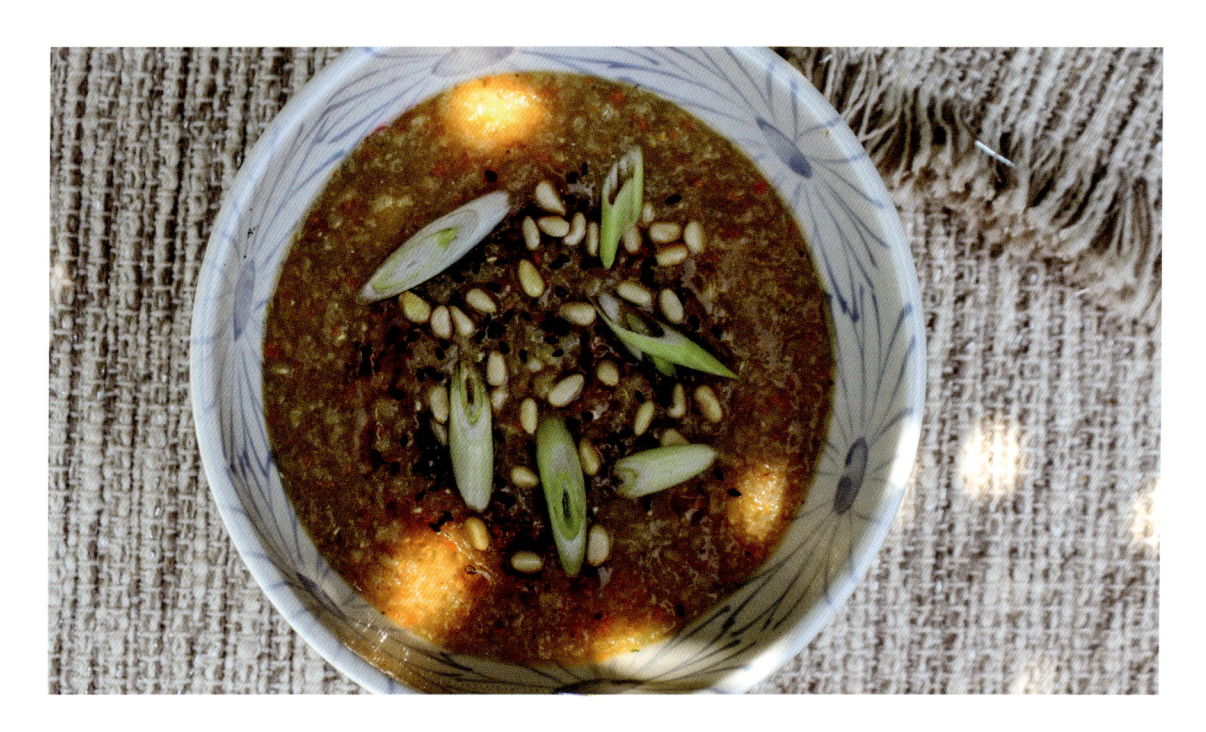

1 cup (190 g) brown rice
3 medium-sized shiitake or baby bella mushrooms
½ small carrot
½ small onion
1 wedge (20 g) green cabbage
3 cups (720 ml) Root and Leaf Magnesium Broth (page 177) or filtered water

FOR GARNISH
1 tablespoon pine nuts
1 small scallion, trimmed
1 teaspoon black sesame seeds
2 teaspoons sesame oil
Soy sauce (optional)

1. Place the brown rice in a bowl, add water to cover, and leave to soak for at least 1 hour. While the rice soaks, roughly chop the mushrooms, carrot, onion, and cabbage (you should have about ¼ cup cabbage).
2. Drain the rice. In a food processor, combine the rice and vegetables. Pulse six to eight times until you achieve a thick, pastelike texture.
3. Place a soup pot over medium-low heat. Transfer the mixture from the processor to the pot and cook, stirring, for 1 to 2 minutes. Add 1 cup (240 ml) of the broth, increase the heat and bring to a boil, then reduce the heat to a simmer, stirring gently but continuously to prevent the porridge at the bottom of the pot from sticking and burning. Add the remaining 2 cups (480 ml) broth and lower the heat to the minimum. Continue cooking for 15 to 20 minutes, stirring every few minutes to avoid burning. When the texture resembles oatmeal, the porridge is done. Remove from heat.
4. To prepare the garnish, place a small pan over medium heat and add the pine nuts. Toast them, stirring frequently, until they turn golden and fragrant, 2 to 3 minutes. Transfer to a small bowl. Slice the scallion at a 45-degree angle into four to six pieces.
5. Serve the porridge in individual bowls. Garnish each bowl by sprinkling with sesame seeds, drizzling on the sesame oil, and arranging the pine nuts and scallions over the top. Add a few drops of soy sauce, if you like, to bring a delicious flavor to the dish.

TIPS

While blending the vegetables in the food processor, if you notice any chunks clinging to the sides or stuck on the surface, turn off the processor and use a spatula to push the chunks into the mixture. Secure the top of the processor and pulse a few more times.

As a variation to help digestive woes, I recommend the combinations of sea greens and radish or mushrooms and oat in place of the carrots and cabbage.

As an aid after fasting, consider making this porridge with twice as much magnesium broth as the recipe calls for. This variation will make your fasting recovery easy, fast, and smooth.

Broths, Porridge, and Soups

Sea Greens and Shiitake Soup

MAKES 2 SERVINGS

Imagine a humble pot of rice that holds within it a secret elixir known as rice water. This magical concoction not only quenches your thirst but also comes with a bundle of benefits. It's a hydration hero, providing a soothing embrace for your digestive system when you're feeling under the weather. Packed with energy-boosting carbohydrates, it provides a quick recharge for your body. Rice water has a nutty, milky flavor, and can be used as a nutritious vegan broth to add to soups, chili, and curries.

Sea greens, often underestimated in Western diets, do more than just support bone health. They're fantastic for your skin, hair, and gut and are packed with omega-3 fatty acids.

This recipe keeps things simple yet delicious, and you will learn a simple technique to preserve the crunchy texture of the sea greens and avoid sliminess.

½ cup (80 g) dried miyeok (wakame)
1 tablespoon black sesame oil
1 garlic clove, minced
½ cup (50 g) thinly sliced shiitake mushrooms
3 to 4 collard green leaves
½ cup (60 g) shredded Korean white radish
4 cups (1 L) rice water (recipe follows), plus more as needed
2 tablespoons liquid aminos
Salt
Cracked black pepper

FOR GARNISH

3 tablespoons microgreens
Cold-pressed black sesame oil
Immortal Root Kimchi (page 132)

1. In a medium-sized bowl, add 5 cups (1.2 L) of cold water to the miyeok. Allow the seaweed to hydrate for 5 to 10 minutes, then drain and firmly squeeze it to remove excess water.
2. In a large pot over medium heat, add the sesame oil and garlic, and sauté for 2 to 3 minutes. Add the hydrated seaweed and sauté for 2 to 3 minutes until almost dry. Add the mushrooms, collard greens, and radish, and sauté for 5 minutes, adding a little rice water if the ingredients get too dry.
3. Pour in half of the rice water and bring the mixture to a simmer. Add the liquid aminos, and season with salt and pepper. Add the remaining rice water and return to a simmer for 3 to 5 minutes. Cover, lower the heat to the minimum, and let it cook for 10 minutes more.
4. Serve in soup bowls. Garnish with the microgreens and a few drops of the black sesame oil on top and the kimchi on the side.

How to Make Rice Water

Place 2 cups (370 g) sushi rice in a large bowl in the sink. Add enough water to cover the rice, gently stir by hand, rinse, and drain. Repeat this process two or three times, then drain all the excess water. Add 4 cups (1 L) filtered or spring water to the rice and gently massage the rice until the water turns milky. Pour the milky water through a strainer into another bowl. This liquid is the rice water. Use immediately or store the rice water in the freezer for a future meal.

And keep in mind that rice water also can be used as a gentle toner, leaving your skin glowing and radiant. It's also a haircare hero, strengthening your locks and giving them a glossy finish.

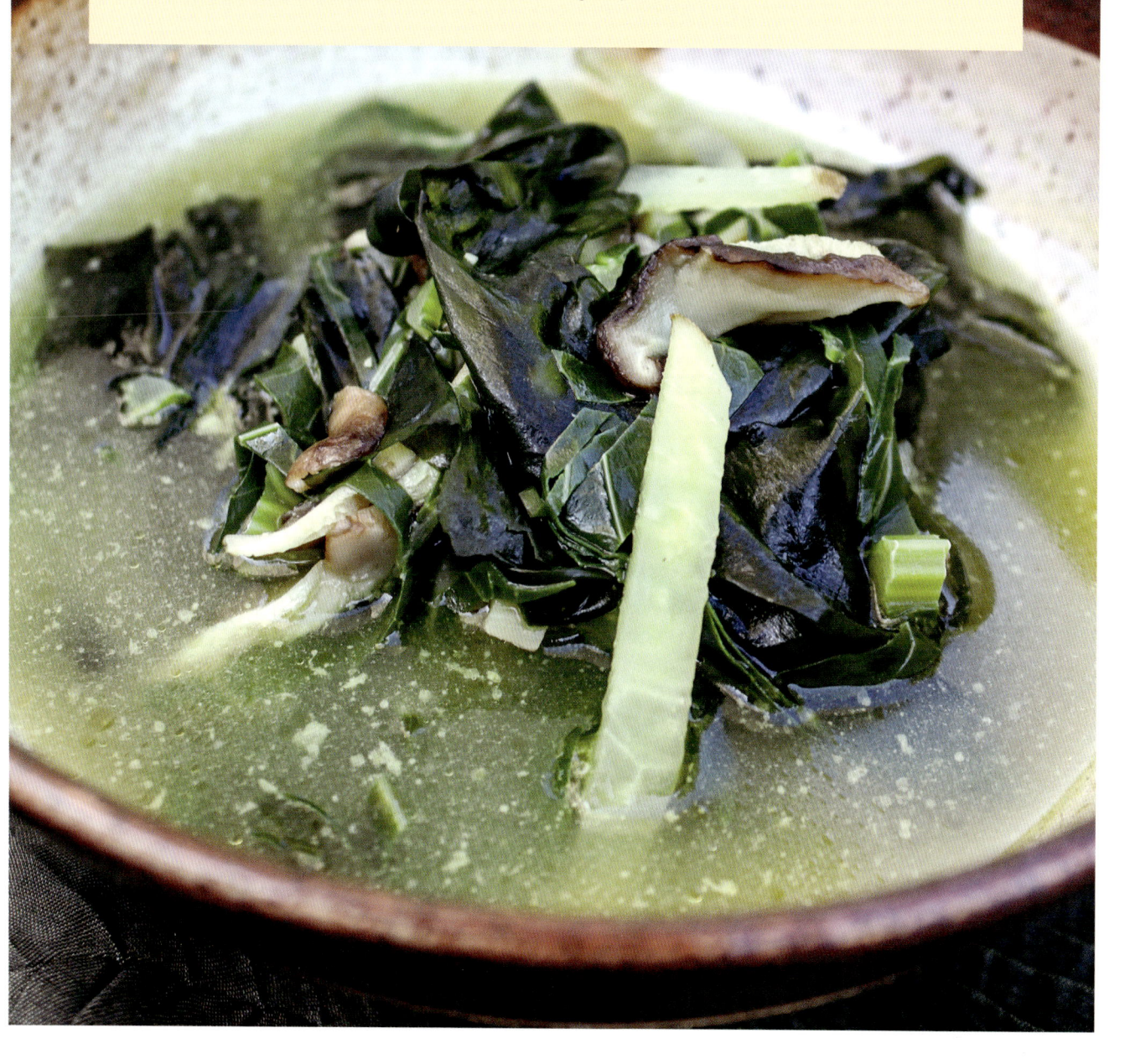

Tomato Soup with Basil and Capers

MAKES 2 SERVINGS

If you close your eyes and sip this soup, you won't believe it's a dairy-free vegetarian dish. The combination of sweet basil, tomato, coconut milk, capers, and a dash of maple syrup creates a rich, classic tomato soup flavor. The capers and maple syrup also help to balance out any bitterness from the tomatoes. Crunchy croutons bring a playful and fun texture, and lava salt adds another layer of smoky complexity to the dish.

According to the principles of Traditional Chinese Medicine's Five Elements, consuming tomatoes during late spring and summer is ideal for cooling the body. If you choose to enjoy them during other seasons, incorporating ingredients like onions and garlic, the fire-food properties, can help neutralize the temperature and maintain balance and grounding.

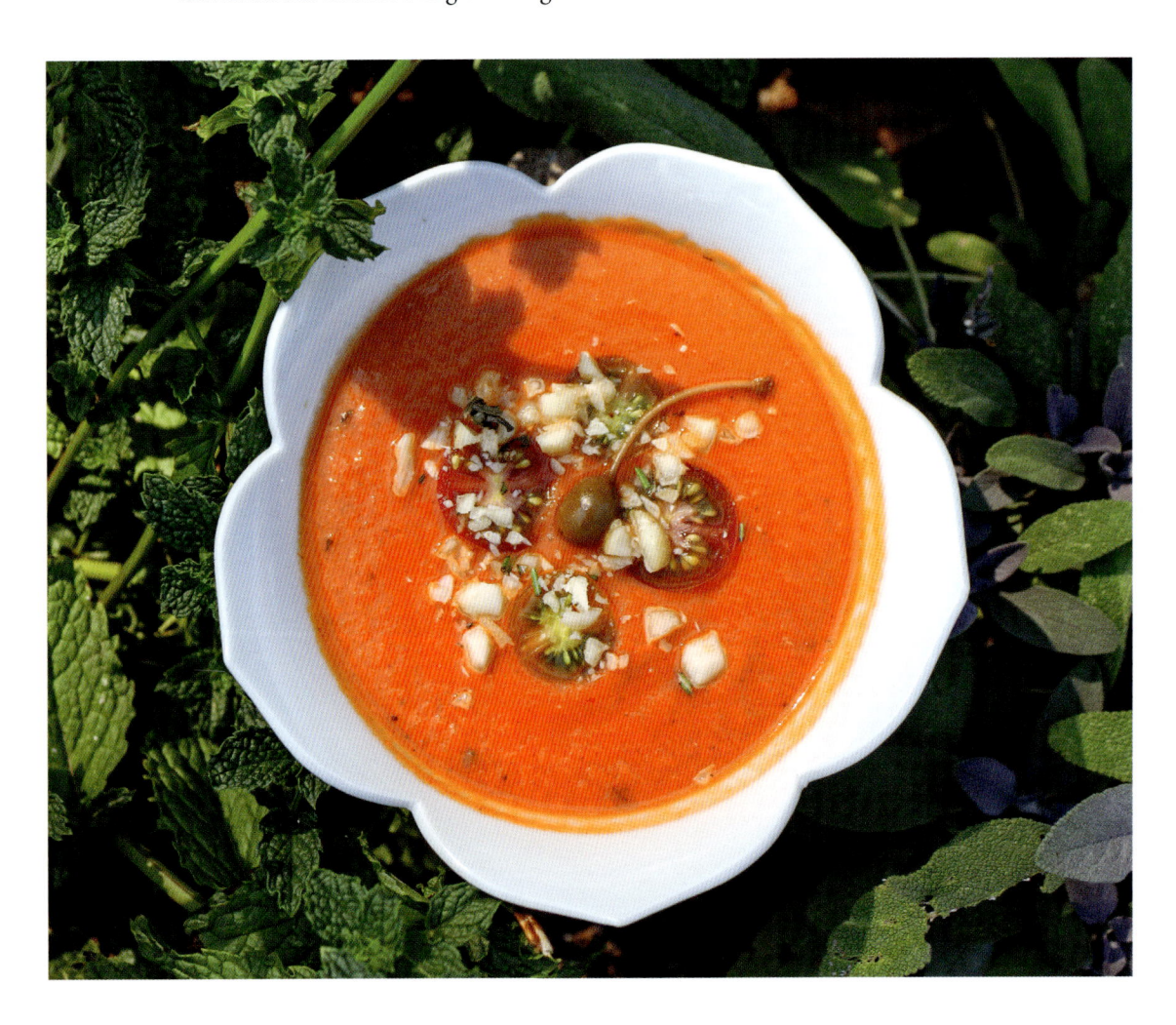

½ medium Yukon Gold potato
½ small carrot
½ celery rib
½ shallot
1 garlic clove
2 teaspoons drained capers
2 tablespoons ghee or extra-virgin olive oil
⅛ teaspoon dried basil
1½ cups (350 ml) canned tomato puree
2 bay leaves
1½ cups (350 ml) filtered water or Root and Leaf Magnesium Broth (page 177)
2 teaspoons tomato paste
3 tablespoons coconut milk or vegan cream
2 teaspoons maple syrup
⅛ teaspoon lava salt
Cracked black pepper
Ground cinnamon

FOR GARNISH

Cherry tomato halves
Crushed macadamias
Finely chopped fresh rosemary
Sourdough croutons (see Tips)

1. Preheat the oven to 400°F (200°C). Roughly chop the potato, carrot, celery, and shallot, and crush the garlic. Mince the capers.
2. In a cast-iron pot over low heat, add the ghee, shallot, garlic, and basil. Allow the herb flavors to infuse into the ghee for 1 to 2 minutes, turn the heat to high, and sauté for another 1 to 2 minutes to create a smoky flavor. Turn the heat to medium, add the potato, carrot, and celery, and sauté for about 3 minutes. Add the tomato puree and 1 of the bay leaves, and bring the mixture to a simmer. Then add the water or broth, capers, tomato paste, and the other bay leaf. Bring it to a simmer again. Stir in the coconut milk and maple syrup and simmer until the liquid is reduced by about two-thirds, 5 to 8 minutes. The longer you let the soup slowly cook over low heat, the richer the flavor will be. When the liquid is reduced, remove from the heat and allow to cool for 10 to 15 minutes.
3. Pour the soup into a large blender and blend. For a country-style soup with rough chunks, 1 to 2 minutes of blending should do. If you prefer a silky and well-blended texture that pairs perfectly with crunchy croutons, blend for 4 to 5 minutes. Season with the salt, and with pepper and cinnamon to taste.
4. Portion into two individual bowls and garnish with the cherry tomato halves and a sprinkle of crushed macadamias and chopped rosemary. Serve the croutons alongside for a delightful accompaniment.

TIPS

To make your own croutons, cut sourdough bread (preferably stale) into 1-inch (2.5 cm) cubes. Transfer the cubes to a baking sheet and drizzle with olive oil. Bake at 425°F (230°C) for 5 to 8 minutes or until they turn golden brown. Remove them from the oven and set them aside to cool down and become crunchy. Sprinkle chopped rosemary over the bread cubes.

For those following a flexitarian diet and seeking stronger bone-health nutrition, adding anchovy paste can be a wonderful choice. It imparts a complex flavor profile while providing high levels of bone-health nutrients. In fact, in Napoli, anchovy paste is considered a secret ingredient for enhancing the flavor of tomato sauce.

Is ghee healthier than butter? According to Ayurveda, yes! Ghee contains healthy fats that support digestion, strengthen the immune system, and provide essential vitamins. It also has anti-inflammatory and potential anti-cancer properties. Ghee enhances the richness of dishes without compromising flavor.

Broths, Porridge, and Soups

Sunrise Carrot-Ginger Soup

MAKES 2 SERVINGS

Carrots are the main star of this recipe, and they deserve more recognition than they get. Not only are they tasty, they also provide fiber, vitamin K1, and potassium. They contain beta-carotene, which converts into the antioxidant vitamin A, and they are a good source of several B vitamins. Fat improves the absorption of beta-carotene, so coconut oil completes the nutritional picture of this bright orange soup, which is sensational when topped with a green olive oil.

1 tablespoon ghee or avocado oil
2 or 3 thyme sprigs
⅛ teaspoon ground cumin
⅛ teaspoon ground turmeric
⅛ teaspoon ground ginger
1 small onion, roughly chopped
½ celery rib, roughly chopped
1 garlic clove, minced
4 medium carrots, roughly chopped
3½ cups (840 ml) filtered water or Root and Leaf Magnesium Broth (page 177)
1 bay leaf
5 tablespoons (75 ml) coconut milk
Salt
Ground black pepper
2 tablespoons sauerkraut (page 130)
1 tablespoon crushed pistachios

1. Heat the ghee in a medium pot and add the thyme, cumin, turmeric, and ginger. Cook for 1 minute, then add the onion, celery, and garlic. Cook for 2 to 3 minutes, then add the carrots. Sauté the mixture for 5 minutes. Pour in 1½ cups (350 ml) of the water or broth and increase the heat to high. Once it's simmering, add the remaining 2 cups (480 ml) water or broth and the bay leaf. Bring to a boil, then reduce the heat to medium-low, allowing the soup to simmer for another 10 to 15 minutes.

2. Watch for the carrots to become translucent. Once you see that change, add the coconut milk and cook for at least 1 to 3 minutes, and perhaps an additional 10 to 12 minutes. Keep an eye on the broth during this time and let it reduce until it barely covers the vegetables. This will give the soup the perfect texture after blending.

3. Pour the contents of the pot into a large blender. Blend the soup, starting at a low speed and gradually increasing to high, for 4 to 5 minutes, or until the mixture has a smooth, silky texture.

4. Ladle the soup into two individual bowls. Place a spoonful of sauerkraut at the center of the soup, and sprinkle the pistachios around the sauerkraut.

TIPS

You can scale up this soup recipe by as many as five times, then freeze the extra portions. The flavors will further develop, resulting in an even more delightful taste after thawing. It's a time-saving and convenient option for a light evening meal.

To add a decorative touch, make some Green Oil (page 143), replacing the walnut oil with extra-virgin olive oil. Drizzle the green oil in a circular pattern over the soup.

CHAPTER 15

Salad Meals

Let's dive into the world of salads—a personal favorite of mine. Sometimes I find myself eating so much salad that I wonder if there's such a thing as too much salad. The answer is no! Salads are the perfect dish to help you eat the rainbow, and as Laura and Helen explained in chapter 4, eating the full rainbow of colors found in veggies and fruits is one of the best ways to ensure that you're taking in the full range of flavonoids and other phytochemical superheroes that your bones and body need for vibrant good health.

This chapter also includes instructions for growing your own sprouts, something that I recommend everyone add to their kitchen routine. Sprouting seeds enhances nutrient availability, making them easier to digest and richer in vitamins and minerals. Sprouts also contain enzymes to promote digestion and contribute to better nutrient absorption. Sprouts, as part of a balanced diet, support overall wellness and provide a source of fresh, living nutrients according to macrobiotic principles.

I have sweet memories of watching my mother diligently cut fresh sprouts from a giant pot of greens every day. These sprouts would find their way into our salads and soups, becoming part of my flesh and bones. Looking back, the entire process of sprouting, all within the confines of our bustling urban household, contributed to our family's strength, health, and resilience.

Most of the recipes in this chapter yield two servings suitable for eating before a main course. But here's a tip: Simply double the portion size, and these salads become a main meal all on their own.

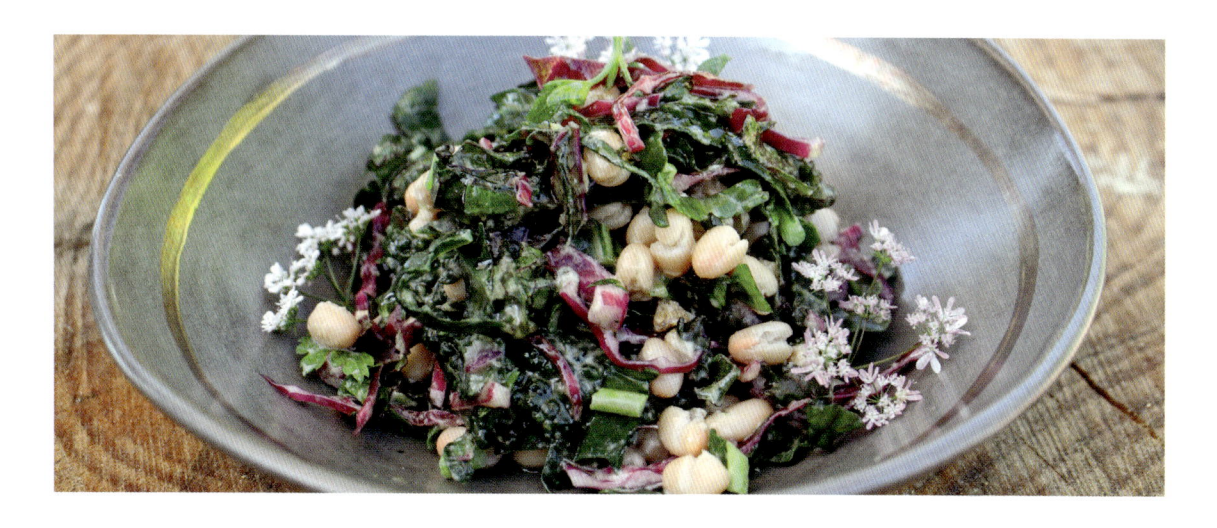

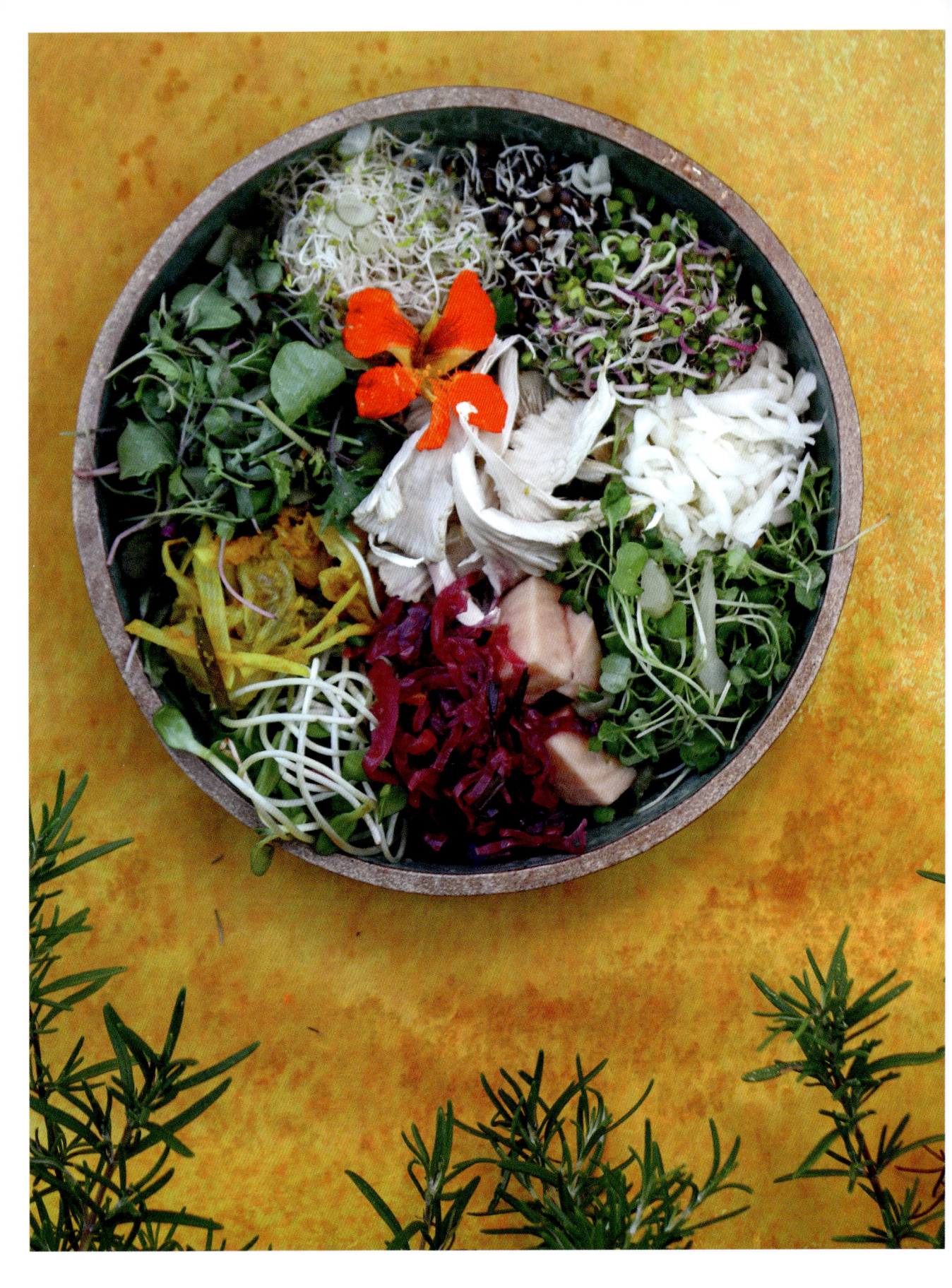

Ageless Macrobiotic Salad

MAKES 2 SERVINGS

This recipe is an example of a beautifully crafted, well-balanced macrobiotic dish, with the addition of slow-aged kimchi and pickles to enhance the vital force of whole foods that help balance the body and mind and increase vitality—thus, this salad can help you feel "ageless." Eating it may guide you toward a Zen-like, calming eating experience, awakening body and soul.

The contrast between extreme simplicity and dense nutrition, combined with the complex vinaigrette, makes this humble dish a perfect fit for busy lifestyles.

Handful sunflower sprouts
¼ cup (10 g) alfalfa sprouts
¼ cup (50 g) black lentil sprouts
¼ cup (10 g) radish sprouts
¼ cup (60 g) Pineapple-Turmeric Kimchi (page 134)
¼ cup (5 g) mixed microgreens
¼ cup (35 g) sauerkraut (page 130)
¼ cup (22 g) hand-shredded sun-soaked oyster mushrooms
1 tablespoon natto

FOR THE MISO-GINGER VINAIGRETTE

3 tablespoons extra-virgin olive oil
1 teaspoon mild white miso paste
½ teaspoon fresh lemon juice or any vinegar
¼ teaspoon grated lemon zest
⅛ teaspoon mustard seed
⅛ teaspoon ground ginger
½ garlic clove, minced
Sea salt
Cracked black pepper

1. Create the salad base by heaping the sunflower sprouts in the center of a large serving plate. Place the alfalfa, black lentil, and radish sprouts around the edges, as well as the kimchi, microgreens, sauerkraut, and mushrooms, forming a ring. Play around with arranging the differently colored sprouts on the plate to create fun contrasts. Sprinkle the natto on top.
2. Make the vinaigrette: In a small glass jar, combine the olive oil, miso, lemon juice, lemon zest, mustard seed, ginger, garlic, and a pinch of salt and pepper and shake well. Transfer the dressing to a separate bowl for serving alongside the salad.

TIPS

To turn this salad into a main dish, try adding Maple Syrup BBQ Tempeh (page 230) with extra mushrooms.

You can boost the bone-health quotient of this salad by garnishing it with protein-rich hemp seeds, sesame seeds, or soaked walnuts.

Salad Meals

Easy Breezy Home Sprouting

There's an incredible sense of preciousness and gratitude when you harvest your own food, transform it into a dish, and serve it to your own body and loved ones. Not only do you experience the joy of witnessing the sprouts' growth, but they also add a touch of beauty and decoration to your kitchen. Growing your own sprouts is cost-effective and a rewarding experience compared to buying them from the store. They grow like a weed and can add a delightful touch to your lunchtime salads, fill wraps and sandwiches, and garnish a wide variety of dishes. Radish sprouts in a glass jar with a sprouting lid can stay fresh in the refrigerator for 5 days.

Best Choices for Homegrown Sprouts

It's important to source high-quality organic seeds for sprouting. You can find these seeds online through organic seed companies or at local farmers markets. There are a wide variety of crops to choose from, making it an exciting time to explore the health benefits of sprouts. Look for:

alfalfa	dill	pumpkin
arugula	fenugreek	radish
beet	kale	spinach
black lentil	lettuce	sunflower
broccoli	mung bean	Swiss chard
cabbage	mustard	turnip
cilantro	pak choi	

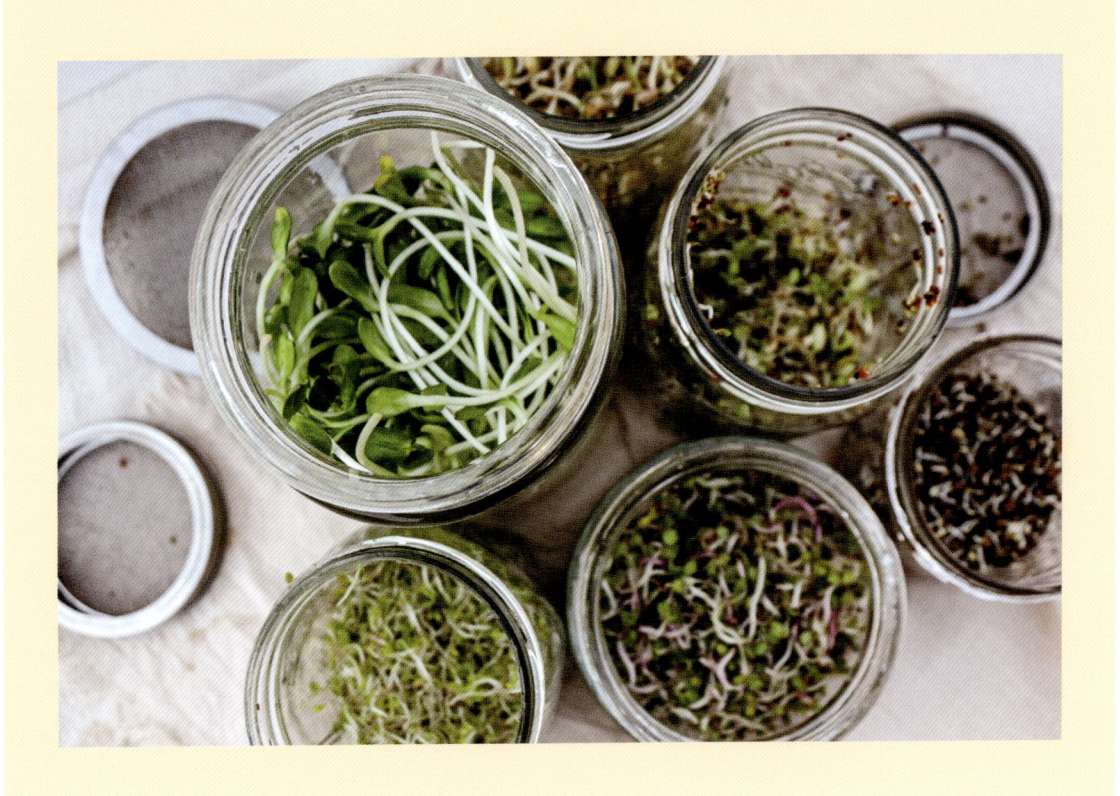

Home Sprouting 101

MAKES FIVE 1-QUART (1 L) JARS

Follow these instructions for growing delicious fresh sprouts. You can use any type of seed listed at left. Five types that sprout easily and grow fast are alfalfa, radish, mung bean, black lentil, and pumpkin.

1. Gather five 1-quart (1 L) canning jars and five airy sprouting lids. Choose five different types of seeds to sprout. Add 5 tablespoons of each seed to its own jar. Add 1 cup (240 ml) water to each jar, close the lid tightly, and label the jar with the date and seed type. Place the jars in a cool, shaded area in your kitchen for 24 hours.
2. After the seeds have soaked for 24 hours, drain the water from each jar. Rinse the seeds thoroughly with water and then drain the excess water again. To facilitate drainage, place the jars upside down at a slight angle. You can use a dish rack to support the jars while they are positioned upside down.
3. Repeat this rinsing and draining process once or twice daily for 3 to 5 days.
4. After 3 to 5 days, you'll notice sprouts emerging from the seeds. At this point, drain any remaining water and move the jars to the refrigerator. Keeps for 5 days.

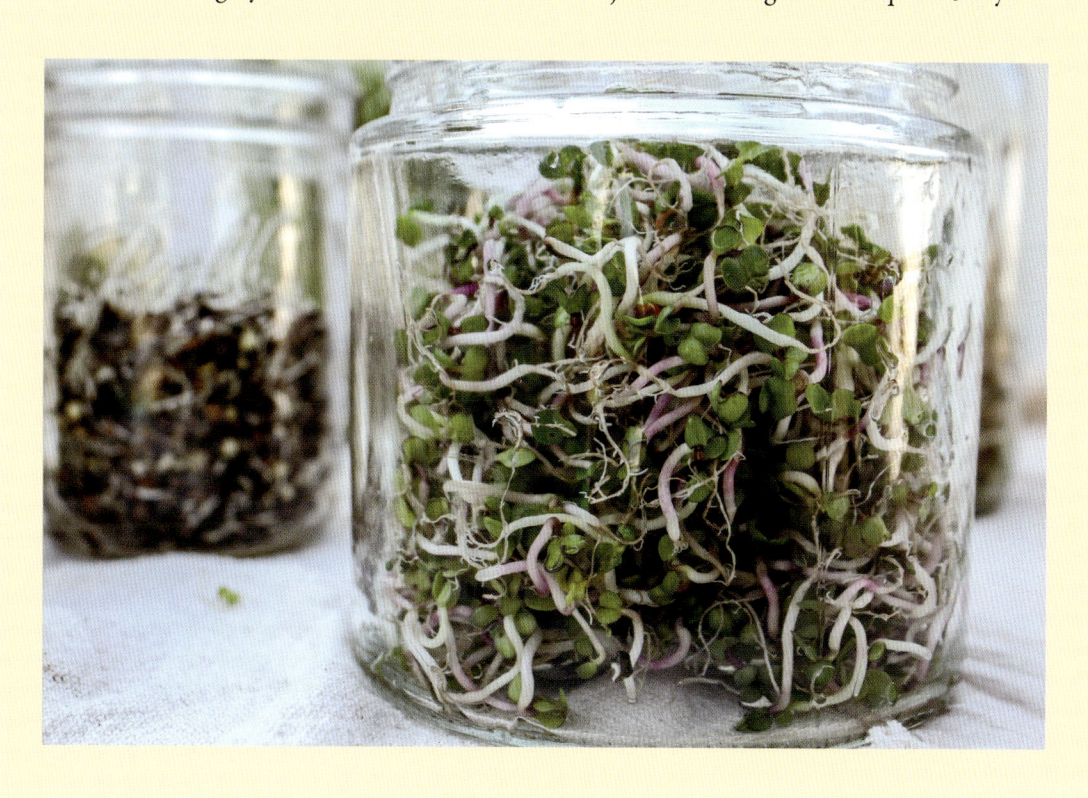

Chickpea-Cucumber Salad with a Hint of Mint

MAKES 2 SERVINGS

Farmers and gardeners have been growing chickpeas for over 7,000 years, making them one of the world's oldest cultivated crops. When this fiber- and protein-rich superfood meets juicy cucumber and apple on a hot day, the result is a perfect midsummer paradise salad that is also a well-rounded and satisfying meal.

This recipe makes two generous portions, so it's an ideal choice for a refreshing lunch in season. The dish's flavors, ranging from sweet to tangy, and its creamy textures come together beautifully, much like a jazz combo.

¼ cup (40 g) raw almonds
1 cup (240 g) canned chickpeas
½ medium apple, cored and cubed
½ cup (75 g) cubed English cucumber
6 red or green pitted olives, crushed
6 to 8 green grapes, halved
2 to 3 mint leaves, roughly chopped

FOR THE GREEN GRAPE VINAIGRETTE

½ cup (120 ml) fresh-squeezed green grape juice
¼ cup (60 ml) extra-virgin olive oil
1½ teaspoons fresh lemon juice
1 medium garlic clove, minced
1 teaspoon chopped capers
1 teaspoon mustard seed
¼ teaspoon grated lemon zest
Sea salt
Cracked black pepper

TO SERVE

Handful chopped mint leaves
3 grapefruit slices

1. Begin soaking the almonds 2 to 3 hours before mealtime (see page 47). After soaking, drain and peel the almonds (if they are not skinless).
2. Rinse and drain the chickpeas. Combine the almonds, chickpeas, apple, cucumber, olives, and grapes in a large bowl.
3. Make the vinaigrette: In a mini blender or small glass jar, combine the grape juice, olive oil, lemon juice, garlic, capers, mustard seed, lemon zest, and a pinch each of salt and pepper. Cover tightly and blend or shake until well mixed.
4. Pour the dressing over the chickpea mixture. Gently mix the ingredients together until they are evenly coated with dressing. At the last minute, stir in the chopped mint leaves. Serve immediately, over the grapefruit.

TIPS

To boost the protein content and make this a main meal, consider adding a poached egg or smoked tofu.

Substituting hibiscus tea or pomegranate juice for the grape juice will result in a vivid, deep red dressing packed with vitamin C.

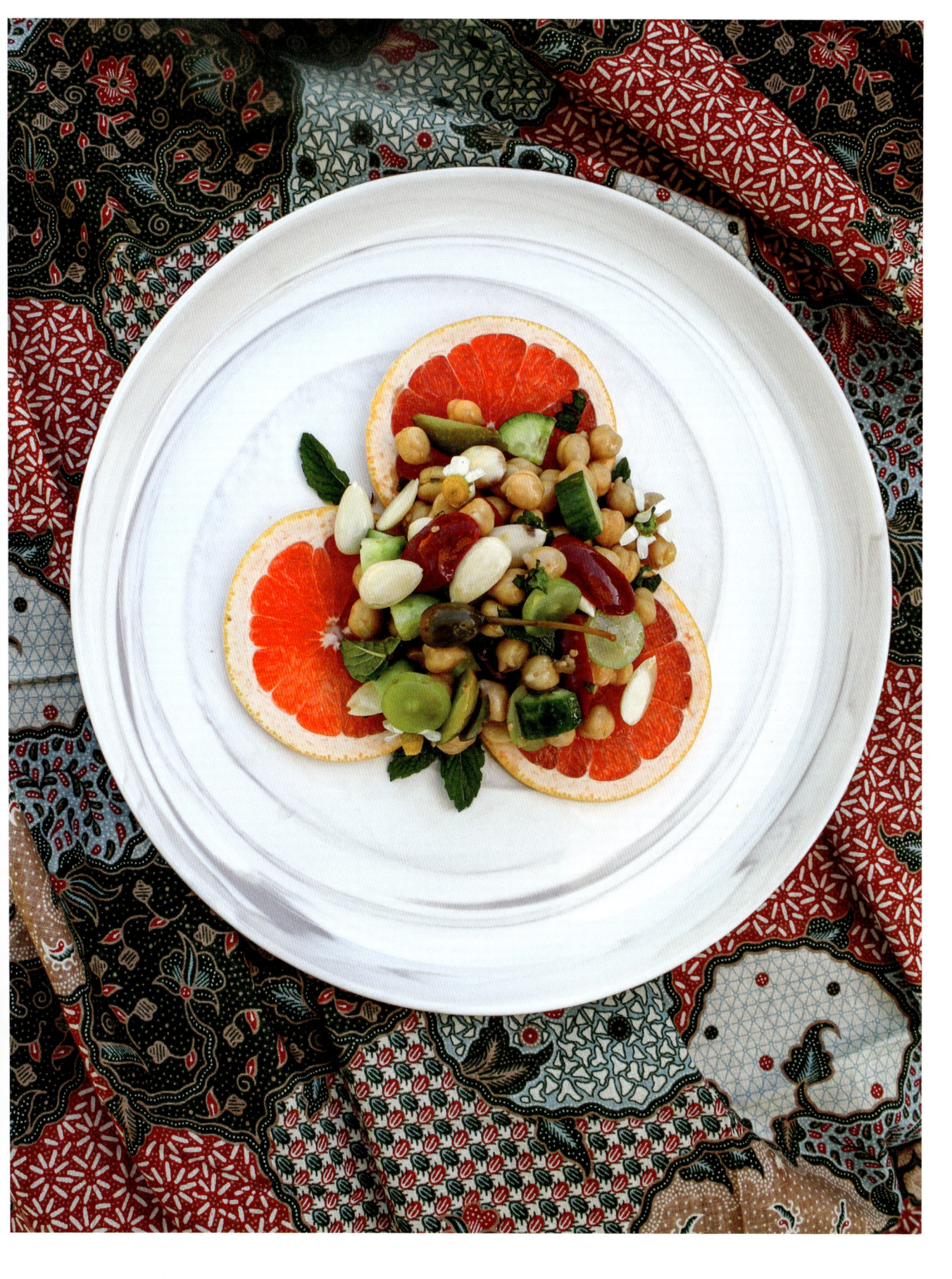

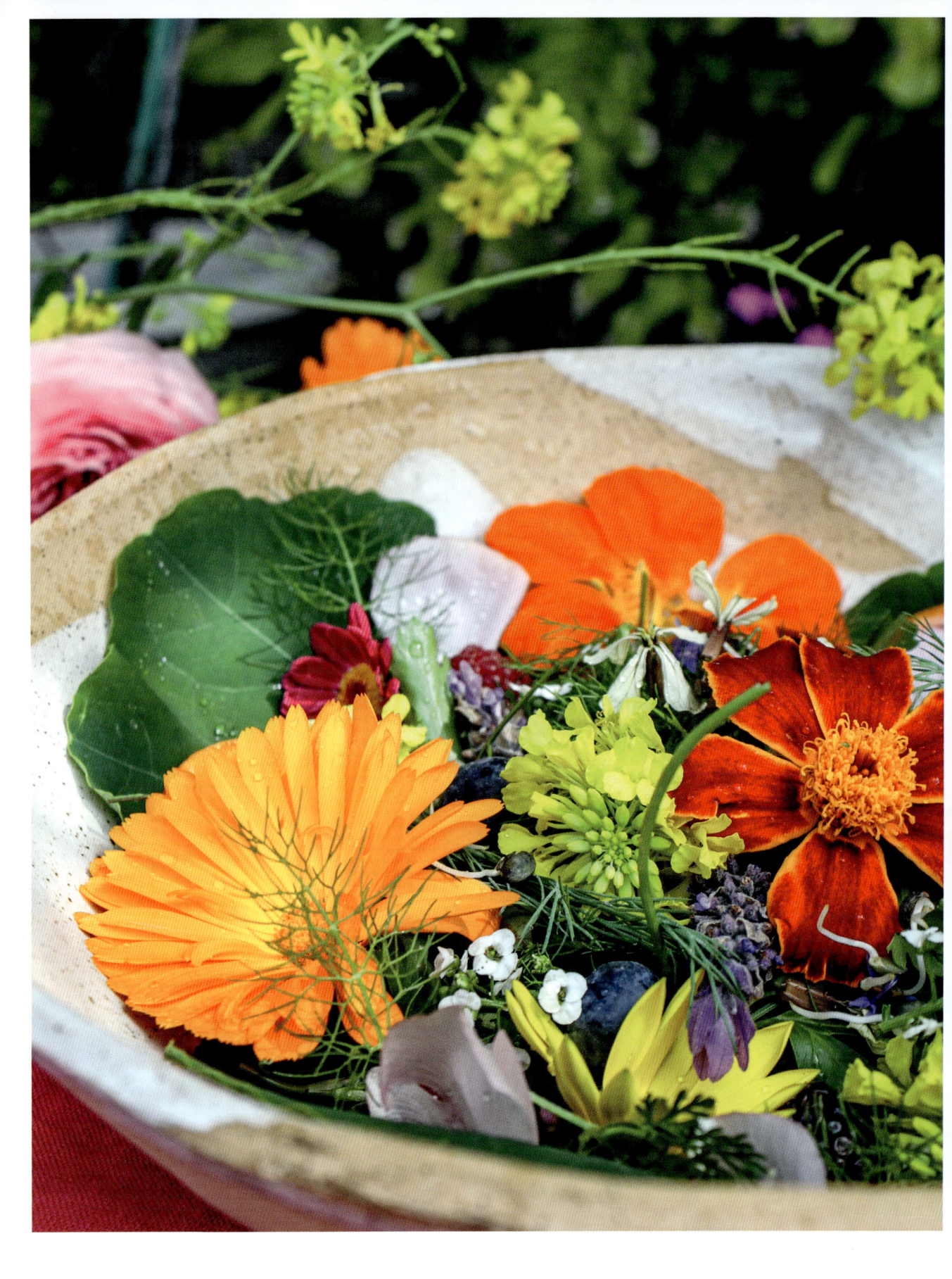

Herb and Wildflower Garden Salad

MAKES 2 SERVINGS

The average American consumes only five to ten types of vegetables. Such a limited diet could lead to nutritional deficiencies, which is one reason I use so many different kinds of vegetables and fruits in my salads.

One day I wondered, what if I created a salad *entirely* from fresh herbs? It turned out to be delicious and I felt incredibly energized and well. And the next day, I had the most impressive "emptiness practice" in the bathroom!

Try using basil, cilantro, parsley, dill, chives, and mint for starters, and add edible flowers such as mustard flowers, arugula flowers, and rosemary flowers. Just looking at the colors and beauty will make you hungry.

As with any fresh salad, be sure to clean off any soil or debris from your garden-fresh ingredients by washing them in water or wiping them with a wet cotton towel.

---

1 cup (25 g) mixed microgreens

A couple handfuls fresh herbs: basil, cilantro, parsley, dill, chives, mint, lemon balm, sage, fennel fronds

A couple handfuls edible flowers: rosemary flowers, calendula blossoms, lemon balm, rose petals, lavender flowers, nasturtium flowers and leaves, mustard flowers, dandelion leaves and flowers

¼ cup (40 g) wild or cultivated blueberries

¼ cup (35 g) blackberries or raspberries

6 blood orange slices

FOR THE BLOOD ORANGE–HAZELNUT OIL VINAIGRETTE

3 tablespoons hazelnut oil

1 tablespoon blood orange juice

1 teaspoon grated blood orange zest

1 teaspoon apple cider vinegar (page 136)

⅛ teaspoon Dijon mustard

Sea salt

Cracked black pepper

1. Arrange the microgreens at the center of a large serving bowl or platter. Distribute the herbs, flowers, blueberries, and blackberries along the edge and on top of the microgreens. Place the slices of blood orange around the edge as well.
2. Make the vinaigrette: Add the hazelnut oil, orange juice and zest, vinegar, mustard, and a pinch each of salt and pepper to a mini blender or small glass jar and blend or shake until well combined.
3. Drizzle the dressing over the salad and serve immediately.

TIP

If you live amid a bounty of wild berries, you are so fortunate. Take a moment to savor nature's gifts, ensure you identify the berries correctly, and be mindful to take only what you need. If wild berries aren't on your doorstep, seasonal farm-grown blueberries and blackberries work just as wonderfully in this salad. Embrace the flavors, whether they're handpicked from the wild or cultivated with care on a nearby farm.

Endive Canoes with Guacamole

MAKES 2 SERVINGS

Imagine a salad of miniature "canoes" you can eat with your fingers, savoring every bit. This creative salad recipe uses a surprising group of fermented and fresh vegetables along with guacamole as a delicious filling for Belgian endive leaves. Endive is a true warrior for bone health, and its high-fiber content aids digestion. When combined with sodium, the nutrients in endive can have a purifying effect for the body and the urinary tract.

The secret of how to make delicious guacamole is ridiculously easy: Add a good-quality unprocessed sea salt or salicornia. Salicornia—also known as salty sea green powder—is a plant that grows near the ocean. Despite its salty taste, it contains almost zero sodium, making it a great substitute for those on a low-sodium or cholesterol-conscious diet.

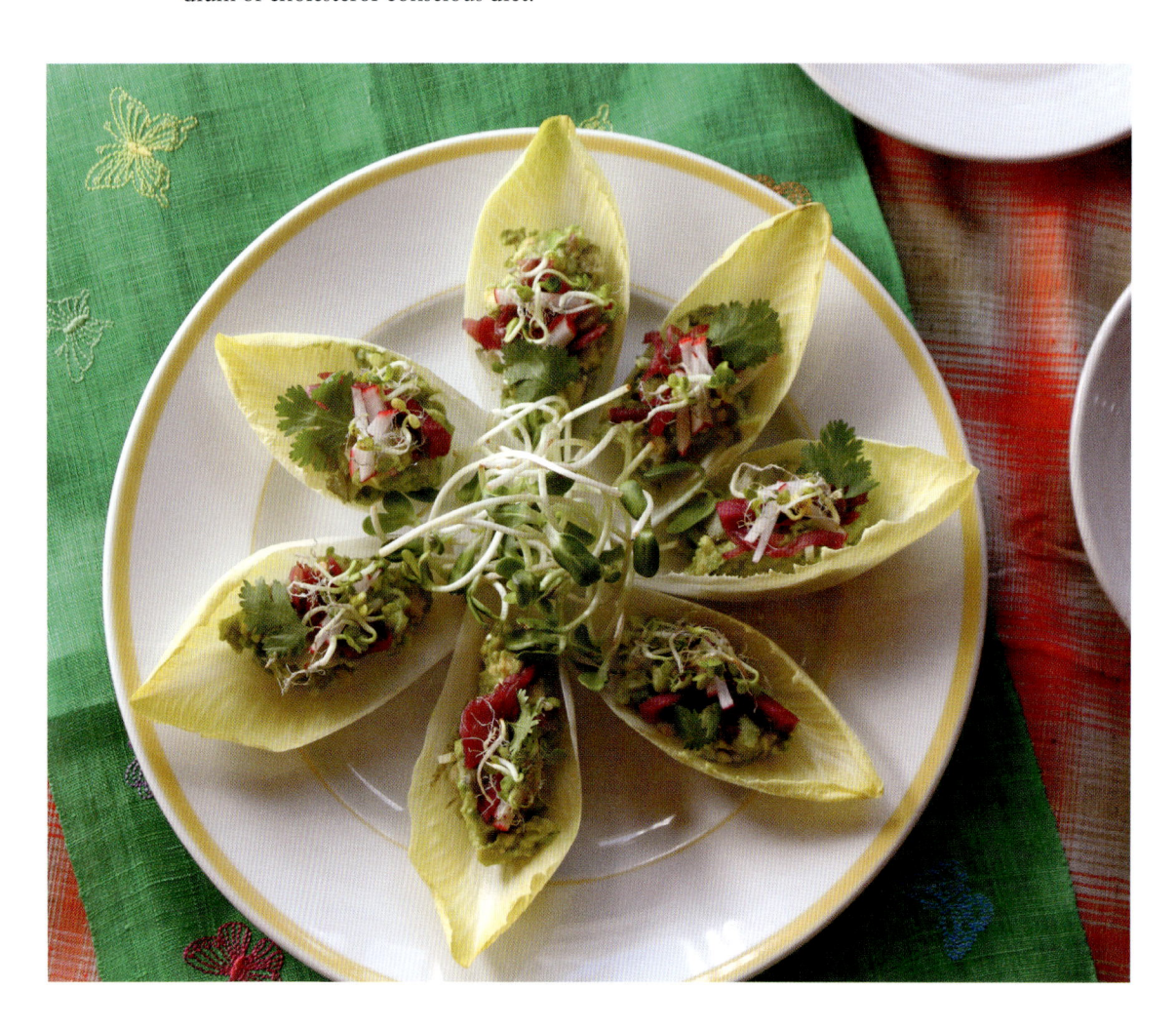

FOR THE GUACAMOLE

1 medium-sized ripe avocado
¼ teaspoon salicornia or salt
3 garlic cloves, minced
3 or 4 drops fresh lemon juice
Cracked black pepper

FOR THE ENDIVE CANOES

3 tablespoons sauerkraut (page 130)
   or store-bought sauerkraut
3 tablespoons radish sprouts
3 small red radishes, sliced thin
2 tablespoons minced pickled cucumber
2 tablespoons thinly sliced scallion
8 cilantro leaves
3 Belgian endive heads
   or small radicchio heads
2 tablespoons vegan sour cream (optional)

TIPS

If you're looking for appetizers or hors d'oeuvres for a dinner party or casual gathering, consider preparing this dish with varied toppings. For instance, you could scatter on some Tofu Sprinkles (page 208) or garnish with edible flowers for an elegant touch.

Endive is a delicate vegetable that needs to be stored in a cool, dark place, wrapped with a damp cloth to maintain its freshness.

1. Make the guacamole: Cut the avocado in half vertically. To remove the seed, gently strike the top of it with a knife, then twist to lift it out. Score the avocado flesh in a 1-inch (2.5 cm) grid, taking care not to pierce the skin. Use a spoon to scoop out the flesh, and place it into a small bowl.

2. Sprinkle the salicornia over the minced garlic and chop them together. The moisture from the garlic will help blend the seasoning. Press well to remove any clumps. Add the garlic mixture to the avocado. Mix and crush the avocado with a fork until you achieve a chunky texture. Sprinkle the guacamole with the lemon juice and the pepper. Set aside.

3. Make the canoes: On a plate, arrange the sauerkraut, radish sprouts, radish slices, pickles, scallions, and cilantro in separate piles. Trim about half an inch (12 mm) off the stem end of the endives and gently separate the leaves, one by one, until you have eight of roughly the same size (two or three leaves from each head). Avoid using the smaller leaves from the inside. (If using radicchio instead of Belgian endive, first clean the leaves as described on page 102.)

4. Take an endive leaf and fill it with guacamole. Place the sauerkraut, sprouts, and radishes on top of the guacamole, add the pickles and scallions, and garnish with a cilantro leaf. Add the sour cream, if using. Repeat this process for the remaining endive leaves.

5. On a serving plate, arrange the endive canoes in a floral or mandala-like pattern. In the center of this arrangement, add any remaining sprouts and pickles. Serve right away.

Fennel-Radicchio Salad

MAKES 2 SERVINGS

Whether in salad or in soup, the sweet licorice taste and fragrance of a fennel bulb can be captivating. In contrast, radicchio, a vibrant red leafy vegetable, has a distinctive bitter flavor. In this recipe, we'll bring together the sweetness and crunchiness of fennel and the bitterness of radicchio with colorful peppery radish sprouts. Finish it off with a drizzle of blood orange vinaigrette, and your salad will be a candidate for Julia Child's catchphrase: "Bon appétit!"

1 small head radicchio
1 fennel bulb
Handful radish sprouts
4 black grapes, halved
4 cherry tomatoes, halved
3 to 5 basil or mint leaves
Blood Orange–Hazelnut Oil Vinaigrette (page 203)
Shaved parmesan cheese (optional)

1. Cut the radicchio head into quarters lengthwise—each piece will have the shape of a small boat. If any soil is trapped between the radicchio leaves, rinse the pieces until there's no sign of dirt in the water. Drain them thoroughly, then transfer to a salad spinner and spin to remove excess water. Place the pieces in a medium bowl and set aside (see Tips).
2. To prepare the fennel, first trim off the root end and fronds. Slice the bulb in half from stem end to root end. Then slice the halves in half, resulting in four wedges. Use a mandoline to shave the wedges as thinly as possible (see Tips). Submerse the fennel slices in cold water to prevent browning. Drain well before continuing.
3. Combine the radicchio, shaved fennel, radish sprouts, and grapes in a large salad bowl and mix well.
4. To serve, place half the salad mix on each of two plates. Arrange the tomatoes freely to create a beautiful red contrast. Garnish with the herbs. Drizzle the vinaigrette over the salad or serve it on the side. Top with a little shaved parmesan, if you like.

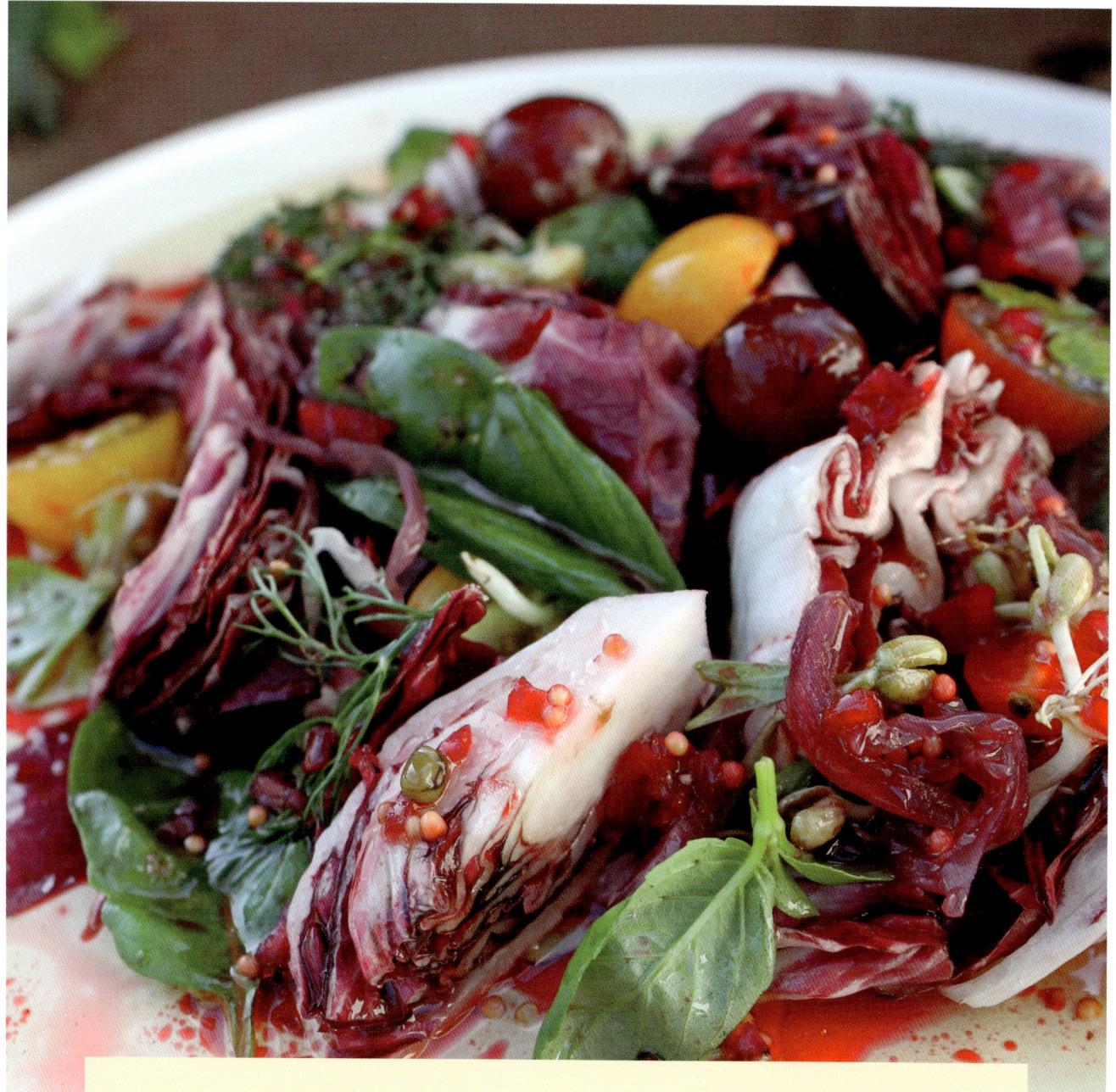

TIPS

Refrigerating the radicchio pieces for 30 minutes after you clean and drain them will enhance their crunchiness.

A mandoline can be one of the most dangerous tools in the kitchen. If you decide to use one, stay present and focused on what you are doing. Ask an experienced cook to show you the proper technique for using this type of slicer.

This is a fantastic base-camp salad. Using this recipe, you can venture in many directions to conquer the world of salads. Instead of radicchio, you can use a Belgian endive. Or you can use arugula or goma-ae (Japanese baby spinach), known for its sweetness and tenderness. Experiment with shredded zucchini, cut in long pieces like noodles, or shredded asparagus. Edible flowers are also a lovely topping for this salad. The possibilities are endless!

Happy-Go-Lucky Caesar Salad

MAKES 2 SERVINGS

Caesar salad is a change from an ordinary mixed greens salad, bringing exciting texture to the table. This recipe uses coconut milk instead of egg as the base of a creamy dressing, and substitutes tofu sprinkles for croutons. I like to do a 15-minute midday workout and then have this salad for lunch.

Instead of the usual small cubes of lettuce, here I cut the romaine into fancy, elongated sections. It is a beautiful presentation that also allows you and your guest to interact with the dish by eating the salad with your hands, like a taco.

FOR THE TOFU SPRINKLES

½ cup (120 g) firm tofu
1 tablespoon extra-virgin olive oil
1 tablespoon crushed soaked raw cashews
⅛ teaspoon dried basil or oregano
⅛ teaspoon ground ginger
Sea salt
Cracked black pepper

FOR THE COCONUT-LEMON CAESAR DRESSING

¼ cup (60 ml) coconut milk
2 or 3 fresh chives
½ garlic clove
¼ teaspoon fresh lemon juice

1 medium-sized head romaine lettuce
¼ teaspoon grated lemon zest

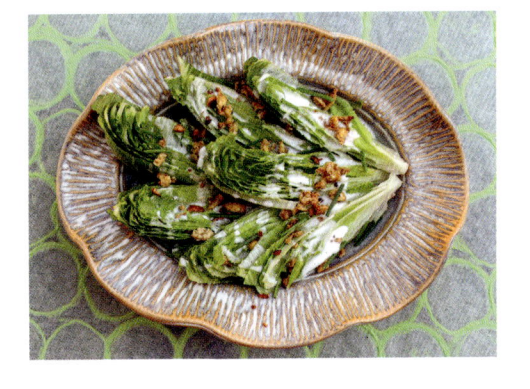

1. Preheat the oven to 425°F (220°C).
2. Make the tofu sprinkles: Wrap the tofu in a cotton cloth, and squeeze to remove excess water. Using your fingers, crumble it into a bowl and add the oil, cashews, basil, and ginger, and toss well. Transfer the mixture to a baking pan and season to taste with salt and pepper.
3. Put the tofu mixture in the oven and check every 5 minutes to assess the color of the tofu. When the tofu is crusty golden brown (which should take 10 to 15 minutes), remove from the oven and let it cool for 10 to 15 minutes.
4. Make the dressing: Combine the coconut milk, chives, garlic, and lemon juice to a mini blender and blend well for a creamy texture. Set aside.
5. Cut the romaine into quarters from stem end to tip end, then cut each quarter in half again to make eighths. On a large serving plate, arrange the narrow boat-shaped lettuce pieces, overlapping each other. Add the tofu sprinkles over the lettuce, then drizzle with the dressing. Sprinkle the lemon zest on top and serve.

> **TIP**
> A granite mortar and pestle is a good tool for crushing cashews thoroughly, almost to a dusty texture.

Kale, Cabbage, and White Bean Salad

MAKES 4 SERVINGS

Kale is my absolute favorite vegetable to grow. For me it's an old friend who always has my back. It thrives in any conditions and practically maintains itself. Grow kale to create a farm-to-table experience in your own backyard.

In this recipe, you will learn how to change kale's texture from rough to tender. Pairing this delicious green with cabbage and beans creates a protein-packed combo that's great for bone health. The creamy, nutty tahini in the dressing is another bone-health superstar. Add highly nutritious pumpkin seeds and goji berries as a garnish and you've got a Himalayan superfood mix.

FOR GARNISH

1 tablespoon pumpkin seeds
1 tablespoon unsweetened dried goji berries or black currants
Edible flowers such as cilantro flowers

FOR THE TAHINI-GINGER DRESSING

⅓ cup (85 g) tahini
6 tablespoons (90 ml) liquid aminos
1 tablespoon roughly chopped radish or celery
1 tablespoon rice vinegar
1 medium garlic clove, minced
½ teaspoon finely chopped fresh ginger
⅛ teaspoon freshly grated nutmeg
Sea salt
Cracked black pepper

FOR THE SALAD

2 cups (135 g) shredded kale
½ cup (35 g) shredded green cabbage
2 tablespoons extra-virgin olive oil
Sea salt
1 cup (275 g) white beans, canned or freshly cooked
1 tablespoon finely chopped fresh parsley

1. Prepare the garnishes in advance by setting the pumpkin seeds to soak in warm water for 30 minutes. Soak the goji berries or black currants for at least 30 minutes as well. After soaking, drain them thoroughly and set them aside.
2. Make the dressing: In a mini blender, combine the tahini, liquid aminos, radish, vinegar, garlic, ginger, nutmeg, and a pinch each of salt and pepper and blend until well mixed. Set aside.
3. Make the salad: Place the kale and cabbage in a large bowl. Add the olive oil, along with a light sprinkle of salt. Gently massage the greens for 5 minutes to tenderize them.
4. If using canned beans, rinse and drain them. Add the beans and the parsley to the greens and stir gently to combine. Drizzle the dressing over the salad and mix everything thoroughly, or you can serve the dressing separately. Serve, garnished with the pumpkin seeds, goji berries, and flowers.

TIPS

For a simple dish of kale and cabbage, marinate the greens in a mix of oil and fresh lemon juice in the refrigerator for a few hours or even a full day. The flavor and texture of the greens will improve as they sit.

By varying the toppings—such as adding tofu, soaked cashews, or hemp seeds—you can add more protein to this salad, making it a balanced main meal.

Salad Meals

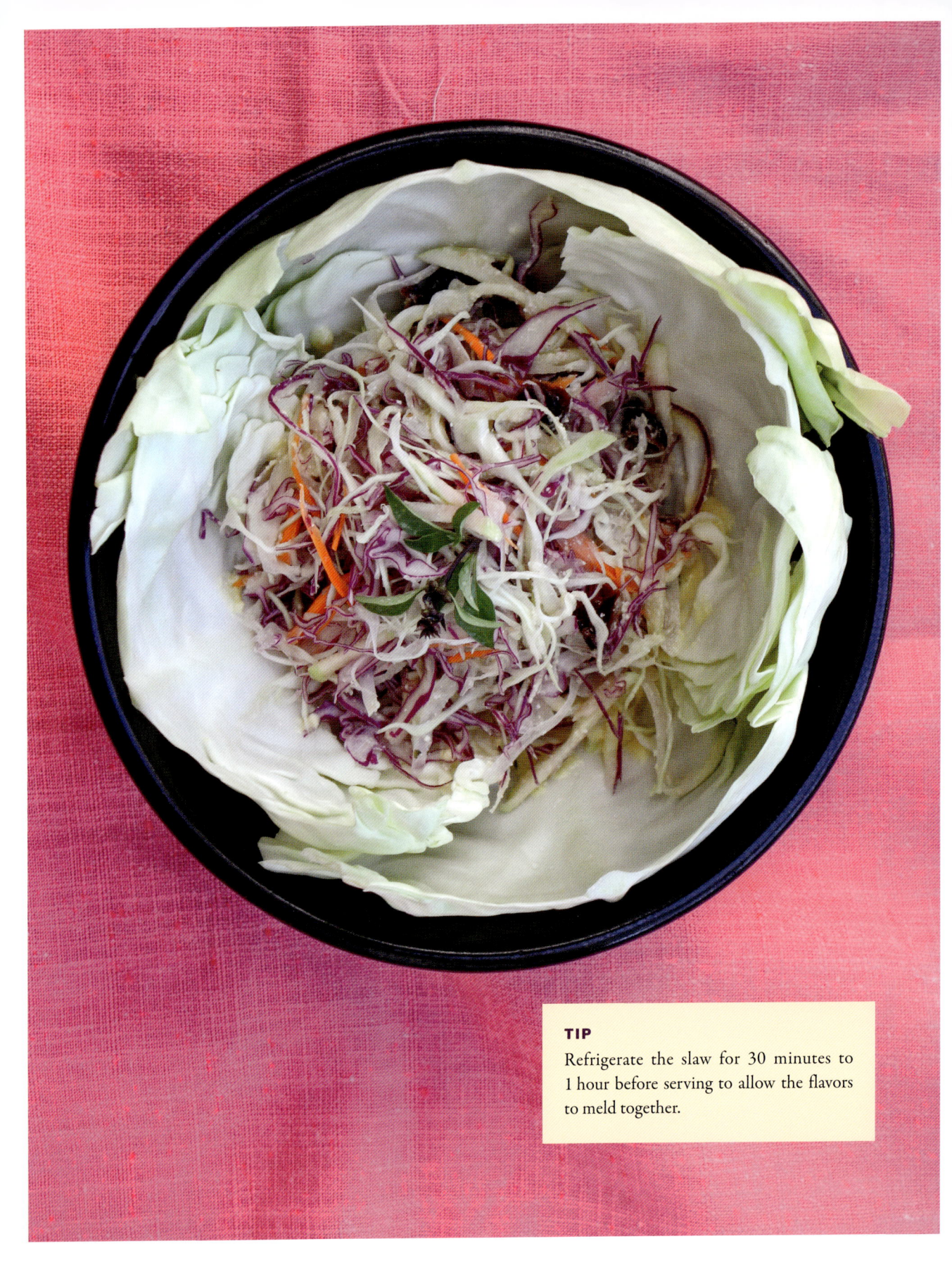

TIP

Refrigerate the slaw for 30 minutes to 1 hour before serving to allow the flavors to meld together.

New Classic Rainbow Coleslaw

MAKES 2 SERVINGS

Did you know that a cup of cabbage contains only about 25 calories? This ancient crop was once the primary food in some cultures due to its rapid growth and low water requirements. However, today cabbage is recognized for its content of vitamin C and vitamin K and because eating it may help reduce the risk of cancer and other health conditions.

Cabbage is the star of this easy-to-make colorful coleslaw recipe. It's a perfect refreshing complement to your summer grill dishes. This slaw can also be used as a filling for sandwiches, burgers, and wraps. A fresh pineapple dressing adds an extra burst of flavor and freshness.

This recipe also includes a great technique for hydrating shredded vegetables to make them extra crunchy. Cabbage can stay fresh for 2 to 3 weeks in the refrigerator, so I recommend you double, triple, or even quadruple the amount of slaw you make, and then you can enjoy it with different dressings at several meals.

½ cup (50 g) finely shredded red cabbage
½ cup (50 g) finely shredded green cabbage
¼ cup (30 g) finely shredded carrot
¼ cup (15 g) finely shredded white or red onion
¼ cup (31 g) finely shredded apple
Fresh lemon juice
2 tablespoons dried cranberries
2 tablespoons hemp seeds
2 tablespoons chopped fresh mint or parsley

FOR THE PINEAPPLE-CASHEW DRESSING

3 tablespoons raw cashews, soaked (see page 47)
⅓ cup (70 g) finely chopped pineapple
3 tablespoons vegan mayonnaise
1 teaspoon Dijon mustard
½ garlic clove
½ teaspoon sea salt
¼ teaspoon fresh lemon juice
Cracked black pepper

1. Fill a large mixing bowl halfway with water and add 1 cup of ice. Add the red cabbage, green cabbage, carrot, and onion to the ice water and let them soak for 15 to 30 minutes. Place the shredded apple on a small plate and drizzle with a squeeze of lemon juice to prevent browning (oxidation). Put the cranberries in a separate bowl with water and let them soak for 15 minutes, then drain them, and set them aside.
2. Make the dressing: In a mini blender, combine the cashews, pineapple, mayonnaise, mustard, garlic, salt, lemon juice, and pepper to taste and blend for 2 to 4 minutes, until smooth.
3. Drain the shredded vegetables and transfer them to a salad spinner. Spin until there's no more water coming out. Add the apples and mix them in.
4. Place the slaw in a serving bowl and top it with the cranberries, hemp seeds, and mint. Serve with the dressing on the side or mix the slaw with the dressing just before serving.

Salad Meals

Beefy Tomato Salad with Cherry Vinaigrette

MAKES 2 SERVINGS

Vibrant heirloom tomatoes and cherries from the farmers market capture the essence of a dreamy, hot summer day. These red fruits are cooling, a symbol of "fire" in Traditional Chinese Medicine, and packed with potent antioxidants, vitamins, and minerals. This recipe is incredibly simple yet delivers a delightful balance of savory and sweet tangy flavors. Pairing these ingredients with arugula can help restore your energy levels during the sweltering summer heat. The garnish of Brazil nuts adds texture and a boost of nutrients beneficial for bone health. With a slice of sourdough bread on the side, this salad is a perfect way to kick-start your meal.

Handful Brazil nuts, for garnish

2 medium-sized ripe heirloom tomatoes

3 baby red radishes

1 cup (20 g) baby arugula

3 tablespoons (32 g) ¼-inch (6 mm) cubes vegan feta cheese

6 basil leaves

FOR THE CHERRY VINAIGRETTE

6 fresh ripe cherries

3 tablespoons extra-virgin olive oil

1 tablespoon rice vinegar or apple cider vinegar

¼ teaspoon minced garlic

⅛ teaspoon mustard seed

Fresh lemon juice

Sea salt

Cracked black pepper

1. Put the Brazil nuts in clean water in a bowl and leave to soak for 30 minutes, then rinse them under running water, drain well, and crush into small pieces. Set aside.
2. Gently slice the tomatoes into ¼-inch-thick (6 mm) slices and slice the radishes thinly. Set these ingredients aside.
3. Make the vinaigrette: In a small bowl, pit the cherries and then crush the fruit. In a blender or small glass jar, combine the crushed cherries, olive oil, vinegar, garlic, mustard seed, a squeeze of lemon juice, and a pinch each of salt and pepper. Secure the lid and blend or shake the ingredients well for 1 to 3 minutes, until the color turns a dark pinkish-red.
4. On a serving plate, arrange the tomato slices in a circle, leaving the center of the plate empty. Place the arugula in the center. Top the arugula with the vegan feta, radish slices, and basil. Garnish with the Brazil nuts just before serving, with the cherry vinaigrette on the side.

TIPS

If you'd like this salad to play the role of a main dish, simply double the portion size and add your favorite protein.

You can substitute 3 to 4 tablespoons blueberries for the cherries in spring and summer, or the same amount of fleshy pomegranate seeds in early fall through early winter.

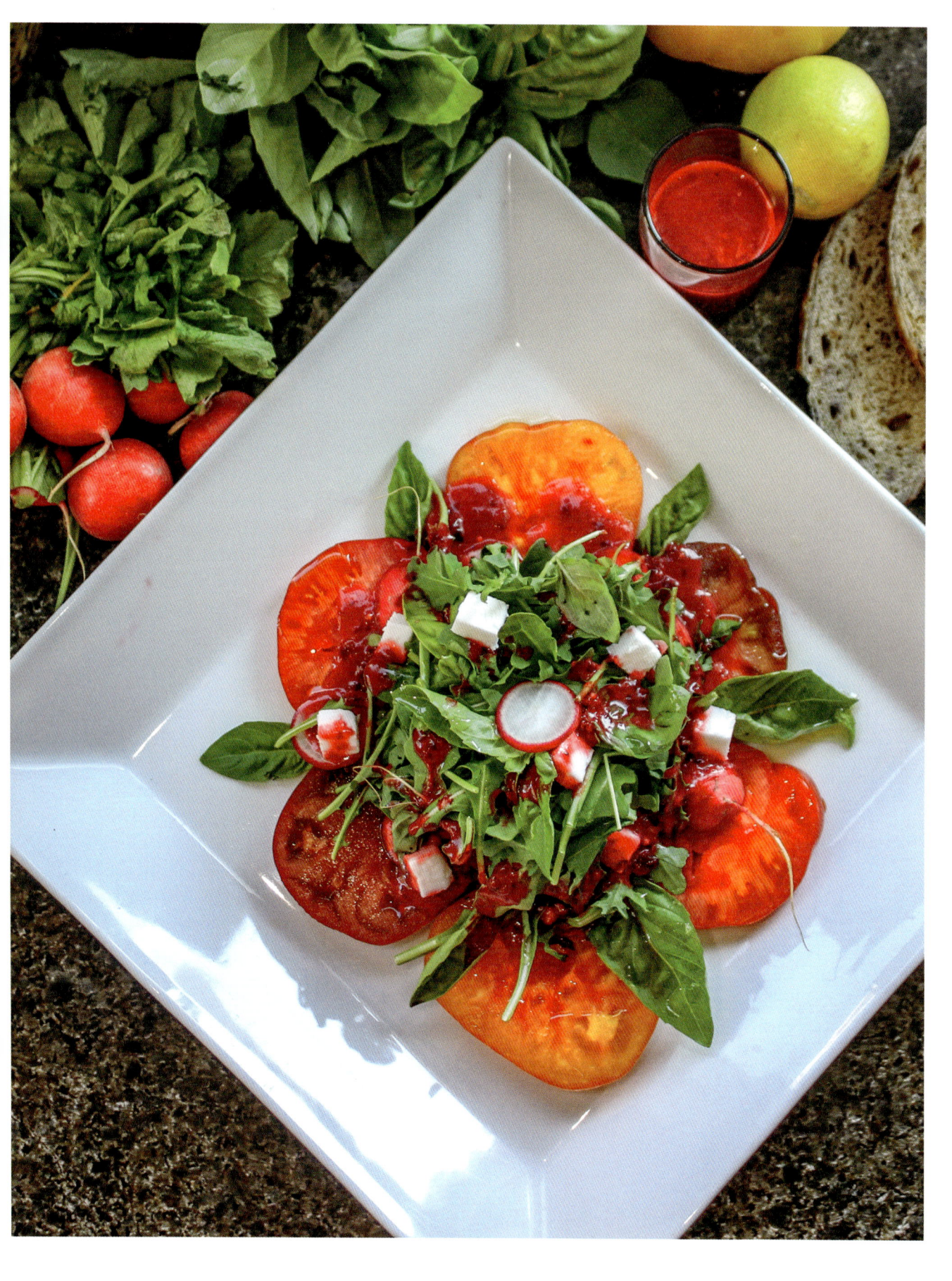

Seaweed Flower Cucumber Salad

MAKES 2 SERVINGS

Here's a fascinating fact. Seaweed, or as some call it, sea greens, can grow 300 times faster than land plants do. So by adding seaweed to your daily meals, you're helping reduce your carbon footprint. It's a win-win for you and our dear Mother Earth.

This recipe features seaweed salad. There are many brands; I like one called Kaneyama Seaweed Flower Salad. These sea greens are perfect for salads because they are light, crunchy, and smooth but never slimy. They are highly nutritious, too, nourishing your skin, hair, and gut.

1 cup (210 g) dry seaweed salad
4 tablespoons (60 ml) rice vinegar
1 Persian cucumber
3 baby red radishes
1 garlic clove
Sea salt
1 tablespoon sesame oil
½ scallion, chopped
2 teaspoons liquid aminos
1 tablespoon hemp seeds
½ teaspoon ground ginger
Green salt
Radish sprouts, for garnish
Immortal Root Kimchi (page 132), for garnish

1. In a medium-sized bowl, add cold water to the dry seaweed. Allow the seaweed to hydrate for 5 to 10 minutes. Drain and firmly squeeze to remove excess water. Place the hydrated seaweed back into the bowl. Add 2 tablespoons of the rice vinegar and massage for 2 to 3 minutes. This process will remove any oceanic smell and prevent the seaweed from having a slimy texture. Rinse the seaweed to remove the vinegar completely, then squeeze out all excess water.

2. Cut the cucumber and radishes into julienne slices: Cut thin slabs at an extreme diagonal across the vegetable. Stack a few of these slabs together and then carefully cut them again into thin strips. Add to the bowl with the seaweed.

3. Smash the garlic clove on a cutting board, remove the skin, and sprinkle with salt. Mince until the garlic turns nearly liquid, then transfer it to a small bowl. Add the remaining 2 tablespoons rice vinegar, the sesame oil, scallion, coconut aminos, hemp seeds, ginger, and a pinch of green salt, and mix well.

4. Top the salad with the dressing and blend well. Garnish with a handful of radish sprouts and some kimchi.

TIPS

To add a touch of sweetness and diversify the texture of this salad, try adding shredded green apple, shredded pear, or thinly sliced persimmon. For a tart flavor, add a few black currants.

CHAPTER 16

Main Meals

You can turn everyday comfort dishes into extraordinary meals in a simple, straightforward way, with a dash of fun and creativity. Many of the dishes in this chapter are remakes of meat-based favorites, including meatballs with no meat and cauliflower roasted with hearty spices to evoke the flavor of a well-cooked steak. Learning to prepare these recipes will boost your culinary confidence with results that deliver outstanding beauty, rich flavors, and a harmonious balance of nutrition on one plate.

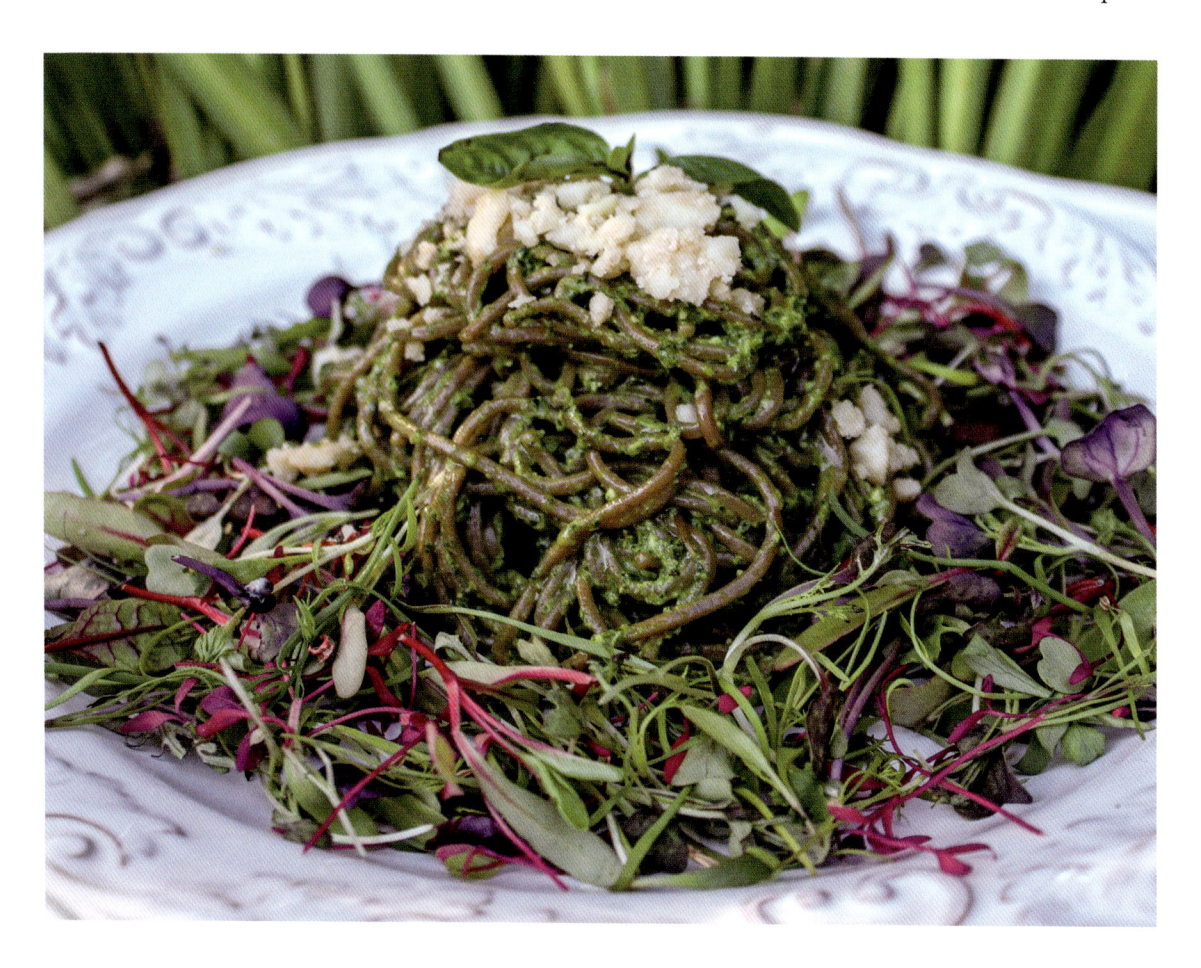

Acorn Squash with Forbidden Rice Stuffing

MAKES 2 SERVINGS

This exquisite dish can be your signature creation, perfect for impressing loved ones and guests during special gatherings. I've nicknamed it the "Falling in Love with Fall" dish.

The initial wow factor of this recipe is its vibrant colors. Sweet and nutty squash pairs wonderfully with high-protein forbidden rice, adding a nice texture. The dish is brought together with a coconut-orange ranch dressing that will undoubtedly make you say yes!

> **TIPS**
>
> I love to take a trip to a pumpkin farm in the fall, and when I do, I turn this dish into roasted stuffed pumpkin, substituting brown rice or quinoa for the forbidden rice in the stuffing. It is equally delicious, and even sweeter.
>
> Adding 2 to 3 tablespoons of Pineapple-Turmeric Kimchi (page 134) to the stuffing makes it both sweet and sour, which is lovely for a cooler-weather dish.

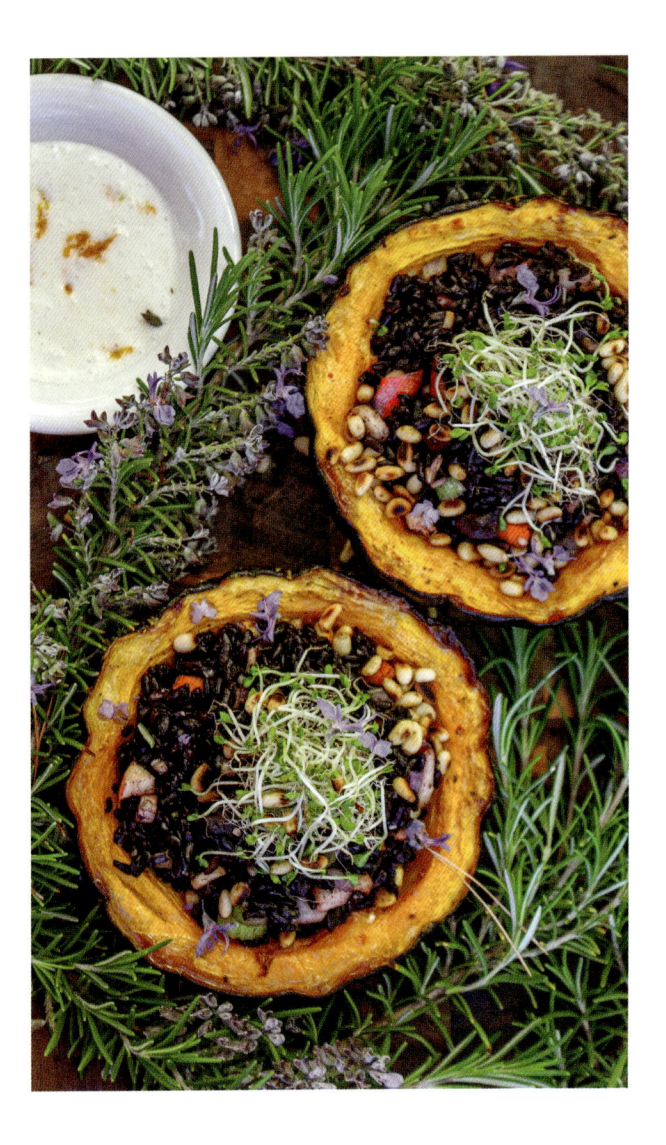

1 acorn squash (about 5 inches [13 cm] diameter)
1 tablespoon sunflower oil
⅛ teaspoon ground cinnamon
Sea salt
Cracked black pepper

FOR THE RICE STUFFING

1 cup (200 g) forbidden rice, soaked for 30 minutes
2 cups (480 ml) filtered water
3 to 4 ounces (90 to 120 g) dried licorice root, sliced
2 tablespoons crushed soaked walnuts
1 tablespoon psyllium
1 tablespoon chopped sun-bathed mushroom
1 tablespoon minced apple
1 tablespoon minced celery
1 tablespoon minced red onion or shallot
1 tablespoon minced carrot
1 tablespoon hemp seed oil
1 tablespoon liquid aminos
1 tablespoon nutritional yeast
Sea salt
Cracked black pepper

FOR THE ORANGE-COCONUT RANCH DRESSING

⅓ cup (80 ml) coconut milk
3 tablespoons fresh orange juice
2 tablespoons hemp seed oil
1 tablespoon hemp seeds or toasted pine nuts
1 medium garlic clove
⅛ teaspoon fennel seed
Lava salt
Cracked black pepper
1 teaspoon grated orange zest

FOR GARNISH

Handful broccoli sprouts
Handful sauerkraut (page 130)
2 tablespoons toasted pine nuts

1. Preheat the oven to 375°F (190°C). Cut the acorn squash in half horizontally, remove the seeds, and place the halves, cut side up, on a baking sheet. Drizzle with the sunflower oil, sprinkle with the cinnamon, and lightly season with salt and pepper. Roast for 20 to 30 minutes or until they turn a beautiful golden brown.

2. Make the rice stuffing: Drain the soaked rice and transfer it to a medium pot. Add the water, licorice root, walnuts, and psyllium. Cook on high heat until it simmers, 10 to 15 minutes, then reduce the heat to the lowest setting and cook for another 5 to 10 minutes. The rice will continue to cook after it is removed from the heat, so stop cooking while there's still some liquid in the rice. Turn off the heat, fluff with a fork, and let it steam, covered, for 10 to 15 minutes.

3. Transfer the warm rice into a medium bowl and add the chopped mushrooms, apple, celery, onion, and carrot along with the hemp seed oil, liquid aminos, and nutritional yeast. Gently stir the mixture a few times and season lightly with sea salt and pepper. Set the stuffing aside.

4. Make the dressing: In a small blender, combine the coconut milk, orange juice, hemp seed oil, hemp seeds, garlic, and fennel seed. Blend for 3 to 5 minutes, until smooth. Stop the blender and season with lava salt and pepper, blending briefly to incorporate the seasoning. Transfer the dressing to a small sauce bowl and top with the orange zest.

5. Place the roasted squash halves on serving plates, fill the cavities with the rice stuffing, and garnish with broccoli sprouts, sauerkraut, and pine nuts. Serve with the dressing on the side.

Main Meals ▪ 217

BBQ Jackfruit Tacos with Mango Salsa

MAKES 2 SERVINGS

Wrapping anything in a tortilla seems to make it taste better, including jackfruit, an exotic fruit with a surprisingly meaty texture. Did you know jackfruit is the largest fruit on planet Earth? Beyond its incredible taste and texture, it is one of the most nutritious fruits, too—it contains more protein than similar fruits, as well as vitamins and minerals. Jackfruit is rich in magnesium, which is important for the absorption of calcium, and helps strengthen the bones and prevent bone-related disorders such as osteoporosis. This meatless taco dish may become a staple in your weekly meal planning.

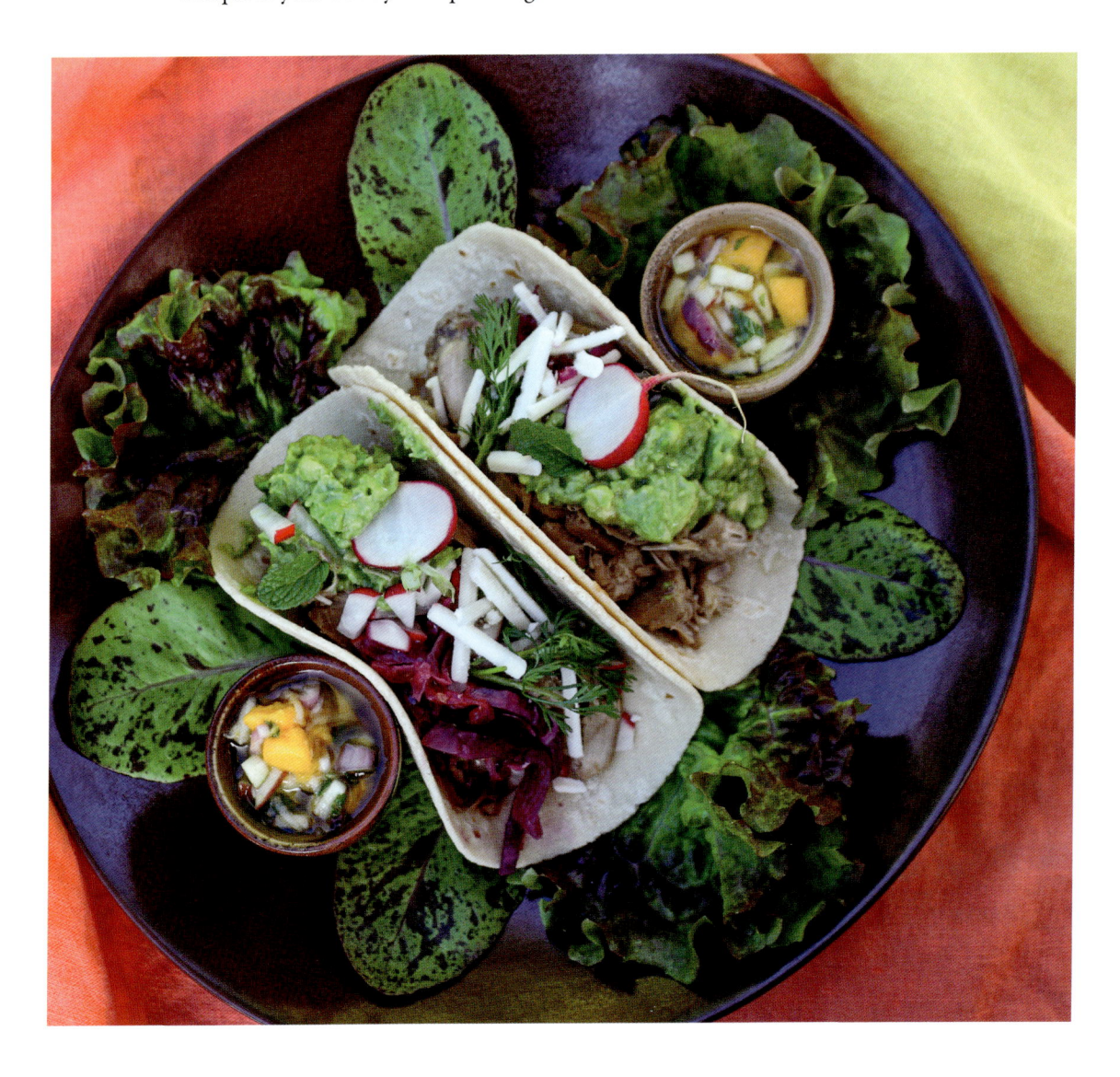

4 gluten-free organic corn tortillas or sprouted wheat tortillas
Guacamole (page 205)
2 baby radishes, shredded
1 tablespoon Pineapple-Turmeric Kimchi (page 134) or sauerkraut (page 130)
1 tablespoon sprouts (page 199)
1 tablespoon natto
Chopped fresh cilantro

FOR THE BBQ JACKFRUIT

2 tablespoons walnut oil
¼ cup (40 g) minced onion
1 medium garlic clove, minced
1½ teaspoons minced fresh ginger
⅛ teaspoon smoked paprika
1 cup (240 ml) filtered water
1 tablespoon liquid aminos
1 tablespoon molasses or coconut sugar
1 (16-ounce [455 g]) can jackfruit
1 teaspoon white miso paste
1 tablespoon sesame oil

FOR THE MANGO SALSA

2 tablespoons chopped mango
2 tablespoons chopped tomato
1 tablespoon chopped apple
1 teaspoon minced shallot
3 tablespoons flaxseed oil
1 garlic clove, minced
3 to 5 mint leaves, chopped
Sea salt
⅛ teaspoon fresh lime juice

1. Preheat the oven to 225°F (110°C). Wrap the tortillas in foil and keep them warm in the oven while you prepare everything else.
2. Make the BBQ jackfruit: Heat the walnut oil in a medium pot over medium heat. Sauté the onion, garlic, ginger, and smoked paprika for 2 to 3 minutes. Add the water, liquid aminos, and molasses and bring the mixture to a simmer. Then, reduce the heat to medium-low and continue cooking for 5 to 8 minutes, until the liquid has reduced to one-third of its original volume.
3. Drain and rinse the jackfruit, then squeeze the fruit to remove any additional liquid. Add the jackfruit to the pot with the sauce, then stir in the miso. Cook for 2 to 3 minutes, until the ingredients blend well and most of the liquid cooks away. Add the sesame oil at the last minute. Remove from the heat and transfer to a medium bowl.
4. Make the salsa: Place the mango, tomato, apple, and shallot in a small serving bowl. Add the flaxseed oil, garlic, and mint. Season with salt. Stir to combine well, and drizzle the lime juice over top.
5. To prepare the tacos, arrange the BBQ jackfruit, guacamole, radishes, kimchi, sprouts, natto, and cilantro on a large plate. Place a warm tortilla on a serving plate, add the BBQ jackfruit, top it with guacamole, spoon some mango salsa over the top, and garnish with the radishes, kimchi, sprouts, natto, and cilantro. Repeat for the rest of the tortillas. Serve the tacos with more salsa on the side.

TIP

To change the flavor of these tacos, experiment with pineapple, plantain, or yucca in place of the jackfruit.

Black Bean and Tofu Scramble Wraps

MAKES 2 SERVINGS

If you're looking for a change from eating eggs every day but still want to maintain your protein intake, this recipe is the perfect fit for you. Scrambled tofu brightened up with turmeric and saffron will become your new go-to egg alternative.

The golden turmeric and saffron make this dish so special and luxurious, yet it only requires a few steps to make. Highly nutritious black bean protein combined with tofu will do the trick. And for almost endless variety, add some of your favorite flavors and textures, from sprouts to pickles or kimchi and seasonal fresh shredded vegetables. Let's get wrapping and rolling!

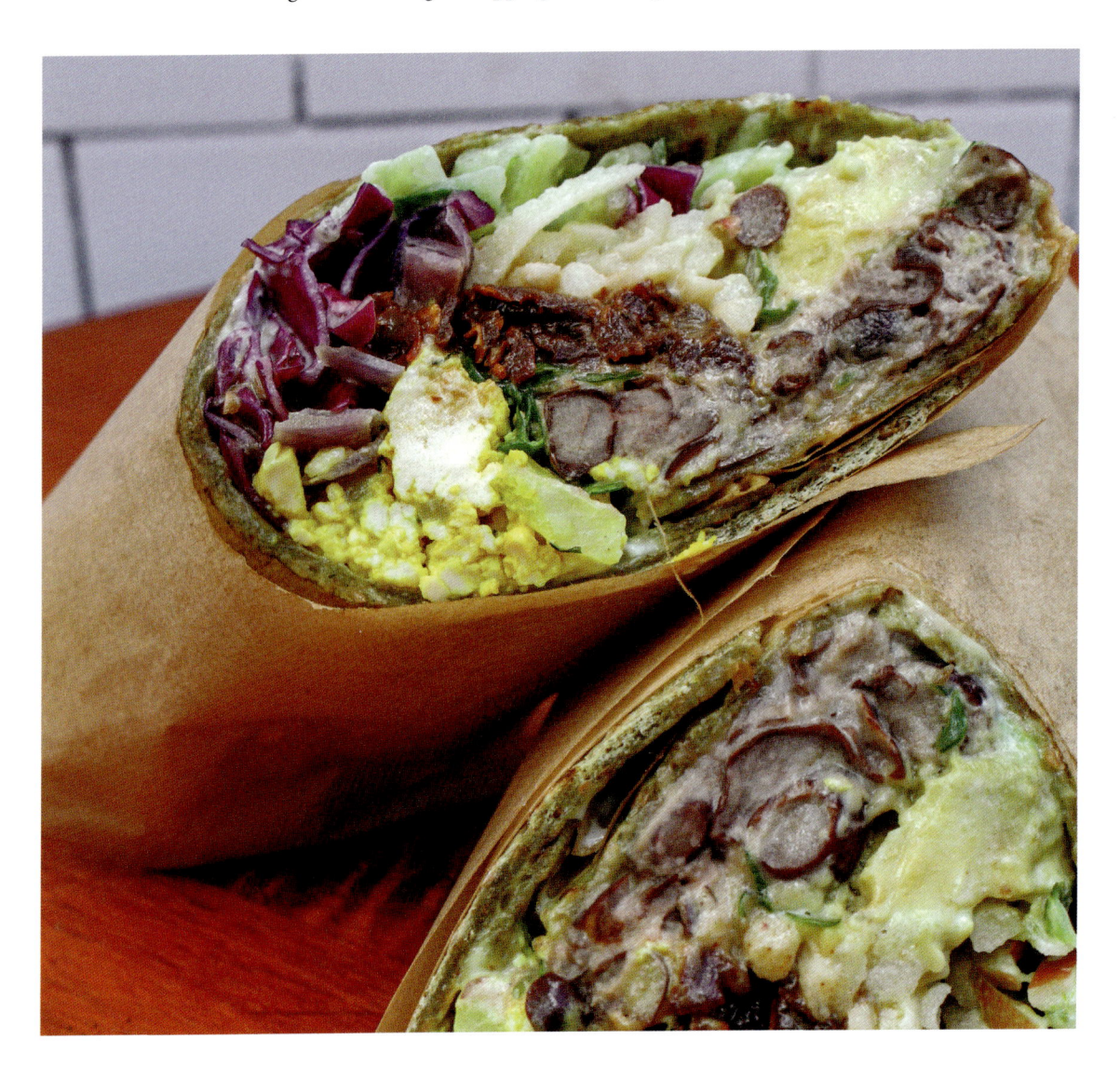

2 (8-inch [20 cm]) sprouted-grain wraps or Red Lentil–Saffron Tortillas (page 150)
1 cup (255 g) crumbled firm tofu
½ cup (130 g) canned black beans
Handful shredded red cabbage
Handful shredded celery
Handful shredded Persian cucumber
Handful grated apple
½ lemon, cut into wedges
Sea salt
Cracked black pepper
1 tablespoon sesame oil
1 medium garlic clove, minced
¼ teaspoon ground turmeric
⅛ teaspoon dried dill
Saffron
1 tablespoon tahini or vegan mayonnaise, plus more for serving (optional)
4 avocado slices
Handful broccoli sprouts
2 tablespoons Pineapple-Turmeric Kimchi (page 134)
1 tablespoon finely chopped onion
Sauerkraut (page 130), kale chips (page 258), or pickles (page 128), for serving

TIPS

You can cook black beans from scratch for this recipe instead of using canned. Be sure to presoak the dried beans as described on page 102 and then cook the beans according to package directions. Feel free to substitute white beans, kidney beans, black-eyed peas, or red beans.

Try the tofu scramble in a breakfast burrito stuffed with roasted bell peppers, sprouts, and avocado for a delicious vegan breakfast option that's high in protein and easy to digest.

1. Preheat the oven to 225°F (110°C). Wrap the wraps in foil and put them in the oven to warm. Rinse the tofu under running water for 10 seconds. Squeeze out excess water and set the tofu in a colander to continue draining. In a fine-mesh strainer, rinse the black beans under running water. Drain completely, 15 to 20 minutes.

2. Place the shredded cabbage, celery, cucumber, and apple in separate piles on a large plate. Squeeze a little lemon juice over the apple. Lightly season all with a pinch of salt and pepper.

3. In a medium saucepan over medium heat, add the sesame oil and garlic. Sauté for 2 to 3 minutes, then add the turmeric and dill. Sauté for an additional 2 to 3 minutes. Add the tofu and a pinch of saffron and cook, stirring, for another 3 to 5 minutes until the tofu turns golden yellow. Do not overcook—remove from the heat when the tofu is still slightly moist. Season lightly with salt and pepper. Transfer to a small bowl and set aside to cool for 15 minutes.

4. To prepare the wrap, place a warmed wrap on a cutting board. Spread one side of the wrap with half of the tahini. Near the bottom edge of the wrap, place half of the black beans, leaving 1 to 2 inches (2.5 to 5 cm) of space around the edges. Add half of the scrambled tofu and half the cabbage, celery, cucumber, apple, avocado, sprouts, kimchi, and onion. Roll the wrap tightly, using the technique described on page 160. Tuck in the ends and cut the wrap diagonally into two pieces. Repeat the process with the second wrap and the rest of the fillings.

5. To serve, place two wrap pieces on a plate along with a lemon wedge and some sauerkraut, kale chips, or your favorite pickles. You can also serve the wraps with extra tahini or mayonnaise on the side.

Buckwheat Linguine with Kale-Macadamia Pesto

MAKES 2 SERVINGS

Buckwheat packs an impressive punch of protein. Just one ounce can fill your daily protein requirement. Whether it's unhulled, hulled, raw, in porridge, or roasted, buckwheat is a nutritional powerhouse. It's loaded with fiber, vitamins, macrominerals, and trace minerals, and it contains no gluten and has a low glycemic load, making it a convenient gluten-free replacement for conventional pasta. Plus, it sprouts like a champ in just a couple of days.

This recipe stands out for its abundance of bone-boosting nutrition and its incredibly rich flavor. The secrets are adding wheatgrass powder and magnesium broth. These ingredients work their magic to elevate the taste to a whole new level, ensuring that every bite is delicious.

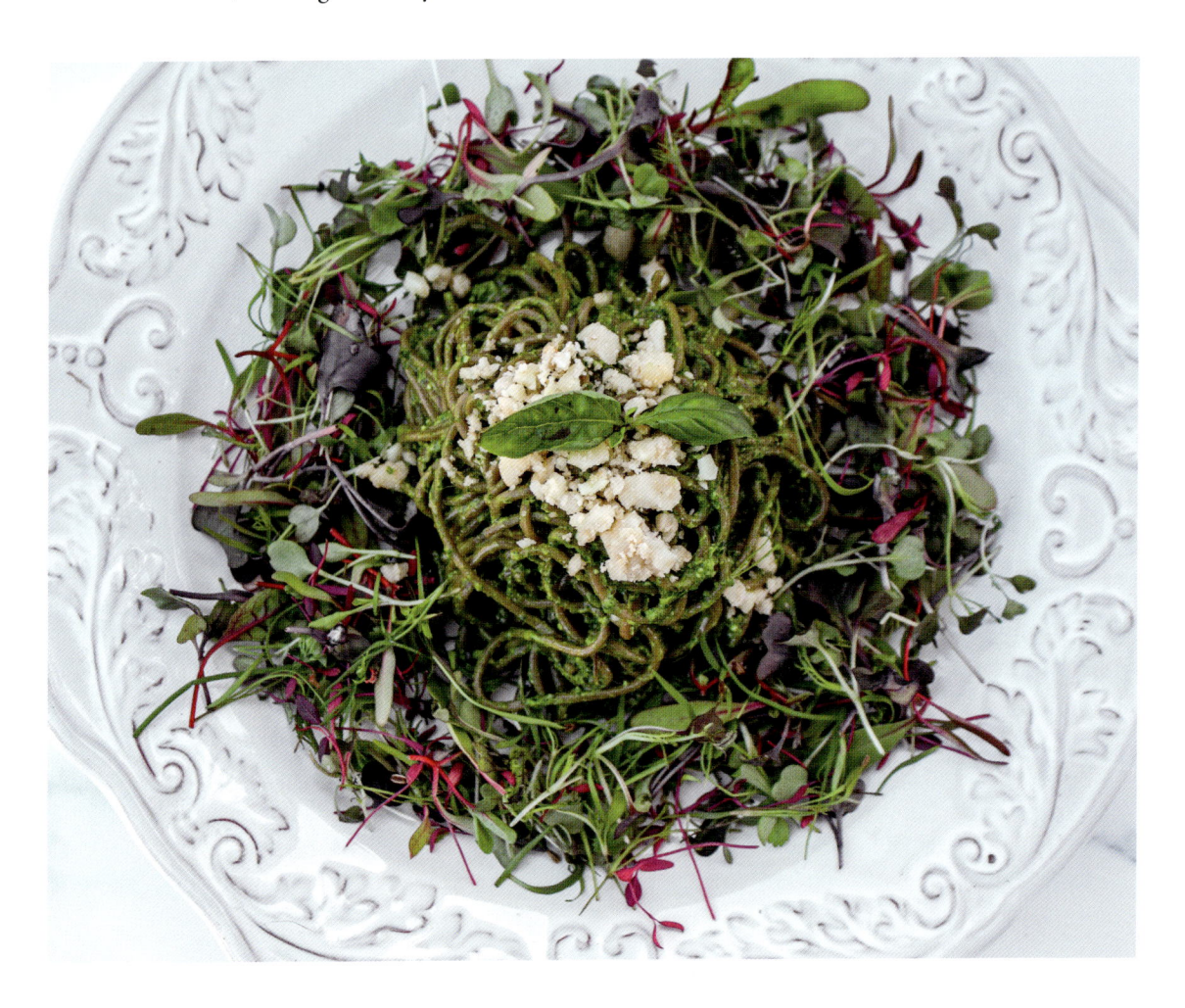

1 rosemary sprig

1 tablespoon cooking oil, such as avocado oil or coconut oil

1 tablespoon sea salt

2 bundles buckwheat noodles (3½ to 4 ounces [100 to 155 g])

2 tablespoons extra-virgin olive oil

FOR THE PESTO

6 tablespoons (90 ml) extra-virgin olive oil, plus more as needed

2 tablespoons finely chopped shallot

1 medium garlic clove

6 to 8 kale leaves, chopped

⅓ cup (45 g) macadamias

6 tablespoons (90 ml) Root and Leaf Magnesium Broth (page 177), coconut milk, or filtered water

4 or 5 basil leaves

1 tablespoon wheatgrass powder

½ teaspoon fresh lemon juice

Sea salt

Cracked black pepper

FOR GARNISH

3 tablespoons finely crushed macadamias

¼ cup (15 g) mixed microgreens

2 to 4 basil leaves

1. In a medium pot, bring 8 cups (2 L) water, the rosemary sprig, cooking oil, and salt to a boil over high heat, then reduce to a simmer. Add the buckwheat noodles and boil for 5 to 8 minutes, or until cooked to your preferred consistency. Drain the noodles in a colander, rinse with running water, and gently massage to remove any slimy texture. Transfer to a large bowl and toss with the olive oil to evenly coat them and prevent sticking.

2. Make the pesto: Heat a medium-sized sauté pan over medium heat. Add the olive oil, shallot, and garlic, and sauté for 3 to 5 minutes. Add the kale and cook for an additional 2 to 3 minutes. Transfer the cooked vegetables to a small plate and let cool for 2 to 3 minutes.

3. Place the vegetables in a food processor, along with the macadamias, broth, basil, and wheatgrass powder. Pulse the mixture for 1 to 3 minutes, until it reaches a thick sauce texture. Add the lemon juice and season with the salt and pepper. Pulse once or twice more.

4. Add the pesto to the noodles and mix gently. If the pesto appears too thick or the noodles seem too dry, incorporate a little more olive oil. Adding oil also will prevent the noodles from sticking together and ensure even distribution of the sauce.

5. Transfer the dressed noodles to serving plates, swirling them creatively—have fun! Garnish with the macadamias, microgreens, and basil.

> **TIPS**
>
> Other dark green leafy vegetables work well for this pesto, too. You can substitute 3½ ounces (100 g) spinach, parsley, or arugula for the kale.
>
> You can also switch things up by using other bone-healthy nuts, like sprouted almonds or sprouted sunflower and pumpkin seeds, or protein-rich hemp seeds, in place of the macadamias.
>
> Try buckwheat noodles with Tahini-Apple-Ginger Dressing (page 122) for a bold, creamy Asian flavor.

Main Meals

Cauliflower Steak with Moroccan Spices

MAKES 2 SERVINGS

Many people think of a steak dinner as a symbol of wealth, masculinity, or stamina, but this recipe turns those perceptions upside down by substituting a big chunk of cauliflower for the beef.

Persian Shirazi Salad, which I think of like a salsa, is a staple in Middle Eastern cooking. With the help of the salad and some Moroccan spices, cauliflower takes a stunningly beautiful turn as a megaflavor steak. This dish is super easy to make, beautiful to behold, and packed with Middle Eastern–inspired flavor, all while it nourishes your body with well-balanced nutrition.

1 medium-sized cauliflower
¼ cup (60 ml) extra-virgin olive oil
1 garlic clove, minced
1 teaspoon minced shallot
1 teaspoon curry powder
½ teaspoon freshly grated nutmeg
½ teaspoon ground turmeric
⅛ teaspoon ground coriander
⅛ teaspoon ground cinnamon
⅛ teaspoon ground cumin
⅛ teaspoon dried parsley
⅛ teaspoon fennel seed
⅛ teaspoon smoked paprika
⅛ teaspoon umami mushroom powder

FOR THE SHIRAZI SALAD
¼ cup (40 g) chopped tomato
1 tablespoon chopped cucumber
1 tablespoon finely chopped fresh parsley
1 tablespoon finely chopped fresh mint
1 tablespoon minced shallot
¼ cup (60 ml) extra-virgin olive oil
⅛ teaspoon fresh lemon juice
Sea salt
Cracked black pepper

FOR GARNISH
2 tablespoons crushed Brazil nuts

1. Preheat the oven to 350°F (180°C). Cut the cauliflower in half vertically, then slice two 2-inch-thick (5 cm) "steaks" from the center. Chop the remaining cauliflower pieces finely as cauliflower "rice"; store the rice in a cotton bag and freeze for future use.
2. Combine the olive oil, garlic, shallot, curry powder, nutmeg, turmeric, coriander, cinnamon, cumin, parsley, fennel seed, paprika, and umami powder in a bowl and mix well.
3. Place the cauliflower slices on a baking sheet lined with parchment paper. Brush the cauliflower evenly with the spice rub. Flip the cauliflower and brush the other side, reserving one-third of the rub. Roast for 20 to 30 minutes, then flip and roast for another 20 to 30 minutes. If the rub hasn't soaked deeply into the cauliflower, brush it a few more times to ensure rich flavor. The cauliflower steaks are ready when they can be easily pierced with a small sharp knife. Remove from the oven.
4. While the cauliflower is roasting, prepare the Shirazi salad: In a bowl, combine the tomato, cucumber, parsley, mint, and shallot with the olive oil and lemon juice. Mix well and season with salt and pepper.
5. To serve, place the roasted cauliflower steaks on individual plates and brush with the remaining spice rub. Spoon the Shirazi salad on top, like salsa, and garnish with the crushed Brazil nuts.

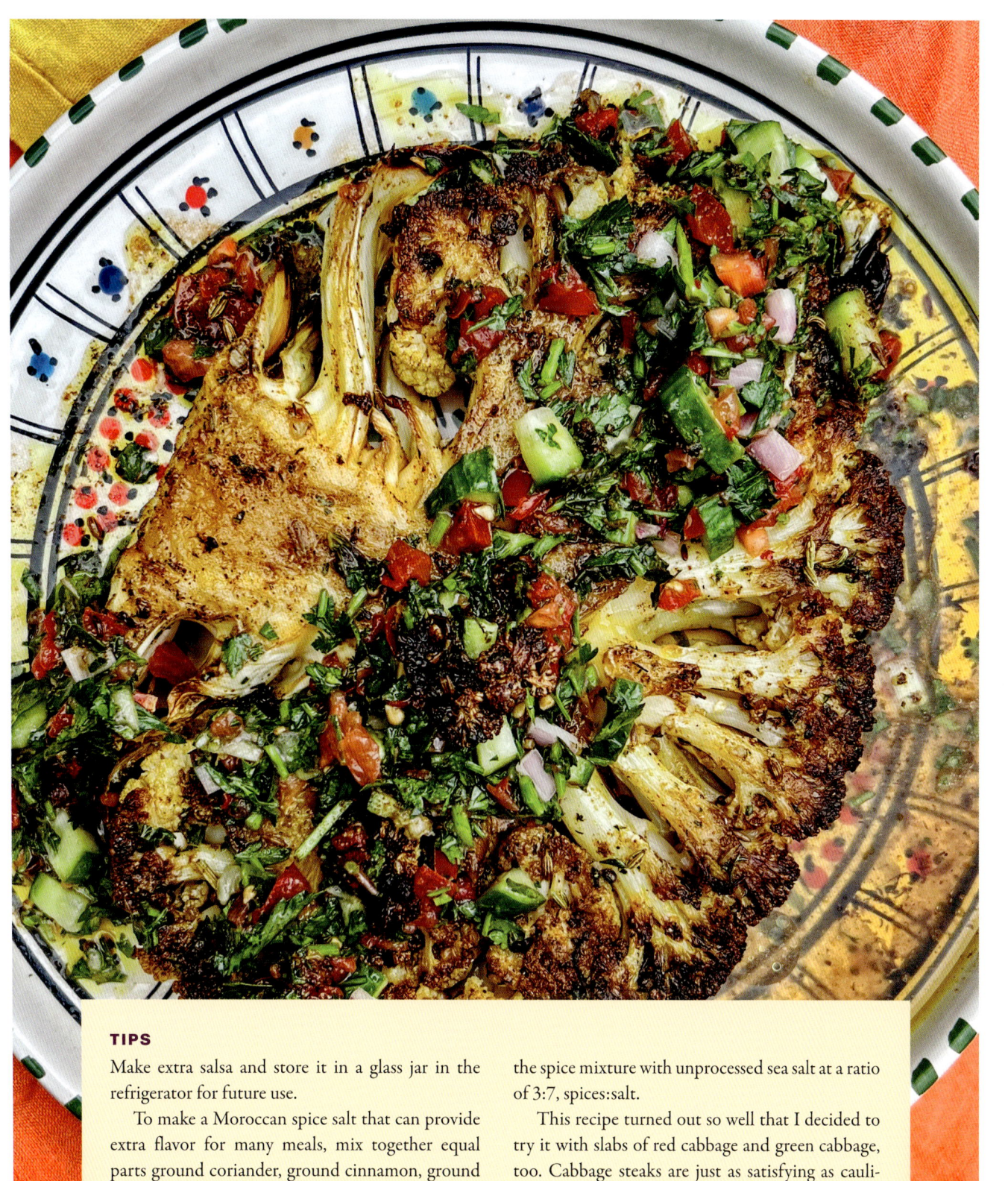

TIPS

Make extra salsa and store it in a glass jar in the refrigerator for future use.

To make a Moroccan spice salt that can provide extra flavor for many meals, mix together equal parts ground coriander, ground cinnamon, ground cumin, fennel seed, and smoked paprika. Combine the spice mixture with unprocessed sea salt at a ratio of 3:7, spices:salt.

This recipe turned out so well that I decided to try it with slabs of red cabbage and green cabbage, too. Cabbage steaks are just as satisfying as cauliflower steaks, and also full of minerals and fiber.

California Sushi Rolls with Licorice Sweet Brown Rice

MAKES 4 ROLLS

Making sushi rolls is quite an art. Rolling up your favorite vegetables, herbs, or cheese, then slicing them into round sushi shapes, is not only enjoyable but also visually captivating. I often teach sushi-making classes for kids, and the excitement they feel when creating their own rolls is contagious. Try it with your own family for a fun team activity.

Through my experiences with private clients, I've realized that, for many people, allergy symptoms or low energy levels often result from consuming the same foods repeatedly. When people transition to a diet rich in diverse, organic, and fresh, local, seasonal foods, their allergies tend to vanish, and they experience a significant boost in energy. This recipe will achieve this key goal of diversity.

You will need a rice cooker and a bamboo sushi roller for this recipe.

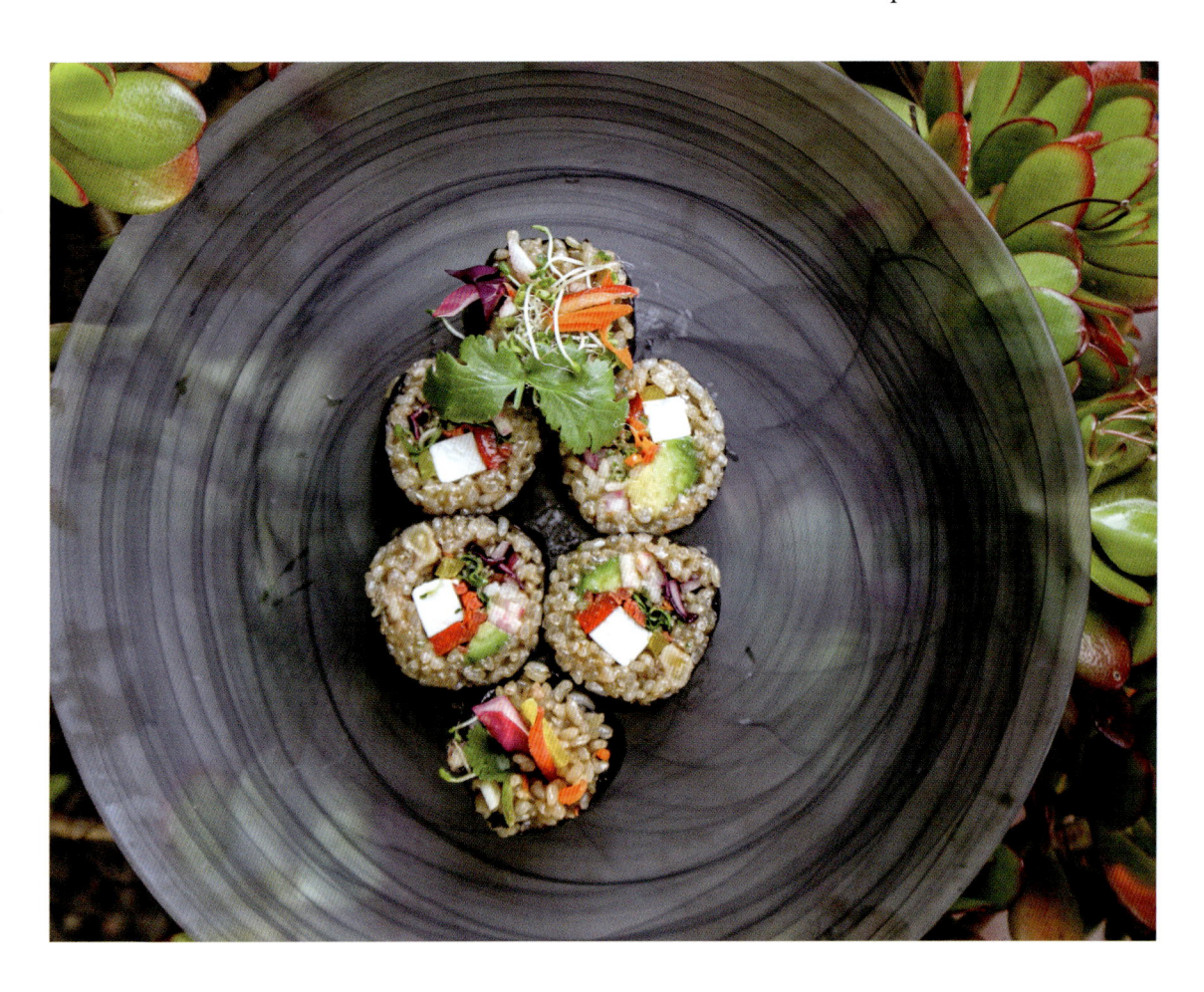

FOR THE SUSHI RICE

1 cup (190 g) sweet brown rice
2 cups (480 ml) filtered water
2 ounces (60 g) licorice root
1 tablespoon crushed macadamias
1 teaspoon psyllium
2 tablespoons toasted sesame oil
2 tablespoons brown rice vinegar
2 tablespoons sesame seeds
1 tablespoon matcha powder
1 teaspoon liquid aminos
1 teaspoon minced fresh ginger

FOR THE ROLLS

½ avocado, cut into strips
Fresh lemon juice
4 (3-inch [8 cm]) sticks vegan feta cheese, cut into cubes
Handful alfalfa sprouts
1 small carrot, shredded
2 tablespoons chopped yellow radish pickle
2 tablespoons chopped red onion
2 tablespoons chopped purple cabbage
2 tablespoons natto
4 strips roasted red peppers
1 scallion, sliced
Brown rice vinegar
Sea salt
2 sheets nori or gim (seaweed)
Toasted sesame oil

TO SERVE

2 tablespoons chopped Pineapple-Turmeric Kimchi (page 134) or Beet-Cauliflower Pickles (page 128)
1 teaspoon black sesame seeds
Tahini-Apple-Ginger Dressing (page 122)

1. Make the rice: In a medium pot over medium-high heat, combine the rice, water, licorice root, macadamias, and psyllium and bring to a simmer. Lower the heat and cook slowly for 15 to 25 minutes, until the rice becomes transparent. Remove from the heat, remove the licorice root, and add the sesame oil, brown rice vinegar, sesame seeds, matcha, liquid aminos, and ginger. Mix the rice well and set aside to cool to lukewarm.
2. Make the rolls: Place the avocado on a large plate and drizzle with lemon juice. Arrange the vegan feta, alfalfa sprouts, carrot, yellow radish pickle, red onion, cabbage, natto, red peppers, and scallion on the plate in separate piles. Lightly season with vinegar and salt.
3. Place the bamboo roller on top of a cutting board, then place a sheet of nori on top with the shiny side facing down. Scoop approximately 1 cup of the rice and spread it out evenly to the edges of the sheet. Gently squeeze to form a firm rice base. Layer the ingredients on top, stacking them together.
4. Roll up the sushi tightly, using the bamboo roller to pull it over gently. Seal the edge with a little water. Coat the surface of the roll with sesame oil to keep it moist and avoid the rolls sticking together. Repeat with the remaining nori, rice, and fillings.
5. Oil a knife blade and slowly and gently cut each roll into pieces. Place the pieces on a plate and garnish with kimchi or pickles and black sesame seeds. Serve with the dressing.

> **TIP**
> Try lightly cooked collard greens or Swiss chard leaves as an alternative to the nori wrap.

Main Meals

Edamame Spread Avocado Toast

MAKES 2 SERVINGS

Avocado toast is one of the trendiest California dishes. The classic version is served on regular bread, but that's not my jam since I'm gluten intolerant. I decided to create my own version using edamame blended with avocado and paired with Ezekiel bread, which is a highly nutritious sprouted bread.

If you're like me and eating too much hummus can lead to bloating, you'll find the edamame paste in this recipe is a game-changer. It has the same creamy texture as hummus and is just as versatile, but it will be easier on your gut. Serve it with fresh veggies as a small plate, with eggs for breakfast, or slathered on grilled zucchini.

I throw in a little spirulina, a type of algae that grows in clean water and is highly nutritious and a great source of protein, copper, and B vitamins. The spirulina cranks up the antioxidants and adds extra iron and minerals. Protein-rich spirulina also lends the paste an awesome vibrant green color.

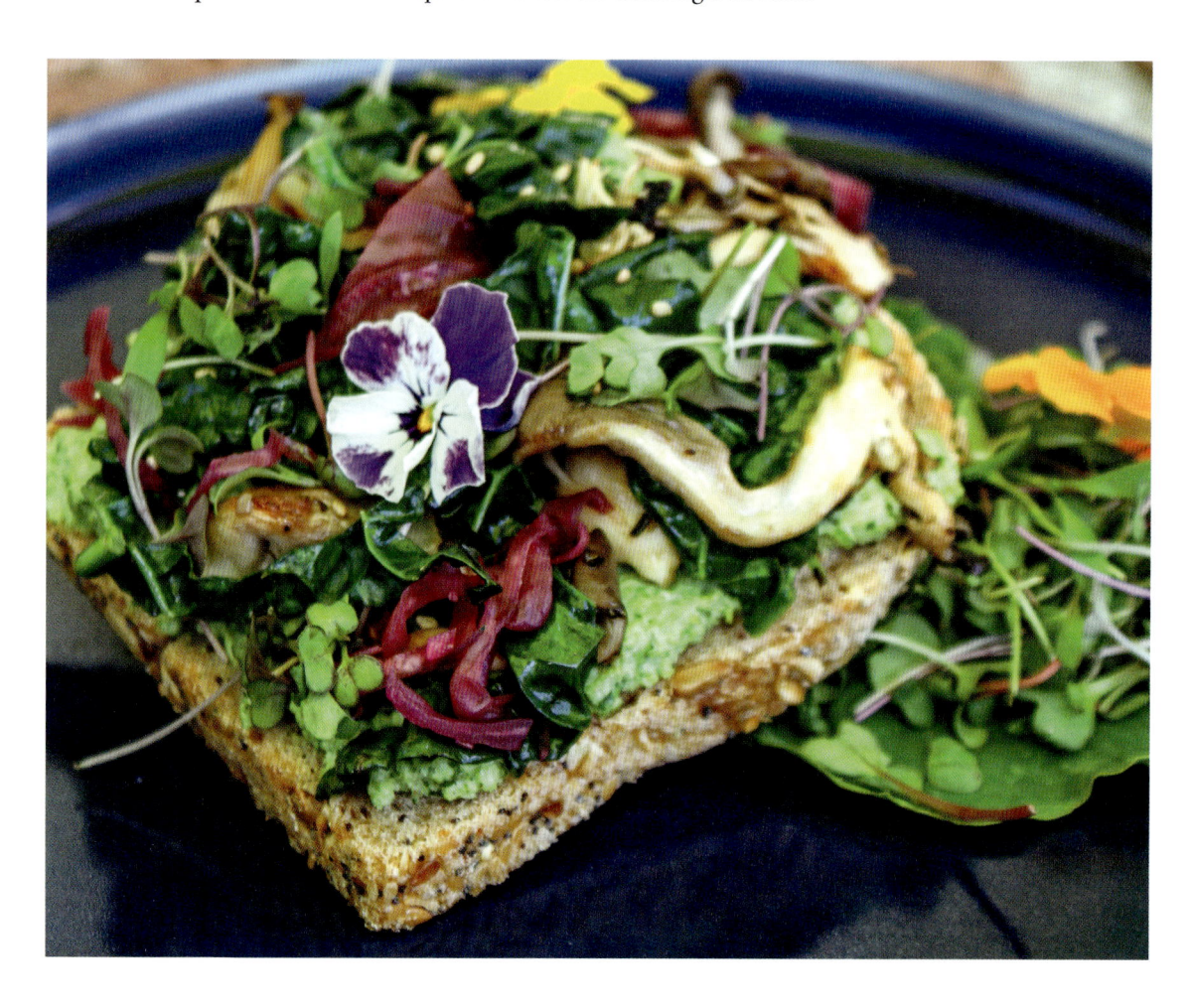

FOR THE EDAMAME-AVOCADO PASTE

1 cup (155 g) frozen precooked edamame, thawed
½ large avocado
2 tablespoons hemp seed oil
1 teaspoon spirulina
⅛ teaspoon ground cardamom
⅛ teaspoon dried basil
⅛ teaspoon dried sage
Sea salt
Cracked black pepper

FOR THE COOKED TOPPING

Hemp seed oil, extra-virgin olive oil, or walnut oil
2 garlic cloves, minced
¼ cup (15 g) finely chopped fresh dill
1 tablespoon chopped fresh rosemary
¼ cup (15 g) chopped onion
1 cup (88 g) hand-shredded oyster mushrooms
4 kale leaves, stemmed and finely shredded
Sea salt
Cracked black pepper

TO SERVE

2 slices Ezekiel seeded sourdough bread
Thinly sliced red onion
Pineapple-Turmeric Kimchi (page 134)
Beet microgreens
Extra-virgin olive oil (optional)
Truffle powder (optional)
Fresh dill leaves

1. Make the edamame-avocado paste: Strain the edamame and rinse under running water. Set aside to drain for at least 5 minutes. Remove the seed and skin from the avocado and slice the avocado.
2. Add the edamame and avocado to a food processor along with the hemp seed oil, spirulina, cardamom, basil, and sage. Pulse on and off until you achieve a thick, hummuslike texture (build this texture gradually). Once you've reached the desired consistency, season with salt and pepper. Transfer to a small bowl and set aside.
3. Make the cooked topping: Heat a sauté pan over medium heat and drizzle in some oil. Add the garlic, dill, and rosemary, followed by the onion. Sauté until the onion becomes transparent, then add the mushrooms and kale. Continue to sauté until the mushrooms turn golden brown. Season with salt and pepper.
4. To serve, place a slice of the Ezekiel bread on a plate. Spread half of the edamame-avocado paste evenly over the bread, followed by half of the kale and sautéed mushroom mixture. Top it off with red onion, kimchi, microgreens, and, if you like, a drizzle of olive oil or a light sprinkle of truffle powder. Garnish with a few dill leaves. Repeat with the second slice of bread. Enjoy your delicious creation!

> **TIP**
> If you are hungry for more about sprouted seeds bread, see page 154.

Main Meals

Maple Syrup BBQ Tempeh

MAKES 2 SERVINGS

The moment I tasted tempeh homemade by an Indonesian friend, I begged her to teach me how to make it. I fell in love with its nutty and earthy texture, and the more I ate it, the more I found my digestion to be smoother and more soothing. Tempeh, a versatile fermented soybean product, is a protein-rich, probiotic-packed food that also supports muscle health. Tempeh is available at most health stores and even mainstream markets.

In this recipe, you'll learn how to create a delicious and simple BBQ sauce that can be used to flavor a variety of ingredients. You will also pair colorful rainbow carrots with a moringa-infused almond oil pesto that is reminiscent of Italian pesto recipes—a delightful combination.

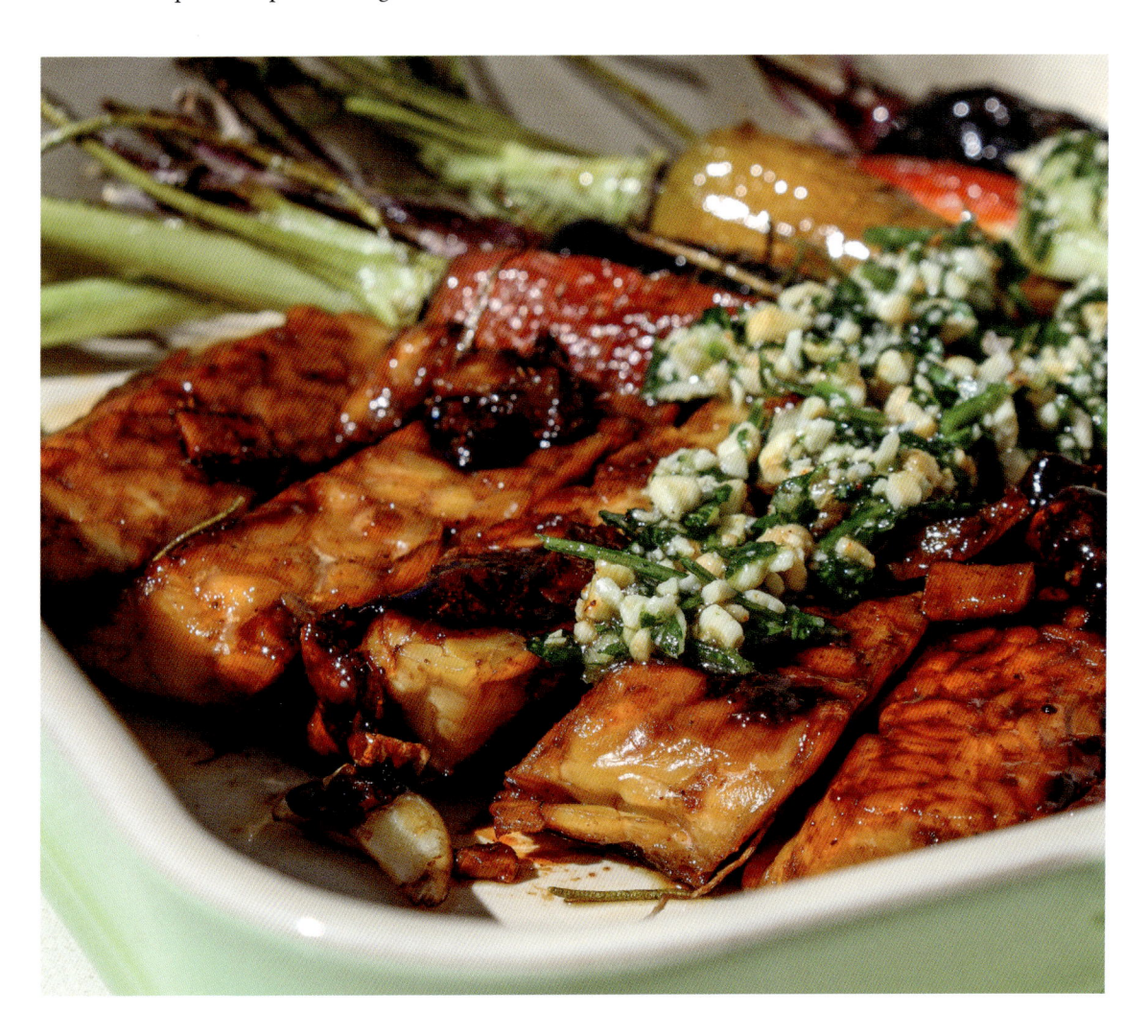

1 (8-ounce [227 g]) block tempeh

FOR THE ROASTED CARROTS

4 small rainbow carrots
2 tablespoons sunflower oil, plus more for brushing
⅛ teaspoon curry powder
⅛ teaspoon dried parsley
⅛ teaspoon dried sage
Sea salt
Cracked black pepper

FOR THE BBQ SAUCE

6 tablespoons (90 ml) filtered water
¼ cup (60 ml) liquid aminos
2 tablespoons maple syrup
2 tablespoons (preferably black) sesame oil
1 tablespoon finely chopped fresh ginger
1 medium garlic clove, minced
⅛ teaspoon ground cinnamon
⅛ teaspoon freshly grated nutmeg
Sea salt
Cracked black pepper

FOR THE CASHEW-PARSLEY PESTO

2 tablespoons raw cashews, soaked
1 tablespoon chopped fresh parsley
1 teaspoon moringa powder
1 medium garlic clove, minced
¼ cup (60 ml) almond oil
Sea salt
Cracked black pepper

FOR GARNISH

⅛ teaspoon sesame seeds
Pineapple-Turmeric Kimchi (page 134), sprouts, or pickles

1. Preheat the oven to 375°F (190°C). Cut the tempeh diagonally into 1-inch-thick (2.5 cm) slices. Place the slices on a plate and set aside.
2. Make the roasted carrots: If the carrots are only 3 to 4 inches (8 to 10 cm) long, roast them whole. For larger ones, halve them, ensuring even-sized pieces for uniform cooking. Arrange the carrots on a baking sheet, drizzle with some of the sunflower oil, and sprinkle with the curry powder, parsley, sage, and a pinch each of salt and pepper. Roast for 25 to 35 minutes, until the carrots become soft and golden. Remove the pan from the oven, then drizzle on more oil and brush it evenly over the carrots to maintain a glossy and moist appearance.
3. While the carrots are roasting, make the BBQ sauce: Heat an 8-inch (20 cm) cast-iron skillet over medium-high heat. Add the water, liquid aminos, maple syrup, sesame oil, ginger, garlic, cinnamon, and nutmeg. Stir to blend well and cook for 2 to 3 minutes, until the sauce thickens.
4. Once the sauce reduces by half, add the tempeh slices and coat them evenly with the sauce. Continue cooking for 2 to 5 minutes, until the sauce forms a glazed, shiny coating on the tempeh. Remove the tempeh steaks from the pan and set them aside on a plate.
5. Make the pesto: In a mortar and pestle, combine the cashews, parsley, moringa powder, and garlic. Crush these ingredients roughly, then add the almond oil gradually, continuing to crush until the mixture reaches a pleasing chunky consistency. Season with salt and pepper.
6. To serve, place the glossy tempeh slices on two plates and sprinkle sesame seeds on top. Arrange the roasted carrots beside the tempeh. Spoon the pesto generously over the carrots. Garnish with kimchi or your favorite sprouts and pickles.

Main Meals ▪ 231

Meaty Meatless Meatballs with Marinara Sauce

MAKES 2 SERVINGS

Eating meatballs is like getting a warm, comforting hug after a long, tough day. But I was very disappointed when I tried to make meatless meatballs using plant-based commercial products. I found the results unsatisfying, and the labels showed that the products contained artificial flavors. That's not my style, so I was inspired to create a rich and meaty meatball without using fake meat products.

These meatballs are simply delicious, and they're medicinal and nourishing, too. In this recipe, you wield the power of flaxseeds, which are brimming with heart-healthy omega-3s and hormone-balancing lignans. Flaxseeds even moonlight as a cholesterol-free egg alternative.

> **TIPS**
>
> Building on the foundation of this recipe, be wild and whip up a variety of vegan, bone-health-friendly meatballs. As long as you stick to the ratio of 2:2:1, protein:veggies:herbs, the possibilities are truly limitless. Try mushroom:carrot:cilantro or tofu:scallion:chives.
>
> Make sure to use flaxseed meal rather than whole flaxseeds for better absorption of their nutrients into the digestive system.

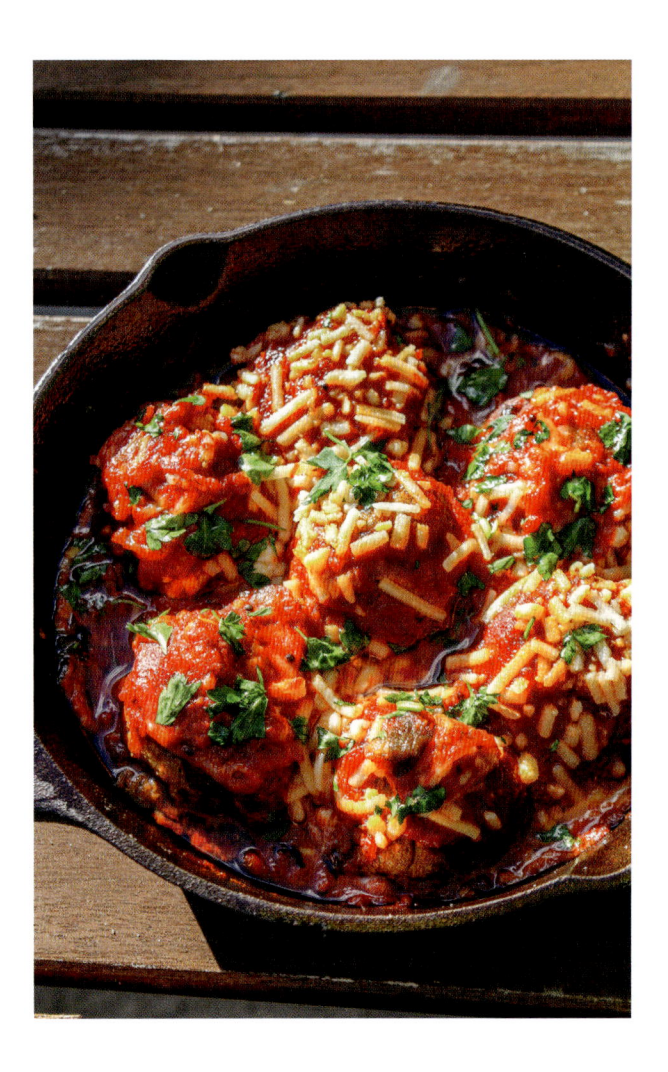

FOR THE MEATBALLS

½ cup (80 g) frozen precooked edamame, thawed
1 cup (250 g) crumbled firm tofu
2 tablespoons chopped onion
2 tablespoons chaga mushroom powder
2 tablespoons flaxseed oil
2 tablespoons flaxseed meal
1 tablespoon nutritional yeast
1 tablespoon chopped fresh parsley
2 or 3 dill sprigs or 1½ teaspoons dried dill
⅛ teaspoon ground cinnamon
⅛ teaspoon ground cumin
⅛ teaspoon dried sage
Fennel seed
½ cup (60 g) cassava flour

FOR THE MARINARA SAUCE

2 tablespoons extra-virgin olive oil
1 rosemary sprig
¼ medium onion, diced
1 garlic clove, minced
⅛ teaspoon mustard seed
1 cup (240 ml) tomato puree
1 tablespoon chopped capers
1 teaspoon tomato paste
1 bay leaf
1 tablespoon maple syrup
Sea salt
Cracked black pepper

TO SERVE

3 tablespoons vegan or dairy mozzarella
2 tablespoons chopped fresh basil or parsley
High-quality extra-virgin olive oil

1. Make the meatballs: Preheat the oven to 325°F (165°C). Rinse the edamame, drain it well, and set it aside.
2. Squeeze the tofu to remove excess water, then add it to a food processor with the edamame, onion, mushroom powder, flaxseed oil, flaxseed meal, nutritional yeast, parsley, dill, cinnamon, cumin, sage, and a pinch of fennel seed. Pulse on and off for 2 to 3 minutes until the ingredients combine into a thick batter. Be careful not to overprocess; I like a chunky texture. Transfer the mixture into a medium mixing bowl.
3. Put the cassava flour on a plate. Scoop out rounded tablespoons of the mixture and roll each in the flour to coat. Place the coated meatballs in a stoneware or glass baking dish.
4. Bake until the meatballs turn golden—20 to 30 minutes, checking after 15 minutes to avoid overcooking. Do not allow the meatballs to dry out.
5. Meanwhile, make the marinara sauce: Add the olive oil to a medium saucepan over medium heat. After 1 to 2 minutes, brush the oil with the rosemary. Add the onion, garlic, and mustard seed, and sauté for 2 to 3 minutes. Add the tomato puree, capers, tomato paste, bay leaf, and rosemary sprig. Bring the mixture to a simmer and continue simmering until the sauce thickens and reduces by half. Stir in the maple syrup and season with salt and pepper.
6. After removing the meatballs from the oven, increase the oven temperature to 400°F (200°C). Pour the marinara sauce over the meatballs and sprinkle with 2 tablespoons of the mozzarella. Return the baking dish to the oven and bake for an additional 10 to 15 minutes until the cheese turns golden and brown.
7. Plate the meatballs, garnish with the basil, and add the remaining cheese on top. Finish with a few drops of olive oil.

Mouthful Quinoa-Carrot Burgers

MAKES 4 SERVINGS

From humble beginnings, with its diversity and innovations, the hamburger has become a beloved classic and an iconic American dish with enduring appeal, symbolizing fast food worldwide as a global staple.

I have a mission to transform this casual guilty-pleasure dish into a nutritious, delicious, and plant-based meal without compromising its richness and meatiness. I achieve this by using a common yet powerful vegetable—the carrot—paired with high-protein quinoa, creating a blend filled with rich aromas and flavors.

With each giant bite, you'll experience the meaty texture of quinoa, followed by the sweetness of carrots, and then the aromatic, licorice-like fennel that harmonizes with the cheese or vegan mayonnaise that preserves the essence of a classic burger.

A gluten-free bun would be an ideal pairing for this burger, but if you want the real all-American burger experience, a sourdough bun would be a good second choice. Enjoy your homemade burger adventure!

TIPS

If you don't already have cooked quinoa on hand, prepare some using a 1:2 ratio of quinoa to water.

You can freeze the patties, whether cooked or raw, for up to 1 year.

Try making a beet burger by substituting grated beet for the grated carrot. The burger will have a similar consistency but a different color and flavor.

For added nutrition, pair these burgers with roasted sweet potatoes or any salad.

FOR THE PATTIES

3 medium carrots
1 cup (185 g) cooked quinoa
½ cup (75 g) flaxseed meal
3 tablespoons extra-virgin olive oil, plus more for the pan
1 tablespoon ground turmeric
½ teaspoon sea salt
½ teaspoon cracked black pepper
⅛ teaspoon ground cinnamon
⅛ teaspoon ground cumin
⅛ teaspoon fennel seed
⅛ teaspoon ground ginger

FOR THE TOPPINGS

2 portobello mushrooms or 4 button or cremini mushrooms
1 small zucchini
3 tablespoons extra-virgin olive oil or coconut oil
1 rosemary sprig
1 medium garlic clove, minced
4 small lettuce leaves
4 basil leaves
2 medium tomatoes, sliced
4 thin slices green apple

TO SERVE

4 gluten-free or sourdough buns
4 teaspoons vegan mayonnaise (optional)
4 slices Swiss cheese (optional)

1. Preheat the oven to 350°F (180°C).
2. Make the patties: Grate the carrots; you will need 4 cups total. Squeeze the grated carrots with a cotton cloth to remove excess water. Add the shredded carrots, cooked quinoa, flaxseed meal, and olive oil to a food processor. Then add the turmeric, salt, pepper, cinnamon, cumin, fennel seed, and ginger. Pulse for 2 to 5 minutes until the mixture becomes smooth and thick. Be careful not to overblend.
3. Brush a baking sheet with olive oil. Divide the patty mixture into four portions, shaping them into patties. Place them on the pan, about 2 inches (5 cm) apart. Bake for 25 to 30 minutes, or until they turn golden brown.
4. Prepare the toppings: Cut the mushrooms and zucchini horizontally, ¼ inch (6 mm) thick, and place the slices on a plate. In a medium frying pan, drizzle some of the olive oil and infuse it with the rosemary for 1 to 2 minutes. Add the garlic and mushroom and sauté; follow with the zucchini slices separately for 3 to 5 minutes, until they become golden brown. Place the zucchini on a wooden plate or cutting board to prevent sogginess. Put the lettuce, basil, tomato slices, and apple slices on a plate.
5. To serve, cut the buns in half. You can toast the buns in the oven, but they will taste better heated in a pan. In a large skillet, toast the buns over medium heat until they're golden brown. Place a bun half on a serving plate, spread with mayonnaise if desired, place a patty on the bun, and top it with a slice of cheese if desired. Add the mushrooms, zucchini, lettuce, basil, tomato, and apple, and top with the other bun half. Repeat with the remaining buns, patties, and toppings. Hold your burger firmly as you bite into your delicious creation.

Mung Bean Pizza

MAKES ONE 10-INCH (25 CM) PIZZA

Pizza must be the most popular food in the world. Americans eat the equivalent of 100 acres of heavily processed pizza each day, or about 350 slices per second.

Historically, mung bean pancakes were a humble person's superfood to endure hunger and build stamina, then they morphed into everyday street food in Korea. In this recipe, we transform the down-to-earth pancake into a healthy, delicious pizza that will leave you feeling energized and amazed by the versatility of mighty mung beans. Using hemp seed pesto as a topping makes this pizza even more irresistible!

TIPS

Make a large batch of the mung bean dough (increase the recipe by three to four times), cut the dough into pieces of your desired size, wrap them with parchment paper, and store in plastic bags in the freezer. To thaw, put a bag of frozen dough in a sinkful of water for 20 minutes. Then it will be ready to spread and bake. It is delicious for use as avocado toast or soup toppings. Bake it in thin slices for a gluten-free flatbread.

You can add a handful of fresh chopped kale, celery, or mushrooms to this dough to create a savory pancake.

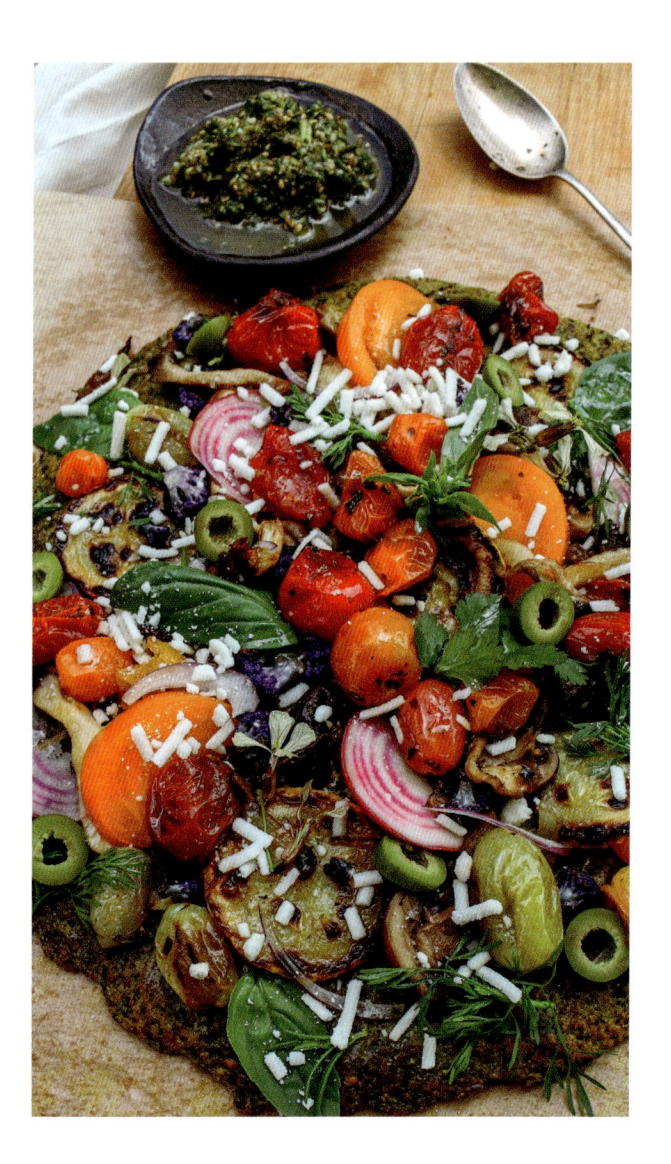

FOR THE MUNG BEAN DOUGH

1 cup (200 g) mung beans, soaked (see page 102 for soaking method)
¼ cup (15 g) fresh basil
3 tablespoons avocado oil
1 tablespoon flaxseed meal
1 tablespoon kelp powder
⅛ teaspoon ground cinnamon
⅛ teaspoon ground cumin
⅛ teaspoon fennel seed
Extra-virgin olive oil, for brushing

FOR THE TOPPINGS

3 tablespoons extra-virgin olive oil
2 garlic cloves, minced
1 cup (30 g) mixed lion's mane and button mushrooms, sliced
5 thin slices red onion
5 medium (round) slices zucchini
¼ cup (15 g) diced purple cauliflower
¼ cup (15 g) sliced onion
10 cherry tomatoes
Few slices heirloom tomatoes
Few slices raw pink beets
3 to 5 pitted olives, sliced
Hemp Seed Pesto (page 125)
Fresh basil
Edible flowers
Handful shredded vegan cheese

1. Preheat the oven to 325°F (160°C). To make the dough, put the soaked mung beans, basil, avocado oil, flaxseed meal, kelp powder, cinnamon, cumin, and fennel seed in a large bowl and mix them well. Transfer the mixture to a food processor. Pulse at first to be sure the food processor can handle the dough. Then blend for 3 to 5 minutes, until the ingredients form a thick dough.

2. Line a baking sheet with parchment paper and coat it with olive oil. Spread the dough evenly on the paper, forming a ½-inch-thick (13 mm) circle about 10 inches (25 cm) in diameter. Brush the top with olive oil, and place another sheet of parchment on top of the dough to keep it moist. Bake for about 30 minutes but begin checking after about 15 minutes, and do not allow the dough to overbake. When the edges start to turn golden, remove the pan from the oven, and set the crust aside on a plate.

3. Meanwhile, make the toppings: Add 2 tablespoons of the olive oil and the garlic to a sauté pan, and sauté over medium heat for 1 to 2 minutes. Add the mushrooms and onion and cook for 2 to 3 minutes, until golden brown. Remove from the pan and set aside. In the same pan, add the zucchini and cook for 2 to 3 minutes, until golden brown. Move the zucchini to a wooden cutting board. In the same pan, add the cauliflower and cook for 2 to 3 minutes, until golden brown, then move to the cutting board. In the same pan, heat the remaining 1 tablespoon olive oil, add the cherry tomatoes, and cook over medium heat until the skins wrinkle and liquid is released. Remove the tomatoes from the pan and place in a small bowl.

4. Cover the crust with the cooked toppings, heirloom tomatoes, beets, and olives, and spoon pesto over the top. Garnish with basil and edible flowers and sprinkles of cheese.

Main Meals ▪ 237

Sweet Potato Boats with Creamy Spinach

MAKES 2 SERVINGS

Spinach and mushrooms make my mouth water, and in this dish the combination looks beautiful and has a silky texture. As you follow this recipe, you'll learn how to prepare boat-shaped roasted sweet potatoes and the creamy spinach filling, which you can use as a stuffing for a variety of colorful dishes by substituting yam, daikon radish, squash, pumpkin, or a large green zucchini for the sweet potatoes.

1 medium sweet potato
2 tablespoons coconut oil
¼ teaspoon ground cinnamon
Sea salt
Cracked black pepper

FOR THE CREAMY SPINACH

2 tablespoons coconut oil
½ teaspoon chopped fresh rosemary
⅛ teaspoon dried sage
⅛ teaspoon chopped fresh thyme
½ small onion, minced
1 teaspoon minced garlic
4 button mushrooms, thinly sliced
¼ cup (60 ml) filtered water
2 tablespoons coconut milk
2 cups (40 g) chopped spinach
¼ teaspoon fresh lemon juice
Lava salt
Cracked black pepper

FOR GARNISH

¼ cup (30 g) crushed walnuts
3 tablespoons pickled red onion
2 tablespoons crumbled vegan feta or grated vegan parmesan
½ teaspoon chopped fresh rosemary

1. Preheat the oven to 400°F (200°C). Wash the sweet potato and trim the ends. Slowly and gently, cut it in half horizontally. Lightly score the potato on the skin side with diagonal slits for a decorative effect. Place the potato halves on a baking sheet, brush them with coconut oil, and sprinkle with cinnamon, salt, and pepper. Flip the potatoes and repeat seasoning, then turn them back to face up. Roast for 15 to 20 minutes, until golden brown on one side. Then flip the potato halves and roast for another 15 to 20 minutes, until they turn golden brown and the score marks are clearly visible. Remove from the oven and set aside.

2. Make the creamy spinach: Heat the coconut oil in a sauté pan over medium heat. Add the rosemary, sage, and thyme, and stir gently to infuse for 30 seconds. Add the onion and garlic and sauté for 1 to 2 minutes, then add the mushrooms and sauté for an additional 2 to 3 minutes, until the mushrooms reduce in size by half. Pour in the water and cook for 3 minutes. When the liquid has reduced by half, pour in the coconut milk. Add the spinach and continue cooking for 2 to 3 minutes. Add the lemon juice. Cook, stirring, until the liquid thickens to a sauce consistency. Season with salt and pepper.

3. Place the sweet potatoes face up on a serving plate. Spoon the creamy spinach and mushroom mixture on top. Garnish with sprinkles of crushed walnuts, pickled red onion, cheese, and rosemary.

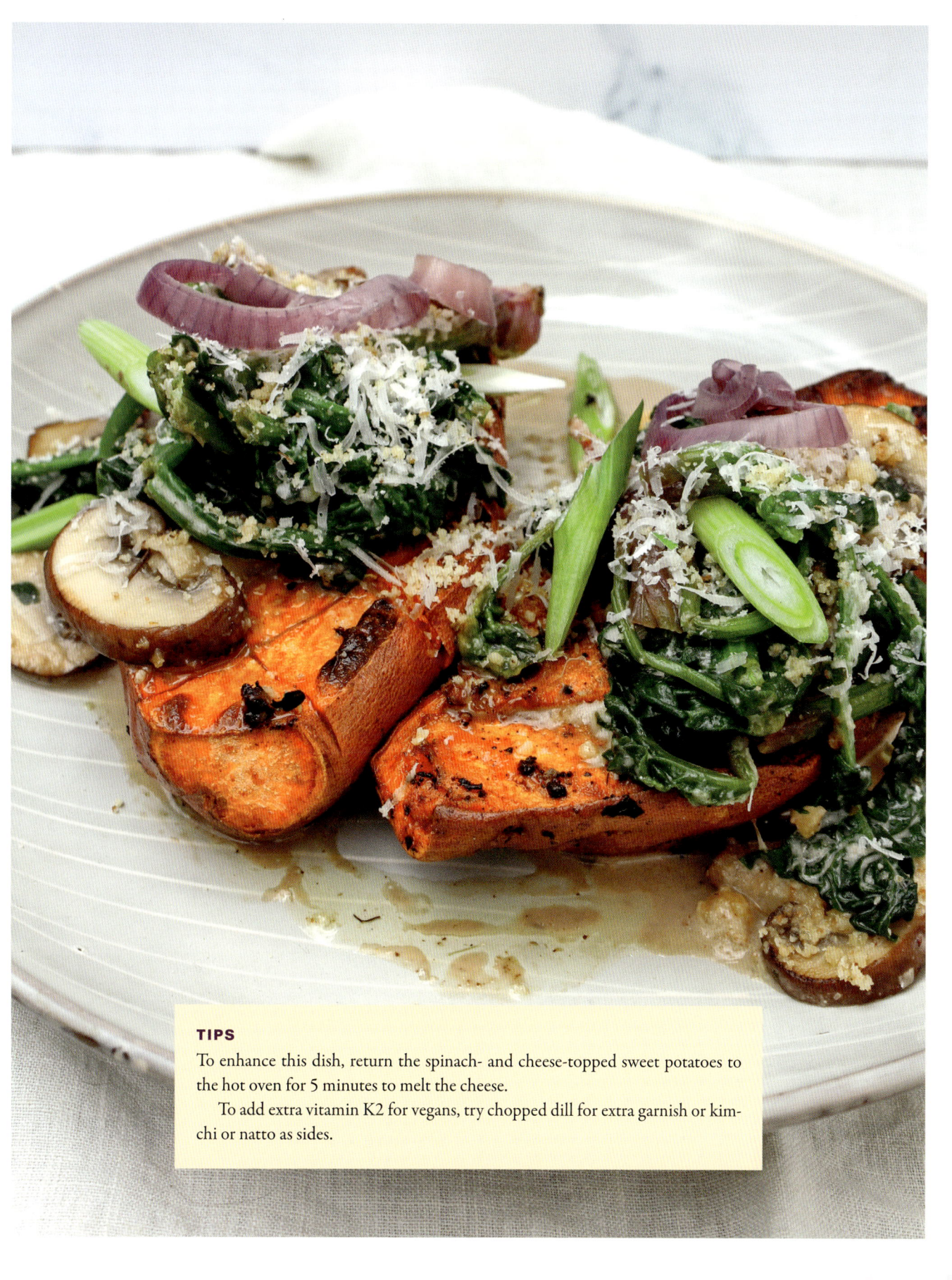

TIPS

To enhance this dish, return the spinach- and cheese-topped sweet potatoes to the hot oven for 5 minutes to melt the cheese.

To add extra vitamin K2 for vegans, try chopped dill for extra garnish or kimchi or natto as sides.

Vegan Delight Matcha Curry

MAKES 2 SERVINGS

Have you ever gotten so many vegetables at the farmers market that you didn't know what to do with them all? This recipe comes to your rescue. You will craft a sauce using wheatgrass and matcha, a unique and delicious combination that makes an extraordinary, vibrant green curry. Instead of traditional wheat flour, this recipe uses gut-friendly medicinal sweet rice powder or arrowroot for thickening, ensuring a creamy and delectable sauce. It is easy to make delicious medicinal food once you tune in to how the colors of fruits and vegetables signify a variety of nutrients that help support good health and strong bones.

You can use brown rice for this recipe, but it requires some advance planning (see Tips).

TIPS

If you prefer brown rice, you can substitute it for the jasmine rice, but plan ahead and soak the brown rice for 30 minutes to 2 hours before the time you plan to start cooking. You'll need to use twice the amount of cooking liquid if you did not soak it and double the cooking time for brown rice compared to jasmine rice.

Always wait until 5 minutes before the end of the cooking time to add light vegetables to a curry sauce. This ensures they maintain their color and texture and won't turn brown or become soggy.

Here's a win-win idea: Make a big batch of this curry and freeze the leftovers. The flavors will intensify when you thaw and reheat, and it's a wonderful easy meal when you don't have time to cook.

Try to make your own seasonal curry, sourcing from your local farmer's fresh vegetables.

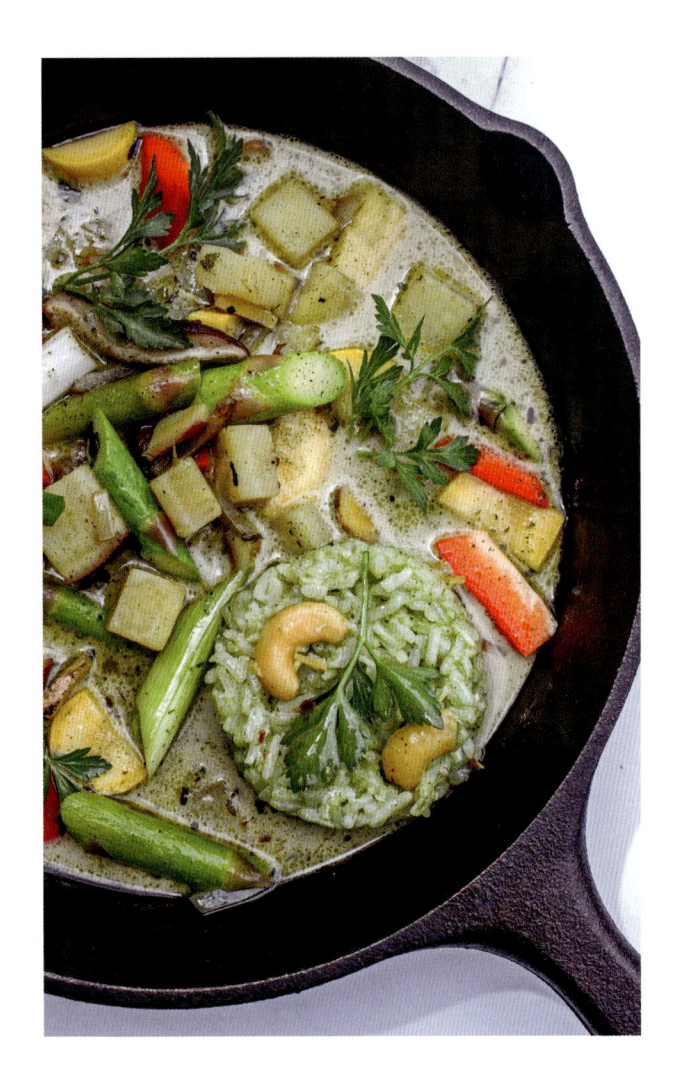

FOR THE RICE

1 cup (190 g) jasmine rice
2½ cups (600 ml) filtered water or Root and Leaf Magnesium Broth (page 177)
2 tablespoons coconut flakes
2 tablespoons crushed raw cashews
1 teaspoon wheatgrass powder

FOR THE CURRY SAUCE

½ cup (120 ml) coconut milk
2 tablespoons curry powder
1 teaspoon matcha powder
1 teaspoon rice powder or arrowroot
1 teaspoon wheatgrass powder

FOR THE CURRY

1 tablespoon coconut oil
1 teaspoon minced garlic
1 teaspoon minced fresh ginger
1 shallot or ¼ small onion, finely chopped
¼ teaspoon cumin
¼ teaspoon fennel seed
1 teaspoon chopped fresh parsley
¼ cup (40 g) coarsely chopped yam or potato
1 cup (240 ml) filtered water or Root and Leaf Magnesium Broth (page 177)
1 bay leaf
¼ cup (40 g) coarsely chopped asparagus
¼ cup (40 g) coarsely chopped bell pepper
¼ cup (40 g) coarsely chopped zucchini
Sea salt
Cracked black pepper

TO SERVE

2 tablespoons pickled ginger
1 scallion, thinly sliced
Fresh flat-leaf parsley or Thai basil

1. Rinse the rice and drain it well. Transfer the rice to a medium pot. Add the water or broth, coconut flakes, and cashews. Bring to a boil and simmer, covered, for 10 minutes. Reduce the heat to medium-low and let it cook for another 3 to 5 minutes, until the water is fully absorbed. Add the wheatgrass powder, gently stirring the rice once or twice to incorporate evenly until the rice turns green. Set aside, covered.
2. Make the curry sauce: In a mini blender, combine the coconut milk and the curry, matcha, rice, and wheatgrass powders. Blend the mixture evenly for 1 minute. Set aside.
3. Make the curry: In a pan over medium heat, add the coconut oil, garlic, ginger, and shallot. Sauté for 1 to 2 minutes. Add the cumin, fennel seed, and parsley and sauté for another 1 to 2 minutes. Add the yam and sauté for an additional 3 minutes. Pour in the water or broth, add the bay leaf, and continue to cook over medium-high heat for 10 minutes, until the liquid reduces by half. Reduce the heat to medium and slowly pour in the green coconut curry sauce from the blender. Add the asparagus, bell pepper, and zucchini, and cook, stirring well, for 5 minutes, until the curry thickens. Season with salt and pepper. Remove from the heat and let cool for 5 to 10 minutes.
4. Serve the rice in two bowls, pour half the curry over each, add a spoonful of pickled ginger on top, sprinkle with scallions, and garnish with parsley.

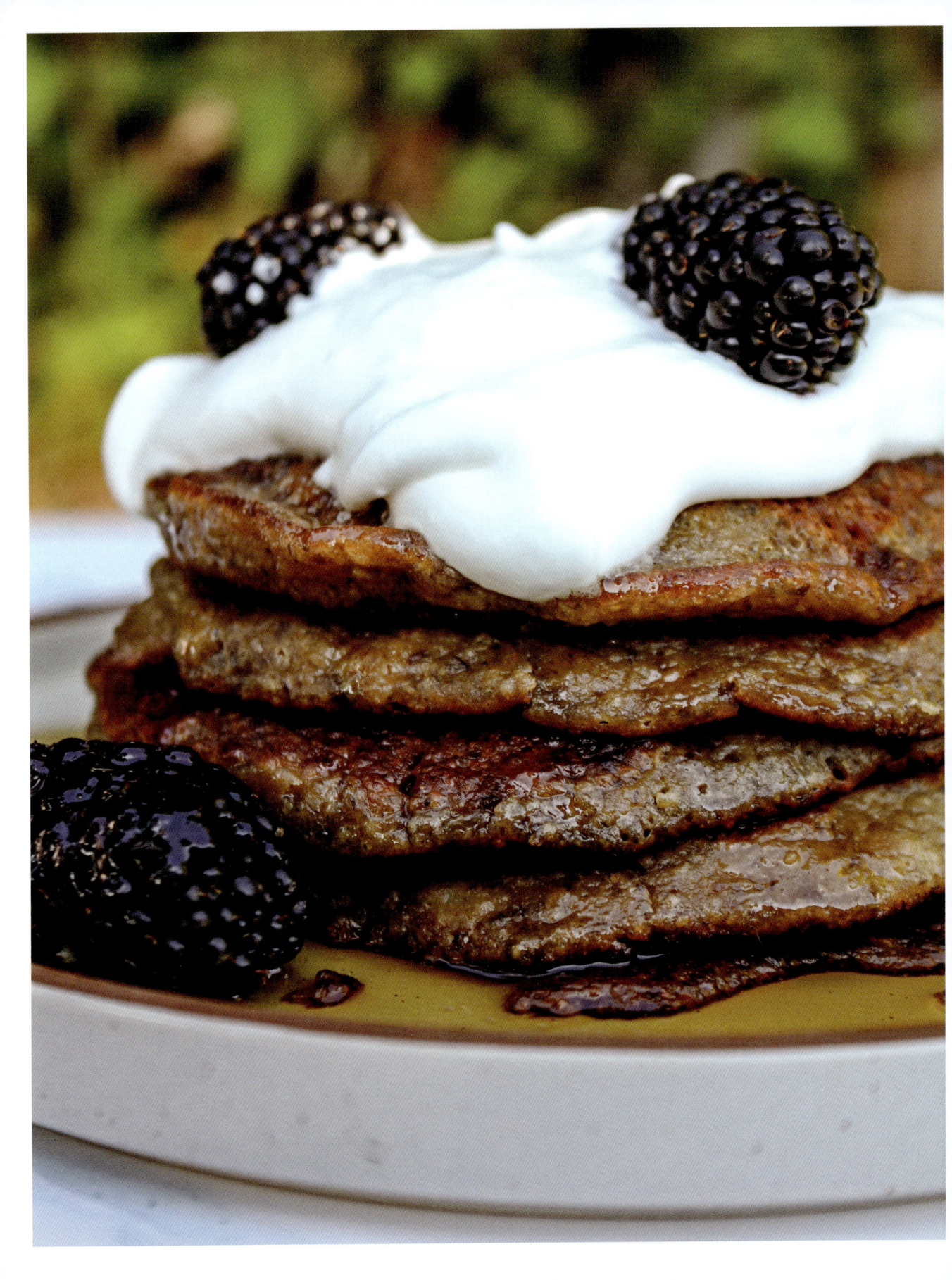

CHAPTER 17

Super Side Dishes

Spain is a foodies' paradise, especially its bustling markets. Anywhere you go, you will find tapas—those cute little dishes that let you experience an extravaganza of flavors without stuffing yourself silly. I remember tapas fondly from my travels, each one a little adventure for my taste buds. Those small but mighty dishes are the unsung heroes of conquering hunger. What amazes me about the power of sides is how they bring together abundant flavors and nutritious, diverse ingredients in one dish. Traditional Korean meals also include lots of small plates, and that's another influence that inspired the recipes to follow.

From broccoli rabe to gazpacho to a veggie frittata, the recipes in this chapter differ widely in appearance, taste, and cooking methods. Alone, they are great solo acts with awesome flavors, but when you put them all together, it's like a fabulous orchestra performance with interwoven themes and moods.

Keep in mind that you can scale up any of these sides to turn them into a major dish on their own. This is a great trick to remember when cooking a full dinner menu feels like a major hassle. Instead, simply double or triple one of these recipes and put it center stage on your dinner table. Throughout the chapter, I offer tips for embellishing these dishes if you want to upscale them to a main meal. Then let a simple salad be the side dish, and dinner is served!

Broccoli Rabe Restaurant-Style

MAKES 2 SERVINGS

Have you tried broccoli rabe? I am obsessed with its crunchiness and its distinctive bitter and peppery flavor. Broccoli rabe also provides plenty of bone-health nutrition, including 112 percent of the bone RDA for vitamin K.

You may have wondered why your attempts at cooking broccoli rabe don't quite match up to the vibrant, crunchy, bright green dishes served at your favorite restaurants. If so, you'll be happy to learn a simple technique through this recipe to make your broccoli rabe just as perfect as those restaurant sides.

Infusing the flavors of cardamom and fennel into this dish creates the perfect culinary marriage. The molasses is optional; if you prefer a complex, rich flavor, there's no need to add it.

2 tablespoons sea salt
1 small rosemary sprig
Extra-virgin olive oil
8 broccoli rabe stems
2 tablespoons hemp seed oil
2 tablespoons minced or thinly sliced shallot
1 teaspoon grated fresh ginger
⅛ teaspoon ground cardamom
⅛ teaspoon fennel seed
1 tablespoon molasses (optional)
Hand-torn fresh parsley leaves
1 tablespoon grated aged parmesan cheese

1. Fill a large pot halfway with water and add the salt, half of the rosemary sprig, and a splash of olive oil. Bring to a boil. Meanwhile, prepare a bowl of ice water.
2. Add the broccoli rabe to the pot and lower the heat to a simmer. Cook for 2 to 3 minutes, then, using tongs or a slotted spoon, remove the broccoli rabe from the pot and place in a colander. Rinse with cold water and transfer to the ice water for 5 minutes. Drain and gently squeeze the broccoli rabe to remove excess water. Set aside.
3. In a skillet over medium-low heat, add the hemp seed oil. Brush the pan with the remaining rosemary to infuse the oil. Add the shallot, ginger, cardamom, and fennel seed and sauté for 1 to 2 minutes. Add the broccoli rabe and sauté while tossing with the other ingredients for 2 to 3 minutes. Add the molasses if using.
4. Plate and garnish with the parsley and parmesan.

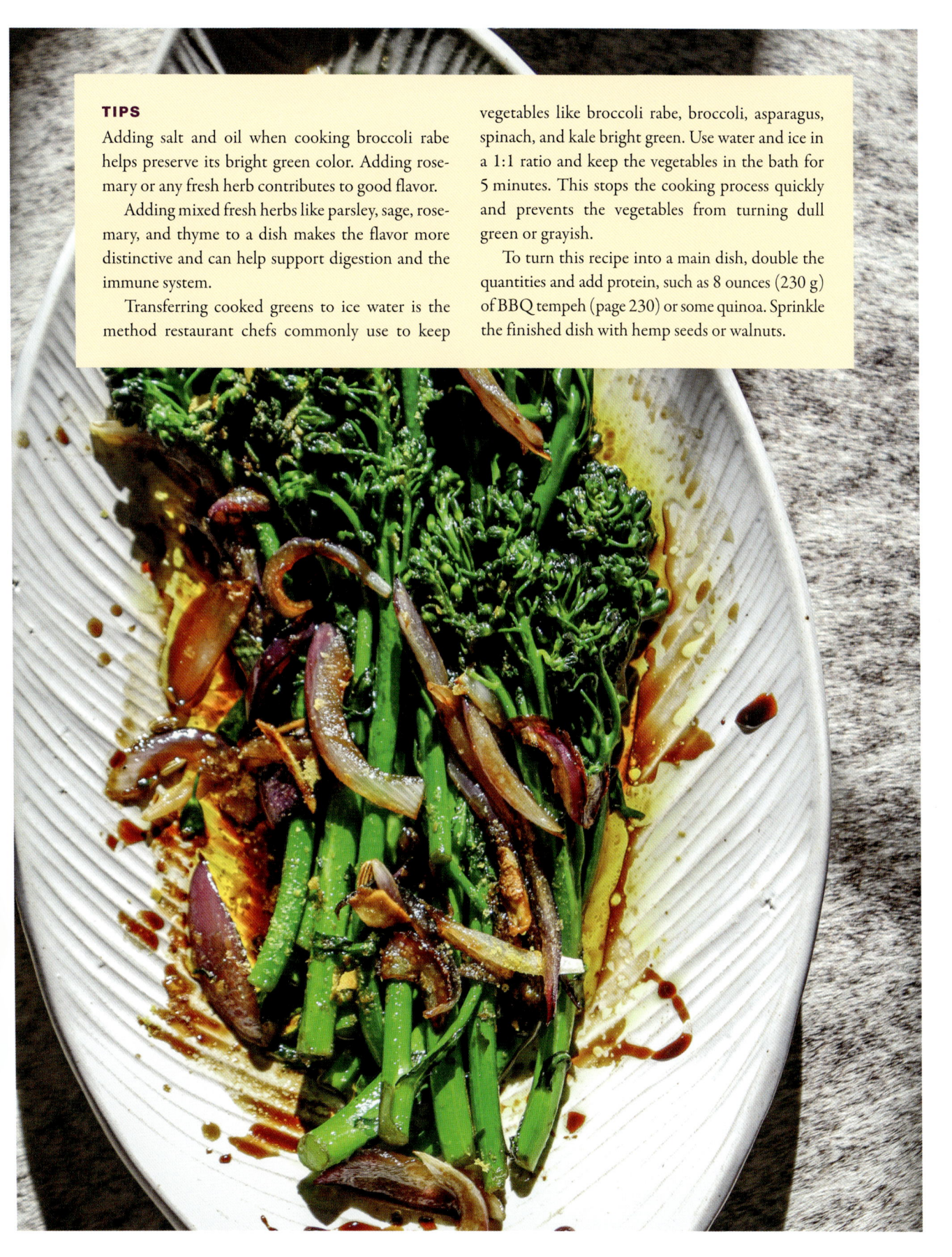

TIPS

Adding salt and oil when cooking broccoli rabe helps preserve its bright green color. Adding rosemary or any fresh herb contributes to good flavor.

Adding mixed fresh herbs like parsley, sage, rosemary, and thyme to a dish makes the flavor more distinctive and can help support digestion and the immune system.

Transferring cooked greens to ice water is the method restaurant chefs commonly use to keep vegetables like broccoli rabe, broccoli, asparagus, spinach, and kale bright green. Use water and ice in a 1:1 ratio and keep the vegetables in the bath for 5 minutes. This stops the cooking process quickly and prevents the vegetables from turning dull green or grayish.

To turn this recipe into a main dish, double the quantities and add protein, such as 8 ounces (230 g) of BBQ tempeh (page 230) or some quinoa. Sprinkle the finished dish with hemp seeds or walnuts.

Go Bananas Flourless Pancakes

MAKES 4 PANCAKES

A pancake topped with berries and sweet syrup is a slice of pure happiness. This recipe satisfies the craving without the heaviness of processed sugar and gluten. These fluffy oat pancakes will take your family Sunday brunch to a whole new level of nutritious goodness—just double or triple the recipe for more people.

This dish is a fantastic choice for kids, too, perfect for breakfast or as a lunchbox meal, paired with a side of nut butter. Add blueberries or strawberries for extra appeal.

Fresh fruits of almost any kind from a local farmers market make a great topping. Add a scoop of coconut whipped cream for a sundae-like pancake experience.

> **TIPS**
>
> If you plan to serve the pancakes with coconut whipped cream, chill the can of coconut cream for at least 4 hours. This step is crucial, as it helps separate the thick coconut cream from the liquid component. Coconut whipped cream is best served right away. But if you have any left over, place it in an airtight container and store it in the refrigerator. Keep in mind that it may firm up, so you might need to rewhip it before using.
>
> You might also enjoy these pancakes as a savory dish by leaving off the sugary toppings. Try drizzling almond or hazelnut butter onto a pancake for extra protein and flavor instead.
>
> Using too much baking soda might make the pancakes bitter, but adding just a bit more than the recipe calls for can yield fluffier pancakes.

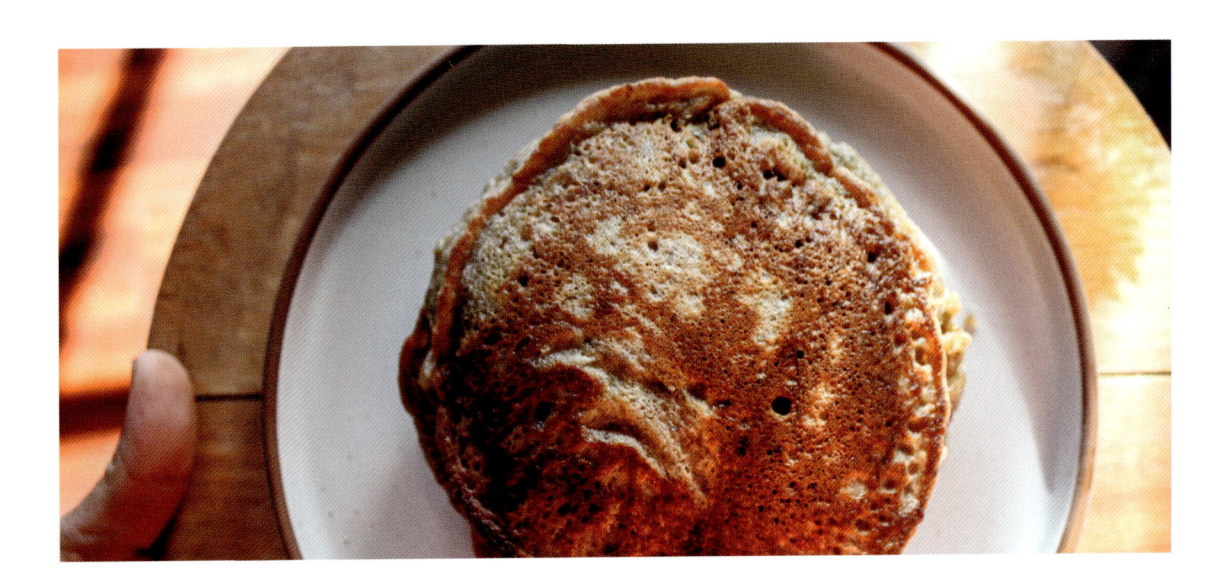

FOR THE COCONUT WHIPPED CREAM (OPTIONAL)

8 ounces (230 g) unsweetened coconut cream
1 tablespoon maple syrup or honey
½ teaspoon vanilla extract (optional)

FOR THE PANCAKES

1 ripe banana
1 cup (120 g) oat flour or freshly ground rolled oats
1 medium egg or flaxseed meal egg substitute (page 146)
2½ tablespoons coconut yogurt
2 tablespoons coconut oil or ghee, plus more for the pan (optional)
1 teaspoon vanilla extract
½ teaspoon baking soda
⅛ teaspoon ground cinnamon
Freshly grated nutmeg

FOR THE TOPPINGS

Fresh berries
Banana slices
Maple or date syrup

1. Make the coconut whipped cream (if using): Remove the coconut cream can from the refrigerator without shaking it. Carefully open the can without tilting it. Scoop out the thick cream into a prechilled mixing bowl, leaving the liquid at the bottom of the can behind. Use an electric mixer or a hand whisk to beat the coconut cream on high speed for 1 to 2 minutes until it becomes fluffy and develops the texture of whipped cream. Add the maple syrup and the vanilla (if using). Beat for an additional 30 seconds to incorporate these ingredients. Put the bowl of whipped cream in the refrigerator until the moment you are ready to top the pancakes and eat them.

2. Make the pancakes: Peel the banana, put it in a medium-sized bowl, and smash it with a fork until smooth. Add the oat flour, egg, coconut yogurt, coconut oil, vanilla, baking soda, cinnamon, and a pinch of nutmeg, and whisk until you've banished all those pesky lumps. If you prefer using a food processor or blender, blend together well for 3 to 5 minutes.

3. Heat a cast-iron skillet over medium-low heat. Add a tablespoon or two of coconut oil or ghee to the pan for that extra yumminess if you wish. Spoon out small dollops of batter, leaving space between them. Watch for tiny air bubbles to form in the top surface of the pancakes and for the pancakes to appear firm from the middle to the edges. Flip the pancakes carefully but swiftly and allow them to cook for 1 to 2 minutes more, until cooked through.

4. Serve the pancakes right away. Bring out the chilled whipped cream, and use berries, banana slices, and maple syrup to dress your pancakes in the way you like best.

Green Pea and Roasted Red Pepper Mash

MAKES 2 SERVINGS

Green peas are packed with nutrients, including vitamins C and E, zinc, and antioxidants that can help strengthen the immune system. Other nutrients, such as vitamins A and B, help reduce inflammation, support heart health, aid digestion, and promote healthy skin. This visually striking recipe pairs the peas with the bright color and smoky flavor of roasted red peppers, and the creamy spinach sauce adds a burst of flavor. Best of all, it's incredibly easy to make, requiring just a few simple steps to achieve green and red nirvana!

The spinach–pine nut sauce is a delightful alternative to traditional tomato sauce for pasta dishes. Adding a hint of lemon juice enhances the flavor and counteracts any potential bitterness. (You can add lemon juice to other green sauces for a similar effect.) The wheatgrass extract boosts the sauce's nutritional value due to wheatgrass's abundance of minerals and vitamins.

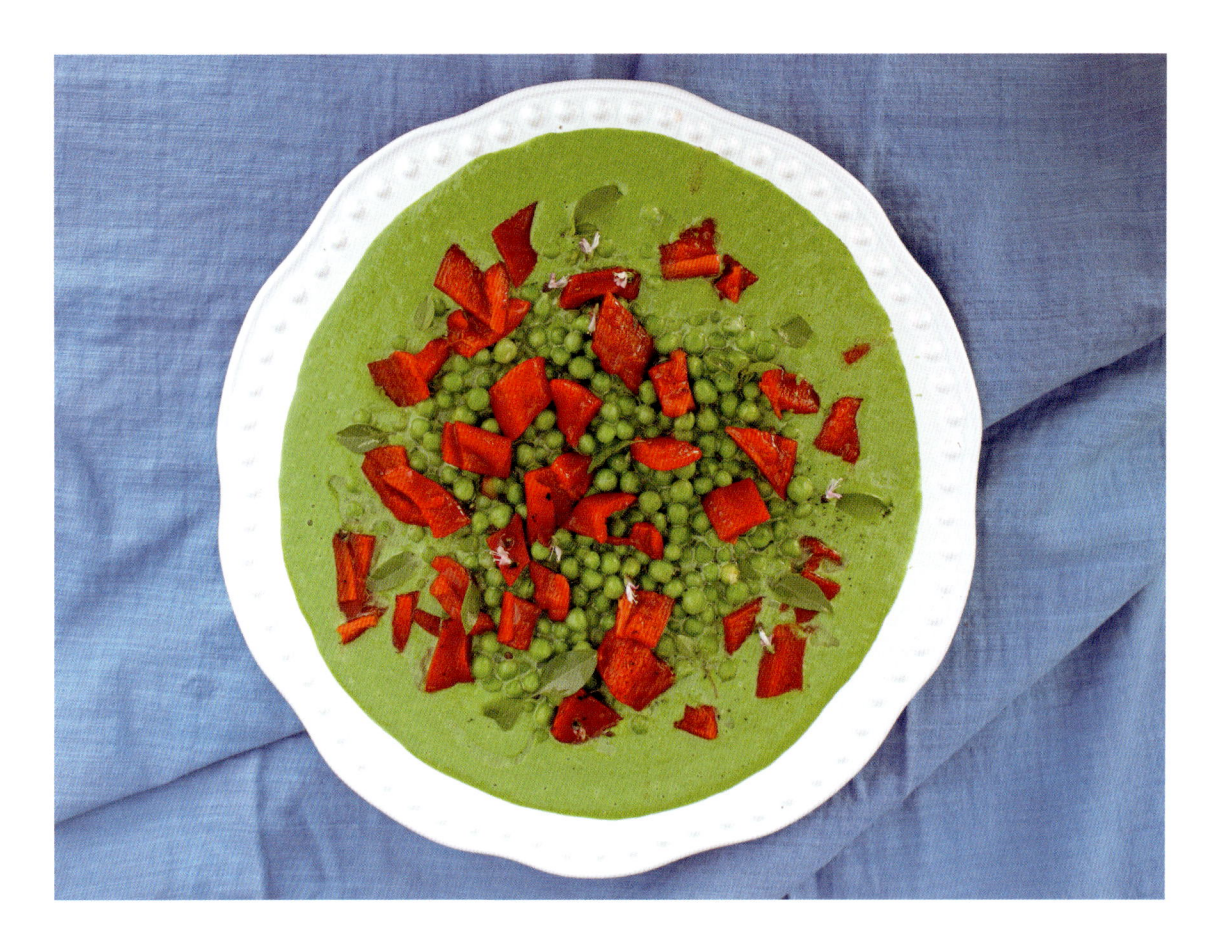

Sea salt

1 rosemary sprig

1 cup (30 g) fresh spinach leaves

2 cups (400 g) frozen green peas

¼ cup (50 g) pine nuts

5 tablespoons (75 ml) avocado oil

2 tablespoons wheatgrass juice (see Tips)

1 garlic clove

2 tablespoons grated parmesan cheese (optional)

Fresh lemon juice

Pink Himalayan salt

Cracked black pepper

1 cup (150 g) chopped roasted red peppers

1 shallot, thinly sliced

Holy basil leaves, for garnish

1. Fill a medium pot about two-thirds full of water and add a pinch of salt along with the rosemary sprig. Bring to a boil and then reduce to a simmer, add the spinach, and boil for 2 to 3 minutes, then remove the rosemary sprig. Using a slotted spoon, remove the spinach from the pot and quickly chill in an ice bath to preserve its bright green color (see page 245). Drain and set aside.

2. To the same pot, add the peas and boil them for 3 to 5 minutes, until warmed through. Then transfer them to an ice bath to preserve their color. Drain and set aside.

3. In a large blender, combine the cooked spinach, pine nuts, avocado oil, wheatgrass juice, garlic, and parmesan, if using. Blend for 2 to 3 minutes, beginning at low speed and gradually increasing the speed until the texture becomes silky and smooth. Then add a squeeze of lemon juice and season with the pink salt and pepper. Blend again at a lower speed for 1 to 2 minutes until the sauce turns bright green.

4. On a serving plate, spread a layer of the spinach–pine nut sauce. Arrange the boiled green peas, roasted peppers, and shallot on top of the sauce, ensuring they are evenly distributed. For added aroma and visual appeal, garnish with the holy basil leaves.

TIPS

Swap in cashews or walnuts for the pine nuts in the sauce. Both options are more affordable and offer their own unique nutritional benefits.

If you don't have wheatgrass juice, you can substitute wheatgrass powder mixed with water.

Super Side Dishes

Immortal Acai Bowl

MAKES 1 SERVING

If kimchi is the reigning fermented staple dish from Korea and South Asia, kefir is its Russian counterpart. Both are iconic everyday fermented staples in their respective regions, celebrated for their fermentation processes, unique flavors, and potential health benefits. Kefir is a fermented milk or coconut water beverage, offering a different taste and texture but sharing the same spirit of harnessing the power of probiotics and fermentation.

This bowl is the perfect dish for a sweet treat, a healthy breakfast, or a midday energy boost. Coconut kefir takes center stage in supporting gut health by promoting a diverse microbiome, aiding digestion, and boosting immunity. Its nutrients and enzymes enhance nutrient absorption and may even have anti-inflammatory effects. When paired with acai berry powder and fresh berries, this dish also provides electrolytes that are crucial for optimal metabolism.

¼ cup (30 g) blackberries
¼ cup (35 g) blueberries
¼ cup (30 g) raspberries
½ cup (120 ml) coconut kefir
2 tablespoons chopped pineapple
1 tablespoon acai powder
1 tablespoon goji berry powder
2 teaspoons chopped pistachios
Fresh lemon juice
1 teaspoon maple syrup

FOR GARNISH
Mint leaves
Ground cinnamon

1. Wash and gently dry the blackberries, blueberries, and raspberries.
2. Spread the coconut kefir in the bottom of a serving bowl. Add the berries, and then spoon on the pineapple, acai powder, goji berry powder, and pistachios. Drizzle a squeeze of lemon juice and the maple syrup over the top.
3. Garnish with mint leaves, dust with cinnamon, and serve.

> **TIPS**
> For added health benefits and texture, soak ¼ cup (40 g) chia seeds in water overnight, and mix into the coconut kefir.
>
> Store leftover pineapple in the freezer for your morning fruit and yogurt smoothie. If you prefer a smoother texture and less sweetness for this dish, try using papaya instead of pineapple.

Crunchy Roasted Brussels Sprouts

MAKES 2 SERVINGS

These little flavor bombs are the epitome of crunchiness and well-balanced nutrition. Don't judge their benefits by size alone. These mini marvels are loaded with vitamins K and C, fiber, and a bounty of antioxidants.

Brussels sprouts are incredibly versatile. You can roast, sauté, or steam them, or shred them to add to salads. The crop thrives in cool and cold weather, making them a fall and winter favorite.

This recipe reveals a supercool technique for making roasted Brussels sprouts extra crunchy.

12 Brussels sprouts (about 10 ounces [300 g])
3 tablespoons extra-virgin olive oil
1 teaspoon red or yellow curry powder
2 tablespoons finely crushed macadamias
1 teaspoon finely chopped fresh rosemary
Parmesan cheese or vegan parmesan
Truffle powder
Fresh chives

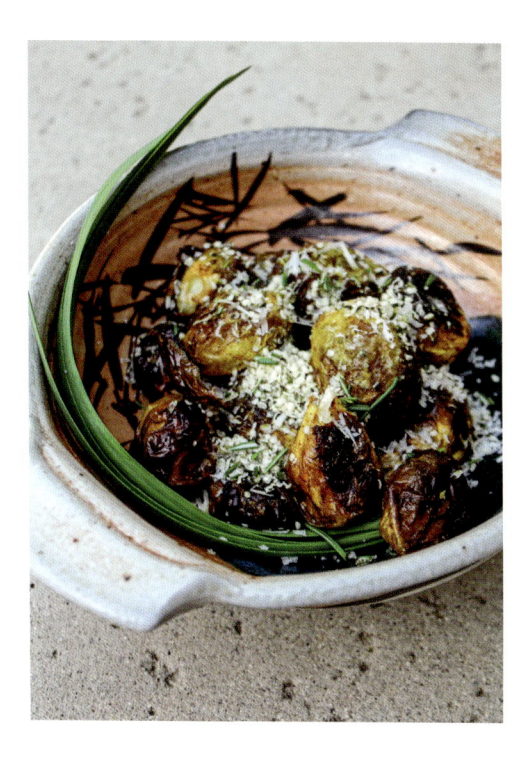

1. Preheat the oven to 350°F (180°C).
2. Place the Brussels sprouts on a baking sheet. Drizzle with the oil and sprinkle with the curry powder, and toss to coat evenly. Bake for 15 to 20 minutes. Test doneness using a wooden skewer to poke a few of the sprouts. When they are al dente, increase the oven temperature to 400°F (200°C) and continue roasting for 5 to 10 minutes more, until the sprouts have browned at the leaf edges. Remove the pan from the oven.
3. Transfer the sprouts to a serving bowl or plate. Sprinkle with the macadamias and rosemary. Shave some parmesan over the top. Finish with a pinch of truffle powder and a graceful arc of chives.

TIP
If you prefer not to use cheese, try Tahini-Ginger Dressing (page 209) as a garnish instead. This gives the dish a nutty, tangy twist.

Super Side Dishes

Rainbow Veggie Frittata with Feta

MAKES 4 TO 8 SERVINGS

In Traditional Chinese Medicine (TCM), each color is associated with an element and organ. Green represents the Wood element and is linked to the liver, symbolizing spring. Red corresponds to the Fire element and is connected to the heart, representing summer. Yellow/orange embodies the Earth element, supporting the immune system and enhancing vision. Earth represents the transition between seasons and is ruled by the gut. White is associated with the Metal element and the lungs, signifying fall. Purple to black represents the Water element and is ruled by the kidneys.

This colorful feta cheese frittata incorporates a variety of rainbow vegetables, reflecting the TCM approach and achieving a balance of essential nutrients by colors. It's sure to brighten up your kitchen and lift your mood.

Using an 8-inch (20 cm) skillet will result in a pizzalike frittata. For a deeper frittata with a quichelike texture, opt for a 6-inch (15 cm) skillet.

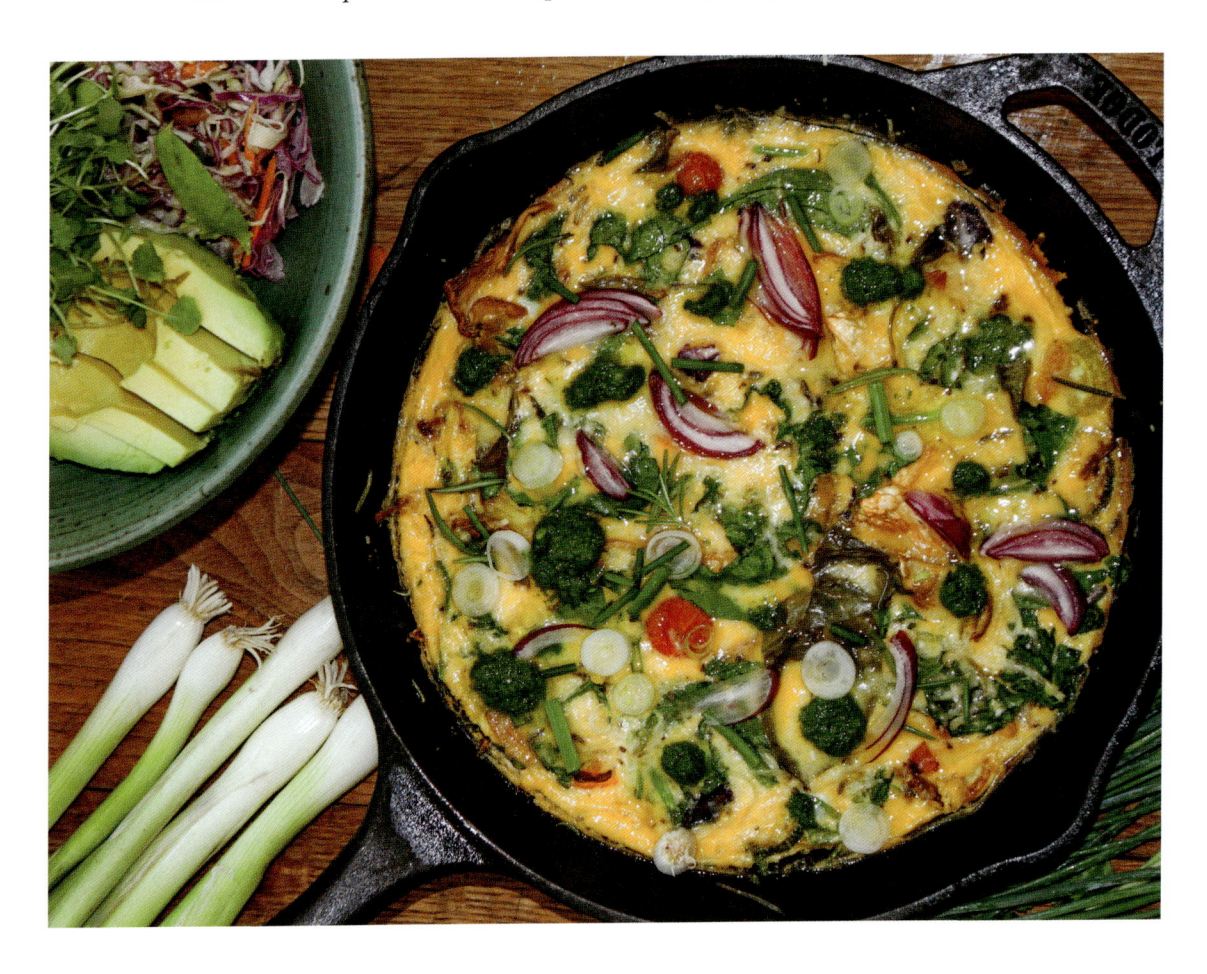

1 small yellow zucchini (3 inches [8 cm])
1 small carrot
Handful spinach leaves
¼ cup (15 g) lion's mane or (10 g) oyster mushrooms
¼ cup (80 g) purple cauliflower florets
¼ cup (40 g) sliced shallot
4 cherry tomatoes
6 medium eggs
2 tablespoons coconut milk
1 teaspoon herbes de Provence
⅛ teaspoon sea salt
⅛ teaspoon cracked black pepper
2 tablespoons pumpkin seed oil
1 rosemary sprig
5 basil leaves
¼ cup (30 g) crumbled feta cheese (optional)

FOR GARNISH

Chopped fresh chives or basil
Green Oil (page 143)

TIP

The versatility of this dish allows you to experiment with various main ingredients. My personal favorite combinations are leek and parsnip, potato and dill, and mushroom and cabbage.

1. Preheat the oven to 325°F (165°C). Slice the zucchini and carrot and roughly chop the spinach. Shred the mushrooms and prep the cauliflower and shallot. Cut the cherry tomatoes in half. Place the prepared mushrooms and vegetables on a plate.

2. In a small bowl, combine the eggs and coconut milk. Add ½ teaspoon of the herbes de Provence, the salt, and pepper and whisk together until well combined.

3. Place a cast-iron skillet over low to medium heat. Add the pumpkin seed oil and brush it with the rosemary sprig. Add the remaining ½ teaspoon herbes de Provence and lightly sauté. Next, add the zucchini, carrot, spinach, mushrooms, cauliflower, shallot, cherry tomatoes, and basil. Sauté the vegetables gently for 2 to 3 minutes, allowing them to soften and release their flavors. Then pour the egg mixture into the skillet. Tilt the pan from side to side so that uncooked egg can spread and contact the pan's surface. After 2 to 3 minutes, the eggs will be mostly set. Remove the pan from the heat. If you wish to make the frittata more creamy, add the crumbled cheese on top.

4. Transfer the skillet to the oven to bake. Begin checking the dish after 15 minutes to gauge the baking progress. Once the surface turns golden, remove the skillet from the oven. Total baking time is likely to be 25 to 35 minutes. Allow the frittata to cool for 10 to 15 minutes before serving.

5. Loosen the frittata in the skillet, then slide it onto a serving plate. Garnish with chives or basil for added freshness and visual appeal. To complete the dish, drizzle the green oil over the frittata; it will complement the flavors of the vegetables nicely. Slice the frittata into four large pieces or eight small pieces for serving.

Saffron Cauliflower Rice

MAKES 2 SERVINGS

Cauliflower is a versatile superfood that can shape-shift into various delicious dishes like meaty vegan steaks (page 224), spicy Buffalo wings (page 156), or even an everyday rice substitute, as here. If eating white or brown rice leaves you feeling heavy, it might be time to try this plant-based alternative.

This recipe is a fantastic option for those looking to increase their fiber, vitamin, and mineral intake, all while enjoying a satisfying texture that doesn't leave one feeling overly full. Cauliflower checks all the boxes!

This dish is enhanced with the anti-inflammatory and antioxidant power of saffron and turmeric. Saffron brings potential mood- and memory-enhancing effects along with its traditional benefits for skin health and digestion.

1 small head cauliflower
3 pitted dates, chopped (optional)
2 tablespoons raw cashews
3 tablespoons pumpkin seed oil
¼ teaspoon dried dill
⅛ teaspoon ground coriander
⅛ teaspoon ground cumin
⅛ teaspoon freshly grated nutmeg
1 bay leaf
⅛ teaspoon saffron
⅛ teaspoon ground turmeric
3 tablespoons filtered water
Soy sauce or sea salt
Cracked black pepper
Minced fresh parsley, for garnish

1. Cut the cauliflower in half and then into large chunks. Use a box grater to grate the chunks into rice-sized pieces. If you prefer to use a food processor, you can cut the cauliflower into small pieces instead, and use the grater attachment. Measure 2 cups (226 g) of the grated cauliflower and put the rest in a sealed container in the refrigerator to use for another recipe.

2. Soak the dates (if you desire to add a little sweetness) and cashews separately in small bowls of water for 15 to 30 minutes, then drain and chop.

3. Heat the pumpkin seed oil in a sauté pan over medium heat. Add the dill, coriander, cumin, nutmeg, and bay leaf, and infuse the spices into the oil for 1 to 2 minutes, until aromatic. Add the grated cauliflower, chopped cashews, saffron, and turmeric. Sauté for 2 to 5 minutes, until the cauliflower becomes somewhat translucent and cooks down in volume. Then add the water and cover the pan with a lid for 30 seconds to steam and further tenderize the cauliflower. Remove the lid and mix well. Continue cooking for 5 to 8 minutes longer, add chopped dates at the last minute, and finish seasoning with soy sauce and pepper.

4. Transfer the cauliflower rice to a serving plate or bowl, and garnish with the parsley.

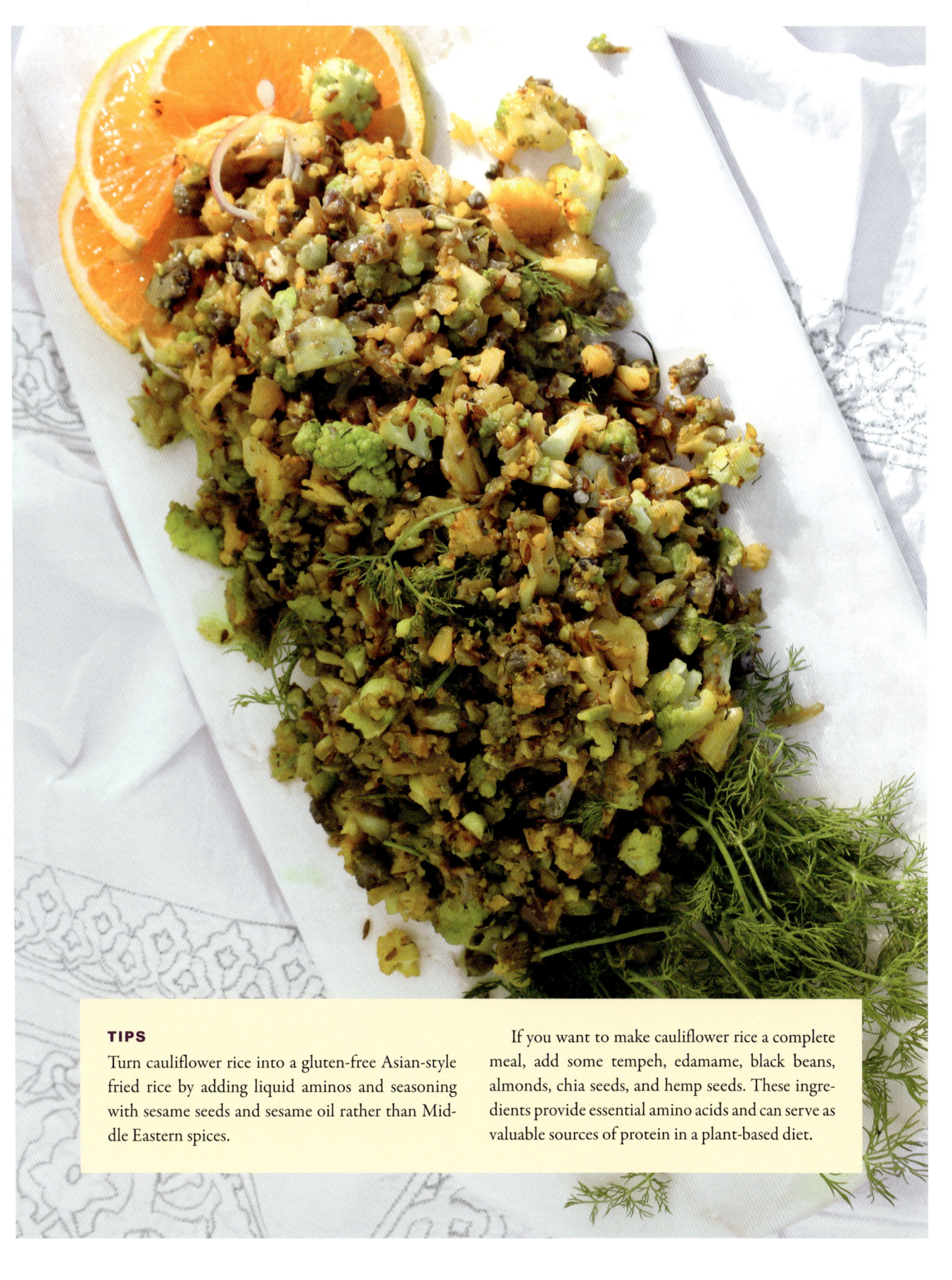

TIPS

Turn cauliflower rice into a gluten-free Asian-style fried rice by adding liquid aminos and seasoning with sesame seeds and sesame oil rather than Middle Eastern spices.

If you want to make cauliflower rice a complete meal, add some tempeh, edamame, black beans, almonds, chia seeds, and hemp seeds. These ingredients provide essential amino acids and can serve as valuable sources of protein in a plant-based diet.

Smoky Roasted Rooty Roots

MAKES 2 SERVINGS

When you pair tender, sweet, and buttery parsnips with other roots, like fingerling potatoes and carrots, you can double the dose of fiber, vitamins, and minerals to boost nutrition. Adding a spinach-based sauce brightens up the dish. This is a hearty winter side dish with roots that will ground you, bringing calm and peace. Parsnips are a great source of vitamins C and K and folate, as well as several other important micronutrients. They are also high in antioxidants that may prevent oxidative stress and health conditions like cancer, diabetes, and heart disease.

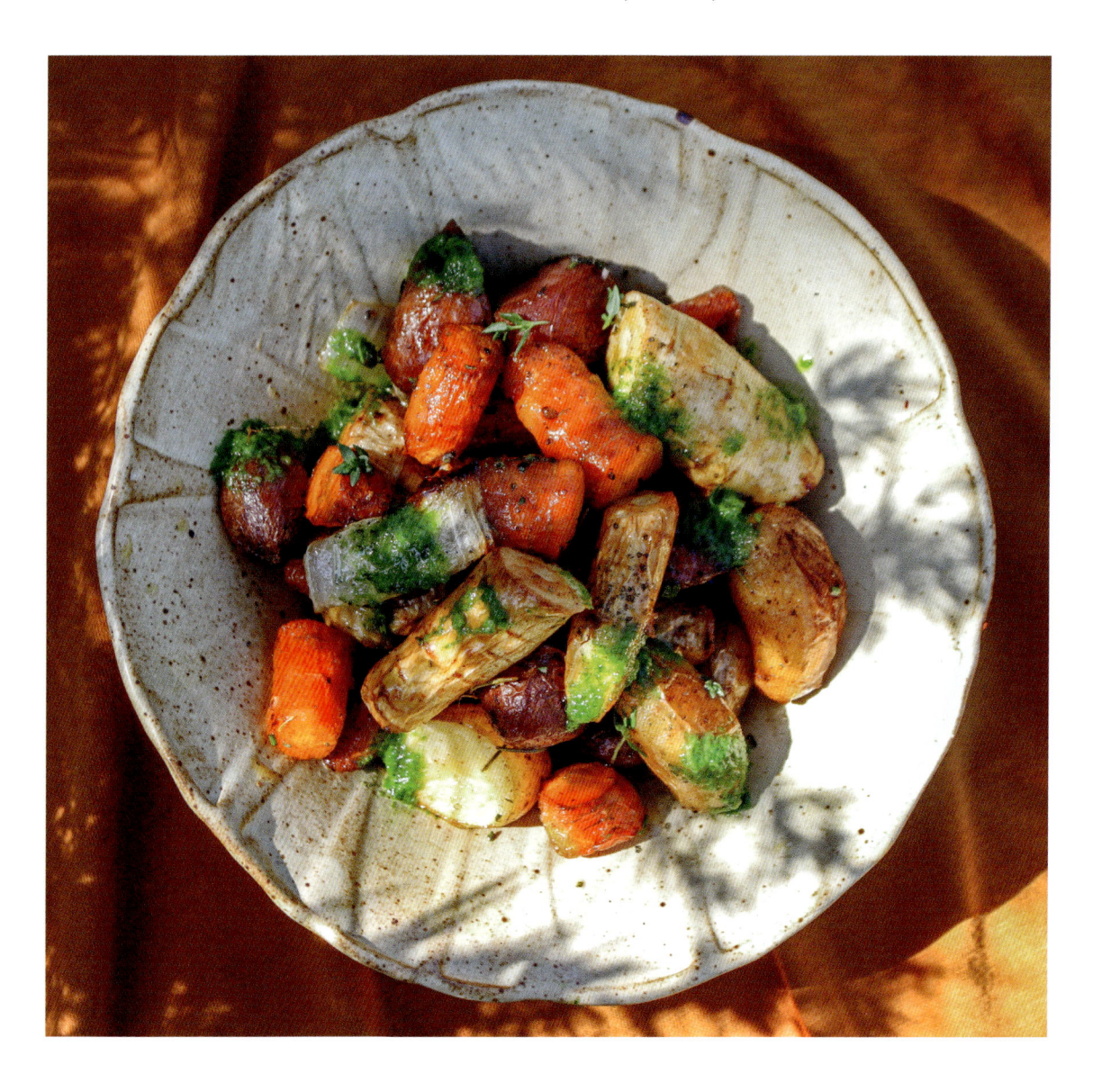

10½ ounces (300 g) red and golden fingerling potatoes
1 medium (60 g) carrot
1 medium (60 g) parsnip
½ onion (30 g)
3 tablespoons flaxseed oil
¼ teaspoon herbal salt (see Tips)
⅛ teaspoon ground cinnamon
⅛ teaspoon freshly grated nutmeg
⅛ teaspoon smoked paprika
Ground black pepper

FOR THE DEEP GREEN SAUCE

3 bunches spinach
3 shallots, sliced
5 tablespoons extra-virgin olive oil
1 garlic clove, minced
Sea salt
Ground black pepper

TO SERVE

2 or 3 rosemary, thyme, or sage sprigs, plus 1 additional rosemary sprig
1 tablespoon extra-virgin olive oil

> **TIP**
>
> Make an herbal salt with fresh rosemary, thyme, and sage. Chop the herb leaves, add them to a small jar, and fill the jar with salt. If you are a garlic lover, add crushed garlic for more flavor and medicinal elements. Cover and store in the refrigerator for up to 6 months. Use the salt in any dressing or seasoning oil. It will save time and increase flavor, and it is a good anti-inflammatory and antifungal remedy.

1. Preheat the oven to 375°F (190°C). Cut the potatoes, carrot, and parsnip into large pieces on a 45-degree diagonal to make the shapes interesting. Make the pieces of potato and carrot approximately the same size so that everything cooks evenly; parsnip pieces should be larger as they will shrink more. (If you want them to cook faster, cut them into smaller cubes.) Slice the onion from root to stem.

2. Place the roots and onion on a baking sheet and drizzle with the oil. Sprinkle with the herbal salt, cinnamon, nutmeg, and paprika. Season with a few grinds of pepper. Mix well to coat the vegetables evenly with the oil and spices. Transfer the baking sheet to the oven and roast for 45 to 55 minutes.

3. Meanwhile, make the sauce: In a mini blender, working in batches as needed, combine the spinach, shallots, oil, garlic, and a pinch each of salt and pepper. Blend well for 1 to 2 minutes. Add salt until it tastes perfectly seasoned.

4. After 20 minutes, check the roots in the oven by poking with a small knife, then adjust the remaining time as needed. Every oven is different, so don't just stick to the recipe time; always check the dish once or twice while it's cooking. Continue to roast until the vegetables are golden brown and a knife goes through smoothly. Remove from the oven and let cool.

5. To serve, remove the herbs from the stems and chop finely. Place the roots on a serving plate and sprinkle with the herbs. Drizzle with the olive oil and add a bit more paprika to increase the smoky flavor. Drizzle with the sauce, garnish with a rosemary sprig, and serve.

Super Side Dishes

Triple Kale Chips

MAKES 4 CUPS [270 G]

Can you guess how many potato chips the average American eats? Ten thousand a year! And many of those chips are loaded with processed chemicals, sodium, and trans fats or seed oils, which can contribute to chronic health conditions.

This number shocked me and inspired me to create this recipe to challenge the supremacy of those non-nutritious potato chips. My kale chips have a fabulous nutty flavor. Combining three different kales and coating them with almond and millet flours gives this chip an insane crunchiness. You can keep a batch on your kitchen table—the more you nibble, the better you will feel.

5 large green kale leaves
5 large lacinato kale leaves
5 large Russian kale leaves
½ cup (120 ml) coconut oil
¼ cup (25 g) almond flour
¼ cup (30 g) millet flour
1 tablespoon nutritional yeast
⅛ teaspoon ground cinnamon
⅛ teaspoon freshly grated nutmeg
Sea salt
Cracked black pepper
3 tablespoons gluten-free panko
Crushed nuts, sesame seeds, or hemp seeds (optional)

1. Preheat the oven to 325°F (165°C). Remove the kale leaves from the stems and tear into large pieces, keeping in mind they will shrink 70 percent when cooked.
2. In a large bowl, add the coconut oil, almond flour, millet flour, nutritional yeast, cinnamon, and nutmeg, and mix well.
3. Add the kale to the bowl and toss evenly with the coating, then season lightly with salt and pepper.
4. Set up two baking sheets with racks on top. Spread the kale evenly on the racks and sprinkle with the panko. Bake for 30 minutes. When the kale is completely dehydrated, remove the pan from the oven. Sprinkle with your favorite nuts or seeds, if desired.
5. Allow the chips to cool for about an hour. After the chips are cooled and crunchy, place in a wooden basket and cover with a cotton cloth to absorb any moisture and keep the chips crunchy.

> **TIPS**
>
> If you'd like to try different flours, I recommend cassava flour or sprouted sorghum flour. Both have earthy, nutty flavors and are gluten-free.
>
> If you want to reduce the baking time for these chips, preheat the oven to 425°F (220°C). The chips will bake in just 5 to 10 minutes.

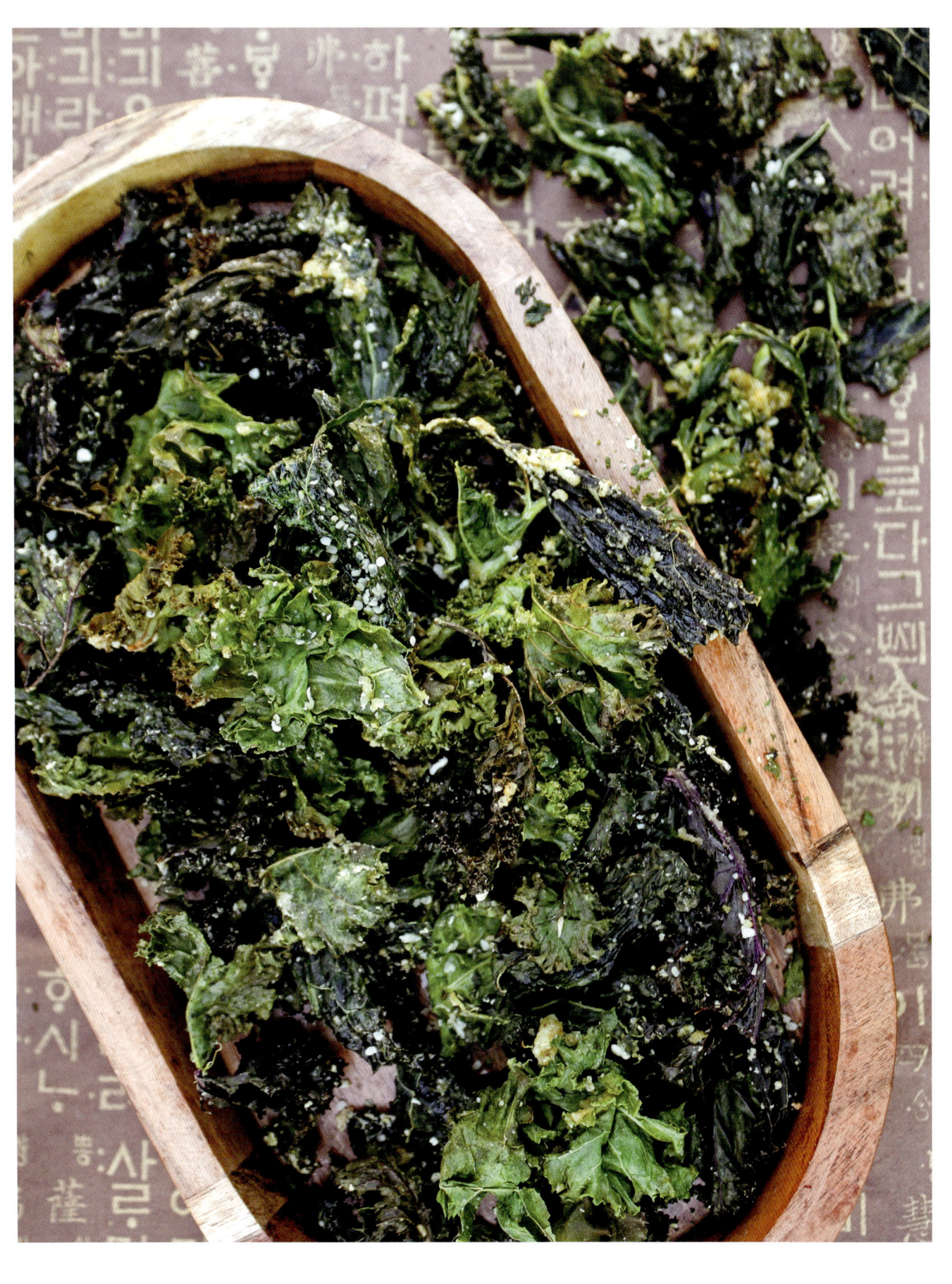

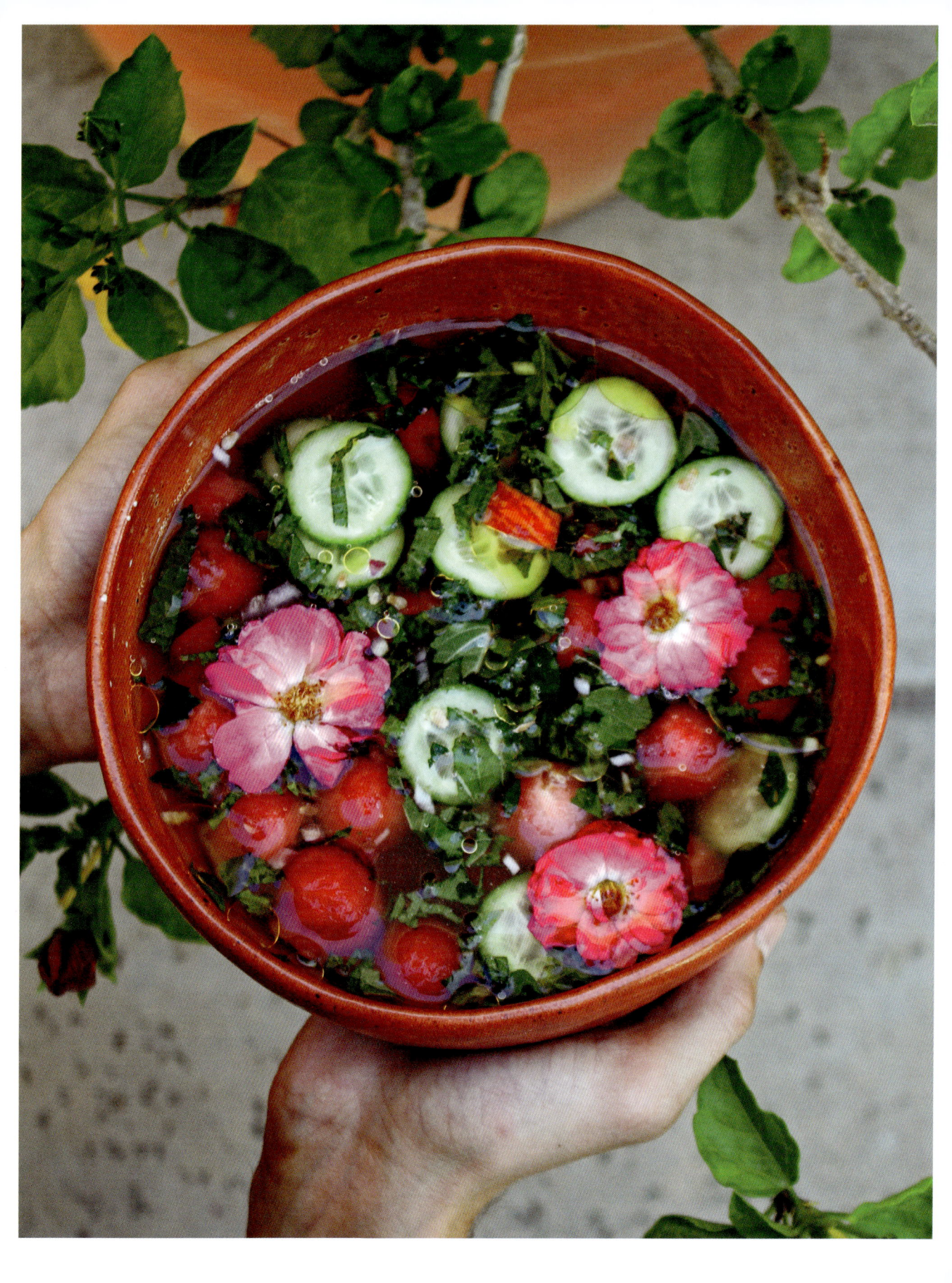

Watermelon-Mint Gazpacho

MAKES 2 SERVINGS

The most summery summer fruit, and one of my favorites, watermelon is a natural thirst quencher. Just a few juicy slices can make you feel wonderfully full. Wait, here's the exciting part—don't toss away that rind! It's packed with antioxidants, vitamins (think C, A, B6), essential minerals like potassium, and even a dash of zinc.

Traditional gazpacho has a creamy, blended base, but this recipe takes inspiration from a type of gazpacho from Portugal, in which the base is a salty, garlicky brine. This chilled soup is the perfect cool-off dish at lunchtime on a hot summer day. Chill the watermelon in the refrigerator for a day in advance if you can.

1½ cups (360 ml) filtered water
1 teaspoon sea salt
1 small garlic clove
Half a small watermelon, chilled
3 tablespoons white vinegar or rice vinegar
2 tablespoons extra-virgin olive oil
¼ teaspoon fresh lemon or lime juice
Sea salt
Cracked black pepper
½ Persian cucumber, sliced
¼ cup (40 g) chopped seeded heirloom tomato
2 tablespoons finely chopped fresh mint
2 teaspoons finely chopped shallot or red onion
½ cup ice cubes
Mint leaves and edible flowers, for garnish

1. In a medium bowl, combine the water and salt, mixing them until the salt completely dissolves. Mince the garlic finely and add it to the salt water.
2. Using a spoon or a melon baller, scoop out rounded pieces of watermelon flesh and rind until you have approximately 1 cup (150 g) of melon flesh plus ¼ cup (20 g) of rind. Place the pieces in a bowl. As you take scoops, pour off the juice that pools into a small bowl until you have ¼ cup (60 ml).
3. In a large bowl, combine the vinegar, olive oil, and lemon juice and season with salt and pepper. The mixture should have a slightly salty taste. Add the watermelon, cucumber, tomato, mint, and shallot. Toss gently to combine.
4. Add the ice cubes, garlic mixture, and watermelon juice, and mix all the ingredients until well combined. Garnish with fresh mint leaves and edible flowers and serve.

TIPS

If you don't have a melon baller, simply cut the watermelon flesh and rind into 1-inch (2.5 cm) cubes.

You can make a refreshing salad using watermelon rind. Cut the rind into thin shreds and add cucumber slices, drizzle with a good-quality olive oil, sprinkle with sea salt, add a squeeze of lemon juice, and finish with chopped mint. It's a super hydrating and delicious combination, perfect for quenching your thirst.

Super Side Dishes

Wok Express Crunchy Green Beans

MAKES 2 SERVINGS

I love the sound of a sizzling wok in a bustling Chinese restaurant filled with fabulous aromas. Yum! Green beans with oyster sauce is a winner. These little green gems are a health superhero packed with protein, vitamins, and minerals, especially manganese to make your bones strong and solid. With my recipe for this classic dish, I will reveal how to make green beans bursting with freshness, crunchiness, and flavor.

2 tablespoons ghee or coconut oil
1 garlic clove, minced
1 teaspoon grated fresh ginger
¼ teaspoon dried chili flakes
½ cup (75 g) thinly sliced onion
2 cups (300 g) green beans, trimmed
1 tablespoon oyster sauce
Lemon peel spirals and fresh lemon juice
1 scallion, finely chopped
1 teaspoon sesame seeds

1. Preheat a wok on high heat for 1 to 2 minutes. Carefully add the ghee, garlic, ginger, and chili flakes. Stir the ingredients for less than a minute to infuse the flavors in the oil. Add the onion, followed by the green beans. Stir-fry rapidly for 2 to 3 minutes, shaking the wok to ensure even cooking. During the last minute of cooking, add the oyster sauce.
2. Transfer the cooked green beans to a serving plate. Drizzle with lemon juice and sprinkle with the scallions, sesame seeds, and lemon curls for added flavor and visual appeal.

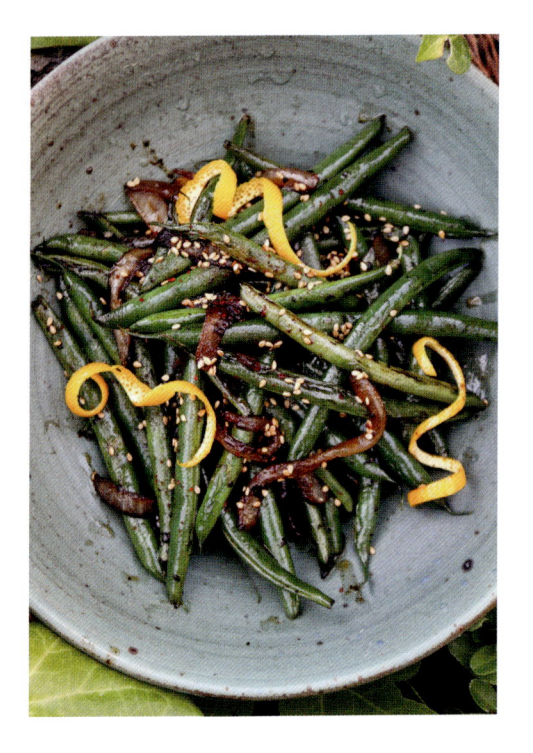

TIPS

This cooking method can also be applied to other vegetables, such as asparagus or broccoli rabe. Any dark green vegetables pair wonderfully with oyster sauce. Since oyster sauce can be quite salty, make sure you gradually adjust the seasoning for this dish. If you're mindful of your sodium intake, consider substituting almond oil and lemon or orange zest, or peanut oil and brown rice vinegar, in a 3:1 oil to vinegar ratio, for the oyster sauce.

For a decorative touch, pare off the lemon skin in long, thin strips. Twist each strip around a long skewer and use the warmth of your hands to shape the peel into a spiral curl. You can also use a citrus peeler or cocktail garnish peeler to make peel curls.

CHAPTER 18

Good Sweets

OK, raise your hand if you have a sweet tooth? My experiences with a majority of my clients who have had some sort of sugar addiction or dependency inspired me to create this chapter, where I share recipes for guilt-free sweet moments that can be a remedy for everyday stress without causing harmful side effects. Let's discover another side of sweet land in this chapter.

Making desserts can be a great opportunity to experiment with different kinds of sweeteners, flours, and even flourless options. My favorite dessert ingredients include coconut sugar, dates, maple syrup, berry powder, acai powder, and goji berries, and for flours, kamut, einkorn, millet, sorghum, quinoa, and amaranth. Sprouted spelt flour (which does contain gluten) has incredible flavor. Try fermented wheat flour, which you may be able to find at a local farmers market. Look for organic, unprocessed, stone-ground flours at natural food stores or online. Oat flours are a great gluten-free substitute for wheat flours, and oats are packed with good protein. Almond flour is nutty, soft, and has a silky texture (but avoid it if you have a nut allergy).

Think of those new ingredients as an opportunity to expand your flavor horizons! See the full list of gluten-free flours and processed sugar substitutes on page 106.

Baking can be a very different animal from cooking, because it can vary greatly based on climate, altitude, and your oven. These differences can affect the shape and texture of cookies and other baked goods. To me, baking is like enjoyable babysitting—you have to keep an eye on your charges! I always suggest checking baked goods in the oven starting at the halfway point. Then you can adjust the remaining time depending on how fast the baking process is unfolding. The bonus? You get to keep smelling the cake, muffins, or cookies up close, and that's a priceless pleasure.

I'm thrilled to share these recipes that use natural sugars and are mainly dairy-free, vegan, and vegetarian, nourishing for both body and soul.

Acai-Yam "Cheesecake"

MAKES 6 SERVINGS

Can we turn the traditional dairy-heavy cheesecake into a divinely smooth, fluffy, no-bake vegan dessert? The answer is yes. In this recipe, we use 100-percent-natural sugar from acai and high fiber from Korean yam, combined with creamy cashew protein and the richness of plant-based coconut milk. Natural sweetness from dates also helps keep this dessert guilt-free.

I like to make a marble pattern on the surface of the cake, but have fun and express your own creativity. Your very first bite of this brand-new cheesecake will leave you feeling good and sweet, just like your first date.

2 or 3 medium white Korean yams or white-fleshed sweet potatoes, peeled
½ cup (120 ml) coconut milk
½ cup (70 g) soaked raw cashews
6 pitted dates
5 tablespoons (75 ml) vegan cream cheese
1 teaspoon vanilla extract
½ teaspoon fresh lemon juice or orange juice
⅛ teaspoon ground cinnamon
⅛ teaspoon ground cardamom
⅛ teaspoon freshly grated nutmeg
½ cup (25 g) acai berry powder
¼ cup (31 g) raspberries
Edible flowers, for garnish

1. In a medium-sized steamer pot, insert the steamer basket and add enough water to almost touch the bottom of the basket. Arrange the yams evenly in the basket. Cook for 20 to 30 minutes over high heat. Remove the basket from the pot and set it aside to cool for at least 30 minutes.

2. Add 3 cups (720 g) cooled cooked yam to a food processor along with the coconut milk, cashews, dates, cream cheese, vanilla, lemon juice, cinnamon, cardamom, and nutmeg. Blend well for 7 to 8 minutes to achieve a thick, smooth, and silky dough.

3. Line an 8-inch (20 cm) springform pan with parchment paper. Spread the yam dough evenly into the lined pan.

4. Using a fine-mesh strainer, dust the dough with the acai powder. Use a toothpick to create the design of your choice in the dusty surface.

5. Refrigerate the cake for at least 1 hour. Remove the pan from the refrigerator, unlock the springform, and remove the ring and base. Peel away the parchment paper, place the cake on a serving platter, and garnish with the raspberries and flowers. Cut the cake into slices and serve.

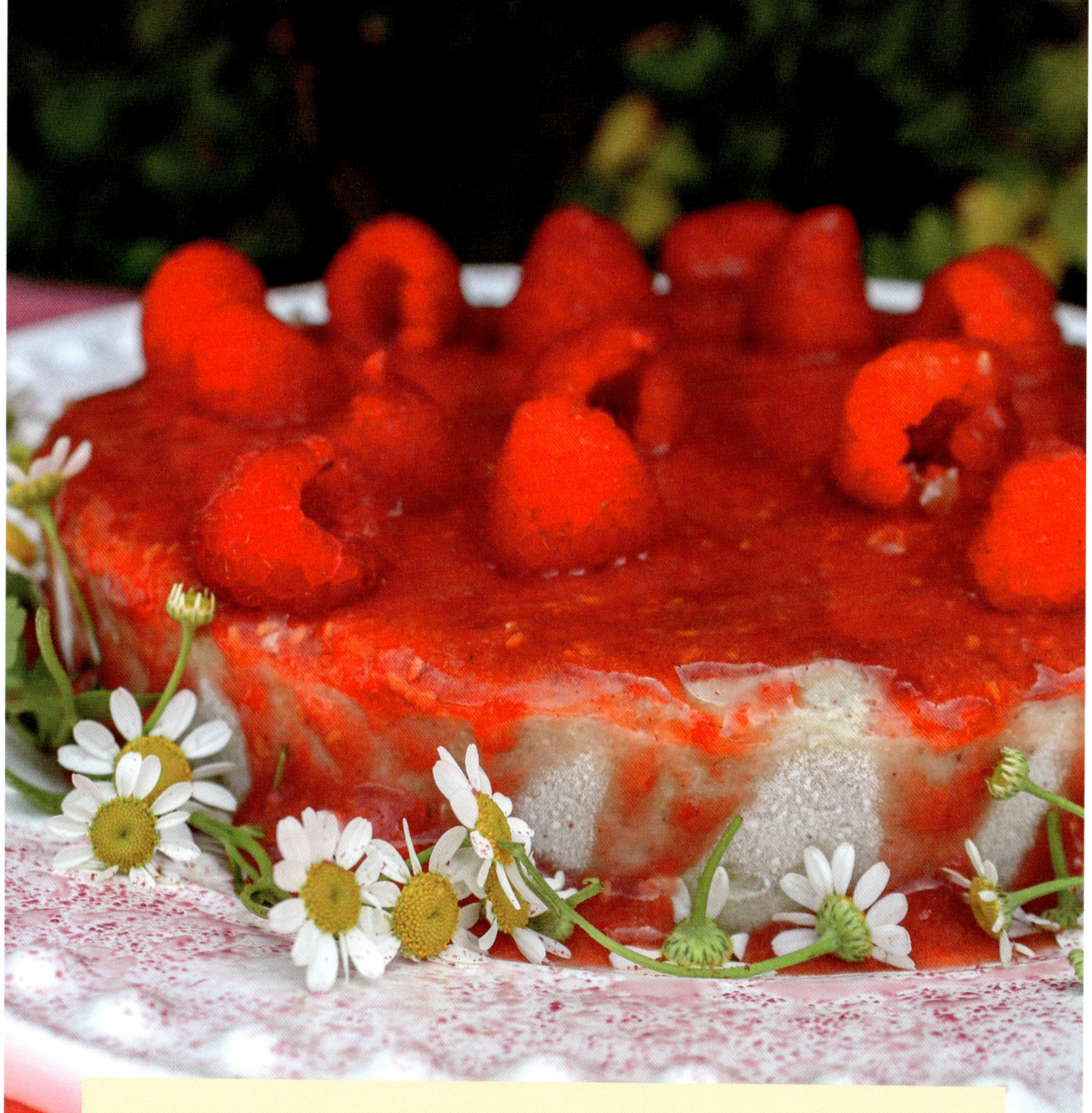

TIPS

To test for doneness, poke the yams with a sharp knife; it will easily penetrate through a fully cooked yam. If you want the yams to cook faster, cut them into 3- to 4-inch (8 to 10 cm) pieces.

Acai powder is highly sensitive to moisture and may start clumping if left unrefrigerated for too long. It is best to return it to the refrigerator immediately after use.

Try swapping in pumpkin for the yams in this cheesecake. You'll be amazed by the vivid color and rich flavors. Another visually stunning substitution to try is matcha powder in place of the acai powder.

Almond-Orange-Cacao Cake

MAKES 8 SERVINGS

How about a slice of heavenly moist chocolate cake when you're feeling down or melancholic? This cake contains chemicals that bring happiness, thanks to naturally mood-enhancing cacao, the origin of chocolate.

The alluring soft, fluffy texture of this almond chocolate cake might surprise you, given that it's dairy-free and wheat-free. Drizzled with flavorful orange syrup for extra moisture, this dark chocolate cake will become your go-to comfort dessert with its fancy flavor profile and a bonus of good nutrition.

Adding finishing touches to a cake is another chance to let your creativity shine! I dressed up my cake by surrounding it with fresh hibiscus flowers from my garden.

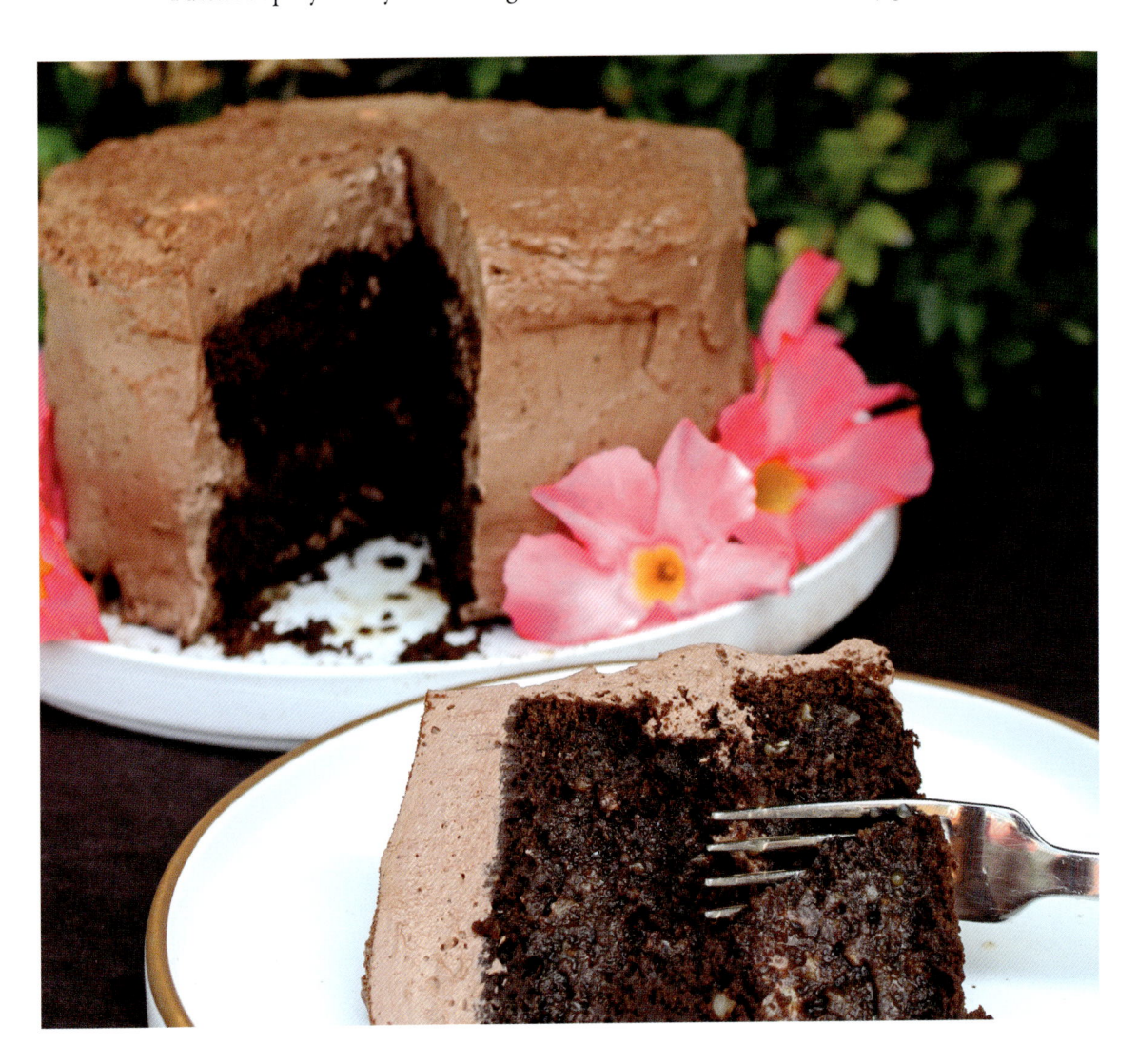

1 cup (240 ml) almond milk (see page 111), at room temperature
1 tablespoon apple cider vinegar or white vinegar
4 cups (400 g) fine almond flour
½ cup (60 g) cacao powder, plus more for dusting
1 cup (240 ml) boiling filtered water
1 cup (200 g) coconut sugar
¾ cup (180 ml) avocado oil or extra-virgin olive oil
½ cup (120 ml) maple syrup or date syrup
⅓ cup (40 g) chopped walnuts (optional)
1 tablespoon vanilla extract
1¼ teaspoons baking powder
1¼ teaspoons baking soda
1 teaspoon sea salt
1 teaspoon chaga mushroom powder
⅛ teaspoon ground ginger

FOR THE ORANGE SYRUP

5 tablespoons (75 ml) fresh orange juice
2 tablespoons maple syrup or date syrup
⅛ teaspoon vanilla extract
⅛ teaspoon ground cinnamon

TO SERVE

2 cups (480 ml) store-bought vegan chocolate buttercream frosting, coconut whipped cream (page 247), or whipped cream
Sliced almonds

1. Preheat the oven to 350°F (180°C). Line an 8-inch (20 cm) springform pan with parchment paper and set it aside.
2. In a medium-sized heatproof mixing bowl, combine the almond milk and vinegar and mix well. In a large mixing bowl, sift in the almond flour and cacao powder. Stir in the milk-vinegar mixture, then add the boiling water, coconut sugar, avocado oil, maple syrup, walnuts (if using), vanilla, baking powder, baking soda, salt, mushroom powder, and ginger. Whisk thoroughly until the ingredients form a thick batter.
3. Pour the batter into the prepared pan, tap a few times to remove any air bubbles, and make the surface even. Bake for 35 to 45 minutes, or until a toothpick or thin knife inserted into the center of the cake comes out clean. Remove the cake from the oven and allow to cool in the pan for 30 minutes.
4. While the cake cools, make the orange syrup: In a blender, combine the orange juice, maple syrup, vanilla, and cinnamon and blend for 2 to 3 minutes. Set aside.
5. Remove the cake from the pan. Using a serrated knife, gently slice the cake horizontally in half. Carefully flip the top half, and let both layers cool completely before applying the syrup and frosting.
6. Use a pastry brush to evenly brush the top and sides of the layers with the orange syrup.
7. Frost the top of one layer with buttercream frosting or whipped cream, then stack the second layer on top and frost the top and sides of the cake. Finish by dusting the cake with cacao powder and some sliced almonds.

TIPS

For a twist, reduce the coconut sugar by half and include several chopped dates instead.

If you'd rather simplify this project and skip the frosting, it will still be delicious! Consider arranging candied orange slices on top of the cake for a decorative touch—it's both beautiful and tasty.

Because it bakes level and is robust enough for stacking, you can double this recipe to create an impressive four-layer cake. This would make an extraordinary gluten-free birthday cake or a standout for any special occasion.

Good Sweets ▪ 267

Upside-Down Apple Pie

MAKES 8 SERVINGS

Baking a pie from scratch has a reputation for demanding lots of time and effort, but with this recipe, you'll discover how straightforward and enjoyable it can be. Let's savor this simpler approach and the sweet, tangy taste of caramelized apples. Apples are loaded with nutrients and fiber as well as antioxidants that may promote heart health and reduce inflammation.

Marinating the apples stimulates them to release liquid, which you will reserve and add to the crumble (dough). This trick helps prevent the pie from becoming soggy during baking.

Sprouted spelt and oats are alternative grains commonly used in baking. Sprouted spelt flour has a smooth texture, making it an excellent substitute for wheat flour. I like to use cashew milk in this recipe, but feel free to experiment with other kinds of plant-based milks for slightly different flavor.

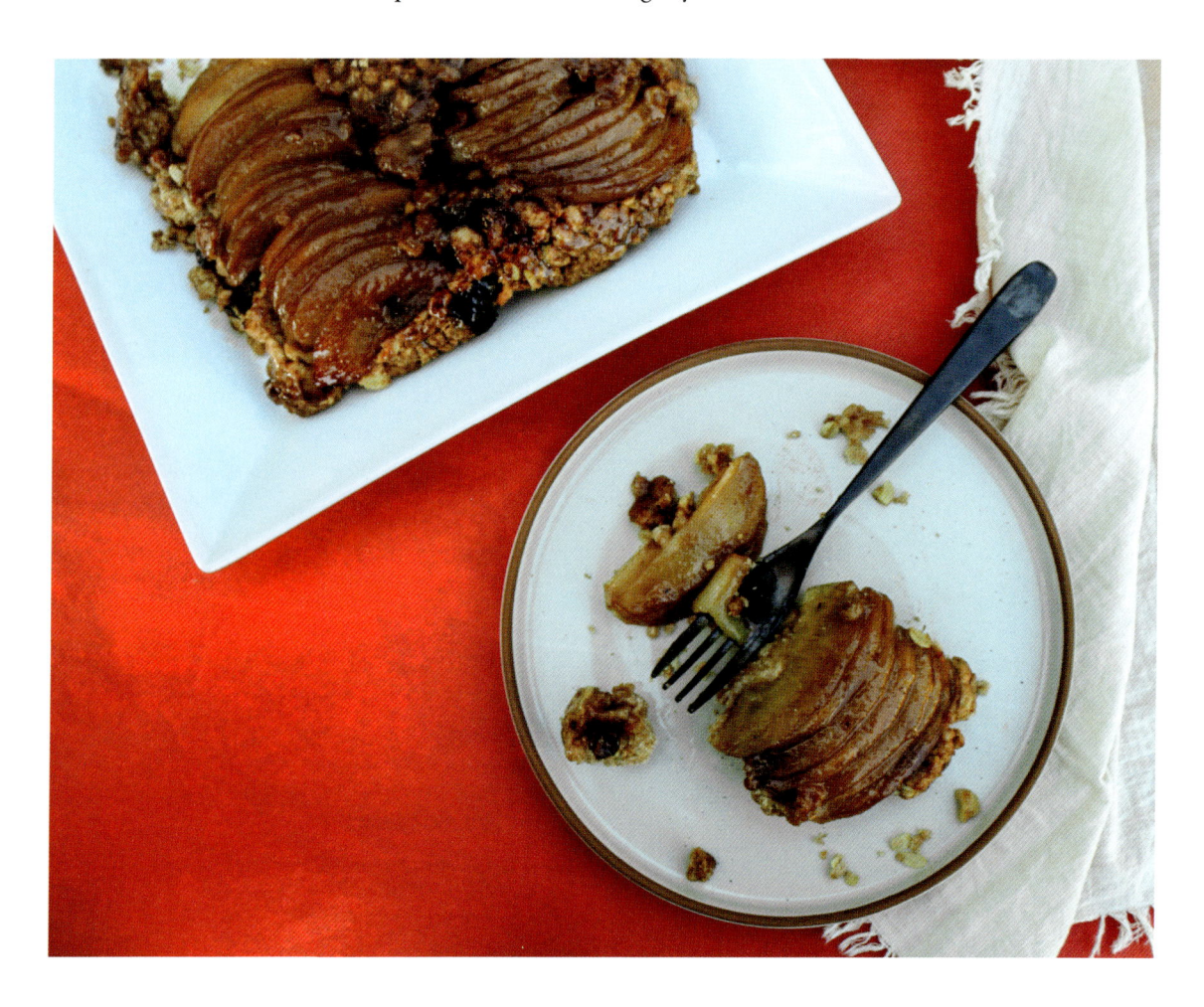

FOR THE MARINATED APPLES

3 cups (360 g) ¼-inch-thick (6 mm) slices Granny Smith apples or any tangy apple variety

7 tablespoons (65 g) arrowroot

¼ cup (50 g) coconut sugar

½ teaspoon vanilla paste

⅛ teaspoon ground cinnamon

⅛ teaspoon freshly grated nutmeg

Pinch of sea salt

3 tablespoons fresh lemon juice

FOR THE CRUMBLE

2¼ cups (160 g) sprouted spelt flour

½ cup (50 g) almond flour

½ cup (50 g) rolled or quick oats

½ cup (120 ml) cashew milk or other plant-based milk (see page 111)

½ cup (120 ml) coconut oil or extra-virgin olive oil

6 tablespoons (90 ml) maple syrup, honey, or agave syrup

¼ cup (30 g) walnuts or pecans

¼ teaspoon salt

5 tablespoons (50 g) soaked goji berries, raisins, or currants

FOR SERVING

Ice cream or coconut whipped cream (page 247) and ground cinnamon (optional)

1. Preheat the oven to 350°F (180°C). Line an 8-inch (20 cm) square baking dish, springform pan, or removable-bottom tart pan with parchment paper, and set it aside.

2. Prepare the marinated apples: Place the apple slices in a large bowl and gently toss them with the arrowroot, coconut sugar, vanilla paste, cinnamon, nutmeg, and salt. Ensure all the apples are evenly coated. Then add the lemon juice (which will prevent oxidation) and leave the apples to sit for 10 to 15 minutes.

3. Make the crumble: In a food processor, combine the spelt flour, almond flour, oats, cashew milk, coconut oil, maple syrup, and walnuts. Pulse the processor on and off several times until the texture resembles coarse dough with a crumbly texture. Be careful not to overprocess. Add the salt and pulse once or twice more. Transfer the crumbly mixture to a bowl and add the goji berries. Stir a few times and set the crumble aside.

4. Arrange the apple slices one by one in the parchment-lined pan. Keep in mind that this arrangement will end up as the decorative top of the pie. Pour the crumble over the apples and pour the leftover liquid from the apples on top. This will keep the crumble moist and tender. Cover the top with parchment paper to retain moisture. Bake for 50 to 60 minutes. Then remove from the oven, remove the parchment paper, and allow to cool for 20 minutes.

5. Place a large flat serving plate on top of the baking dish, flip it upside down, and gently shake. Remove the pan and parchment paper. Slice and serve the pie on individual plates, along with ice cream or coconut whipped cream and a dusting of cinnamon if you wish.

TIPS

You can also make this recipe with fresh June strawberries or summer peaches, cherries, or blueberries. Ripe pears in fall are a wonderful choice, too. For a more complex flavor, try a combination of tangy and sweet apples.

If you prefer a traditional-style apple pie, start by placing half of the crumble in the bottom of the pan, then add the apples and liquid, and cover the apples with the remaining crumble.

Experiment as you arrange the apples in the pan. For instance, you might try making a spiral, starting from the outer edge and working your way in.

Good Sweets

Avocado-Date Chocolate Mousse

MAKES 2 SERVINGS

What if you make silky, chocolatey mousse with scrumptious avocados? What if you use only dates to level up the sweetness and coconut milk to make it creamy on top? Your friends will find it hard to believe that this recipe is vegan, paleo, and gluten-free.

Avocados provide not only their unbelievable smooth texture but also a bonus of great nutritional benefits. This mousse contains 100 percent cholesterol-free good fats that supercharge your body's nutrient absorption, and they are loaded with almost twenty vitamins, minerals, and phytonutrients. Plus one more secret ingredient: lemon juice. It may seem like an odd ingredient for a mousse recipe, but in this case, it's the perfect touch to brighten the overall flavor, since avocado can sometimes taste dull.

1 large, ripe avocado (see Tip)
⅓ cup (35 g) cacao powder
3 tablespoons coconut milk
3 to 7 medium pitted dates, soaked
2 tablespoons maple syrup or 1 tablespoon honey
1 teaspoon vanilla extract or seeds scraped from half a vanilla bean
⅛ teaspoon freshly grated nutmeg
⅛ teaspoon ground cinnamon
Fresh lemon juice
Salt

TO SERVE

Hulled strawberries, raspberries, or blueberries
Mint leaves or edible flowers
Maple or date syrup (optional)
Goji berry powder or ground cinnamon (optional)

1. Pit the avocado and scoop the flesh into the bowl of a food processor. Add the cacao powder, coconut milk, 3 or 4 of the dates, maple syrup, vanilla, nutmeg, and cinnamon, and blend for about 5 minutes, until the texture becomes smooth. Taste to check for sweetness. If you want it sweeter, add more dates, and blend again for 2 to 3 minutes until there are no lumps of date. Add a squeeze of lemon juice along with a pinch of salt to complete the flavor. Blend again for a few seconds.
2. Spoon the mousse into two dessert cups or bowls and decorate with the berries and mint leaves and/or edible flowers. If you prefer a glossy shine, brush the top with some maple syrup. Or you can sprinkle on some goji berry powder or dust the mousse with cinnamon.

TIPS

To test an avocado for ripeness, press gently on the skin. It should be firm but yield a bit to the pressure. Based on my experience, Hass avocados work best for the desired texture in this recipe.

If you prefer a totally creamy dessert, top your mousse with coconut whipped cream (page 247) instead of berries.

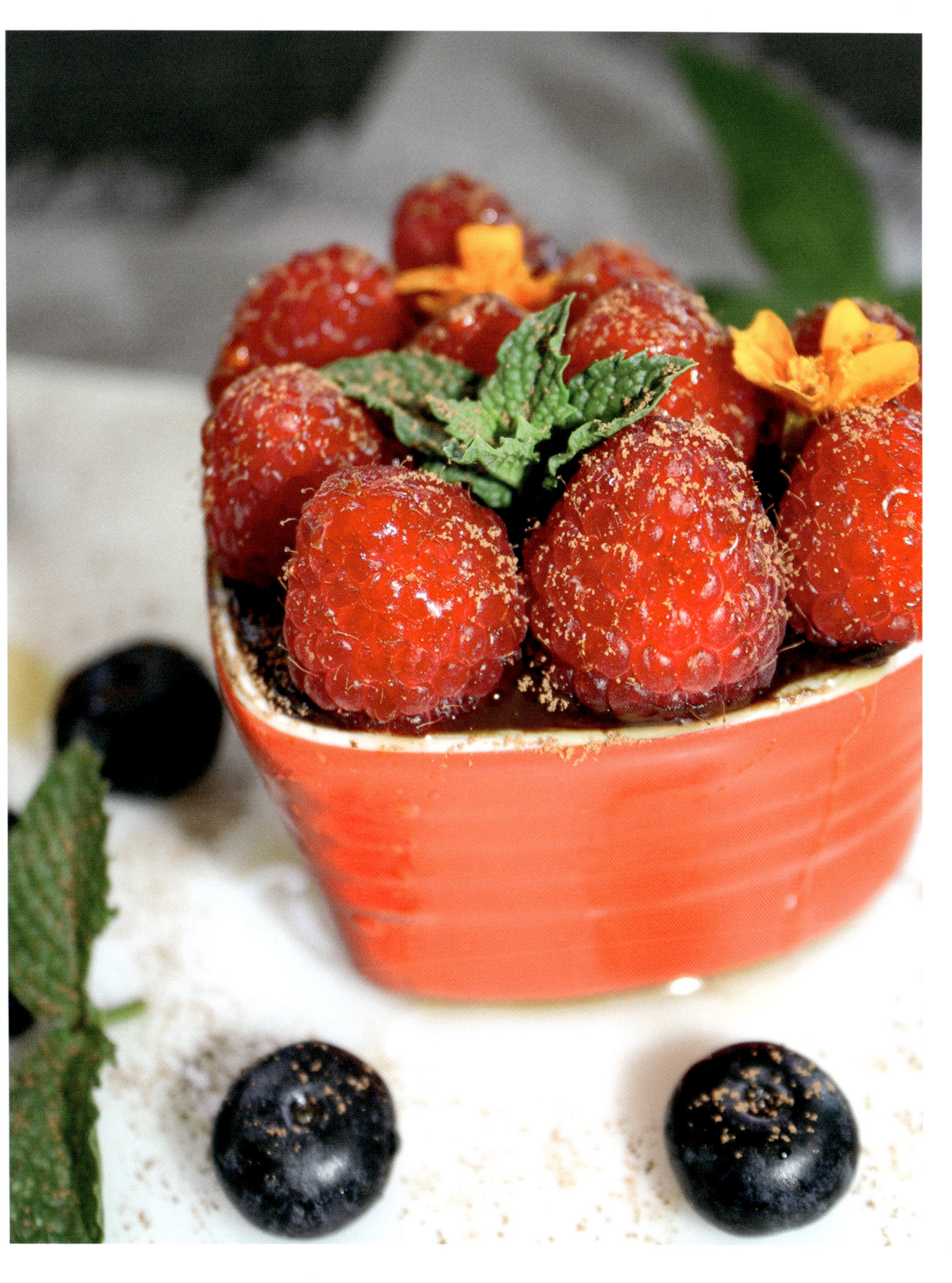

Chia Berry Cup

MAKES 2 SERVINGS

Chia seeds have become one of the most popular superfoods in part because they are packed with giant nutrition and health benefits. Ancient Mayan people called chia *chiabaan*, which means "strengthening," and they cultivated it in South America as an endurance food for warriors.

In these chia cups, you will also taste nutty pistachios, which help provide stamina and endurance support, along with tangy orange zest and sweet maple syrup.

This is a great choice for breakfast, Sunday brunch, or a midday snack, but be sure to plan ahead and start the chia seeds soaking at least 2 hours before you want to enjoy this treat.

¼ cup (35 g) chia seeds
½ cup (120 ml) coconut milk, coconut yogurt, or cashew yogurt
⅛ teaspoon ground cinnamon
⅛ teaspoon grated orange zest
⅛ teaspoon vanilla extract
Handful blackberries, blueberries, or a combination
1 tablespoon maple syrup or date syrup

FOR GARNISH

1 orange slice, cut into small pieces
1 fresh strawberry, halved
2 tablespoons crushed pistachios or almonds
2 tablespoons goji berry powder
1 tablespoon sunflower seeds
1 tablespoon maca powder
Fresh mint leaves
Edible flowers

1. Combine the chia seeds and 2½ cups (600 ml) water in a bowl and mix well. Leave the seeds to soak for at least 2 hours, then drain any remaining water.
2. Add half of the coconut milk or plant-based yogurt, along with the cinnamon, orange zest, and vanilla, to each of two decorative drinking glasses or dessert cups. Divide the chia seeds, berries, and maple syrup between the glasses; the cups will be nearly full.
3. Top each with more berries, some orange pieces, half a strawberry, half of the pistachios, the goji berry powder, sunflower seeds, and maca powder. Garnish with the mint leaves and edible flowers.

TIPS

Chia seeds can absorb up to twenty times their volume in water, so be sure to use enough water when soaking them. The seeds will turn transparent as they soak.

If you follow a strict keto diet, try creamy coconut kefir in place of the coconut milk. Because it's a fermented food, kefir also improves gut health through beneficial bacteria.

Crazy Nutty Nut Bark

MAKES 10 SERVINGS

If you're in search of a snack that will conquer your midday hunger or fuel your weekend adventures, give this recipe a try. Unlike many store-bought energy bars that are loaded with processed sugars, these nutty treats reside in the zero-processed-sugar zone, thanks to the natural sweetness provided by goji berries and cranberries. They also feature dark chocolate chips, which add a burst of flavor and are rich in antioxidants. A blend of seeds brings a wholesome and crunchy delight to every bite.

This recipe is perfect for creating sweet family moments. Your kitchen table will become a creative playground filled with playful laughter and joy.

1 tablespoon crushed walnuts
1 tablespoon pistachios
1 tablespoon hemp seeds
1 tablespoon pumpkin seeds
1 tablespoon sesame seeds
1 tablespoon unsweetened dried cranberries
3 tablespoons filtered water
1 tablespoon coconut flakes
1 tablespoon goji berries
½ cup (90 g) sugar-free dark chocolate chips

1. Soak the walnuts, pistachios, hemp seeds, pumpkin seeds, sesame seeds, and cranberries for at least 30 minutes. Drain and rinse.
2. In a medium-sized bowl, combine the soaked nuts, seeds, and cranberries with the water, coconut flakes, and goji berries.
3. Line an 8-inch (20 cm) square baking pan with parchment paper. Pour the mixture into the pan, and spread it evenly over the paper.
4. Melt the chocolate chips using the technique described on page 277.
5. Pour the melted chocolate over the pan of ingredients. Cool the pan in the refrigerator for 1 to 2 hours. Break the hardened chocolate-nut-seed sheet into individual pieces, and pack in parchment paper for storage in the refrigerator for up to 6 months.

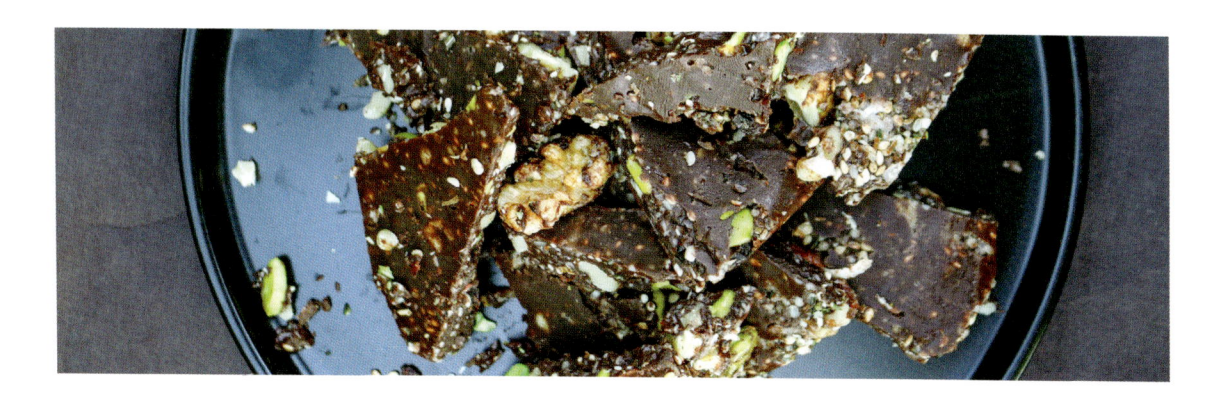

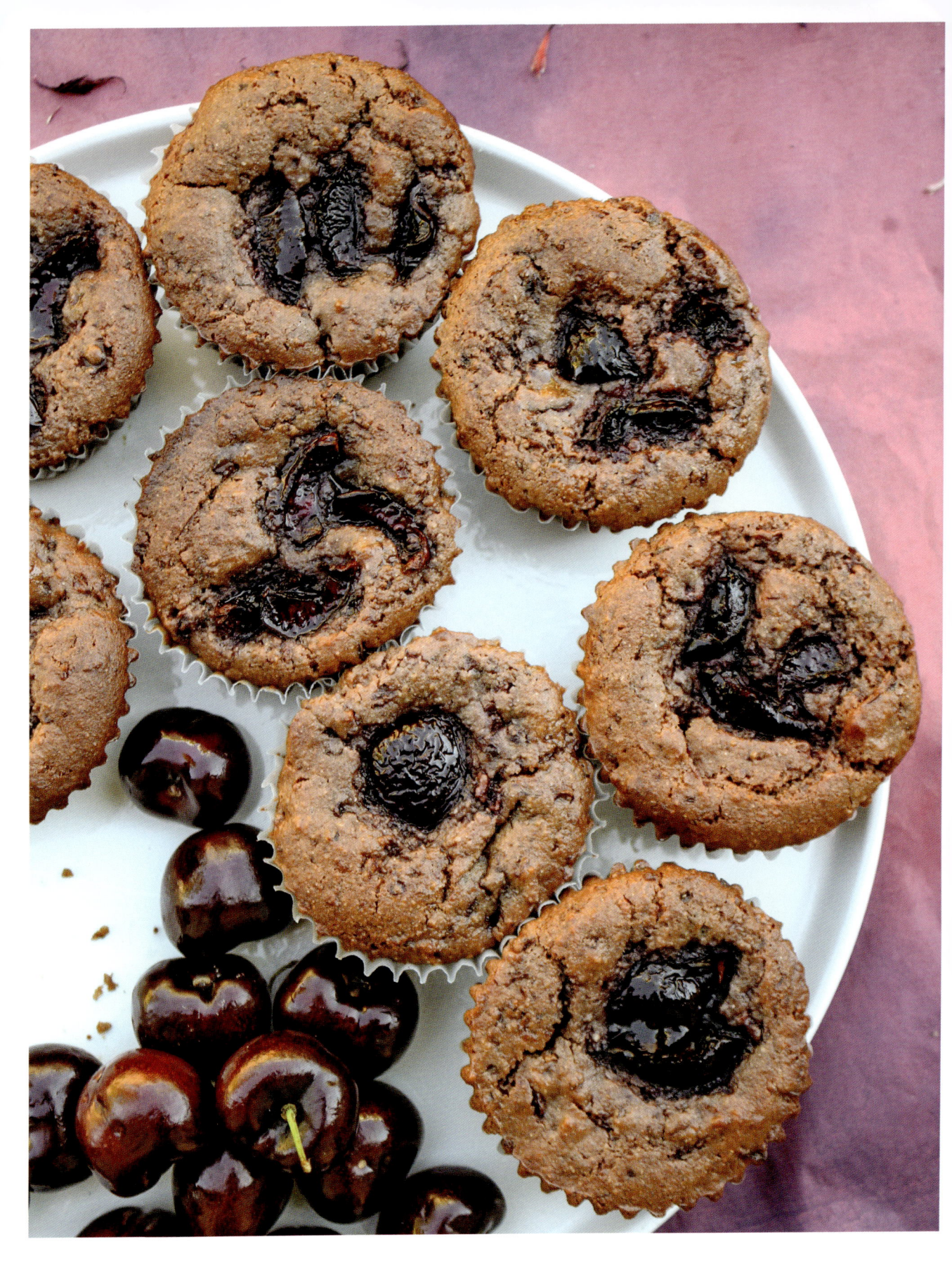

Cherry Velvet Muffins

MAKES NINE 3-INCH (8 CM) MUFFINS

These striking cherry muffins, inspired by red velvet cake, may become your favorite choice when you want something rich yet naturally sweet and refreshing. I eliminate processed sugar by using dates, fresh cherries, and healing spices. You could also add mushroom or dandelion root powder to boost immunity, if you wish, so you can eat sweets and treat your body well at the same time. Cherries are a bone lover's ingredient, too, high in antioxidants and anti-inflammatory compounds.

½ cup (90 g) pitted dates
1½ cups (155 g) red cherries
1 cup (100 g) almond flour
1 cup (140 g) gluten-free flour blend or (120 g) cassava flour
⅓ cup (70 g) coconut sugar
2 teaspoons baking powder
2 teaspoons dandelion root powder (optional)
1 teaspoon baking soda
¼ cup (60 ml) mild olive oil, plus more for the pan
4 teaspoons coconut milk
1 teaspoon vanilla extract
⅛ teaspoon ground cinnamon or freshly grated nutmeg
Sea salt

1. Preheat the oven to 375°F (190°C).
2. In a small bowl, soak the dates in water for 5 to 10 minutes. Drain the dates, chop them roughly, and set aside.
3. Clean and pit the cherries, and chop roughly, saving any cherry juice left over on the cutting board in a small bowl.
4. In a large mixing bowl, add the almond and gluten-free flours, coconut sugar, baking powder, dandelion root powder (if using), and baking soda, and stir to thoroughly combine.
5. Add the olive oil, coconut milk, vanilla, and cinnamon, and stir well for 1 to 2 minutes. Add the dates, 1 cup (104 g) of the chopped cherries and the juice, and a pinch of salt. Stir well.
6. Brush 9 cups of a muffin pan with oil or insert a cupcake paper into each cup. Fill each cup with batter up to three-quarters full. Sprinkle the remaining ½ cup (52 g) chopped cherries over the top.
7. Put the muffins in the oven, and begin checking for doneness after 20 minutes (see Tip). The muffins may take as long as 40 minutes to fully bake.
8. Allow the muffins to cool for in the pan 30 minutes. Remove from the pan and transfer to a cloth-lined basket to serve.

TIPS

You can check the muffins visually for doneness—they should rise to at least the top of the muffin cup. To confirm, poke a muffin with a small knife. If the knife blade comes out clean, with no batter streaks on it, then the muffin is done.

For a different flavor, substitute vegan chocolate chips for the dates.

Good Sweets • 275

Sweet and Salty Chocolate Strawberries

MAKES 2 SERVINGS

Fire up your passion with this classic recipe for chocolate-covered strawberries, transformed with "love dusts." The pistachio dust brings a nutty texture and heart-healthy fats, while coconut flakes add a tropical flair.

In this recipe, I focus on the tricky technique of melting chocolate in just the right way to achieve a smooth, shiny coating. Get ready to dip some strawberries into delicious chocolate and love dusts to dust off an ordinary day and turn it into an extraordinary affair!

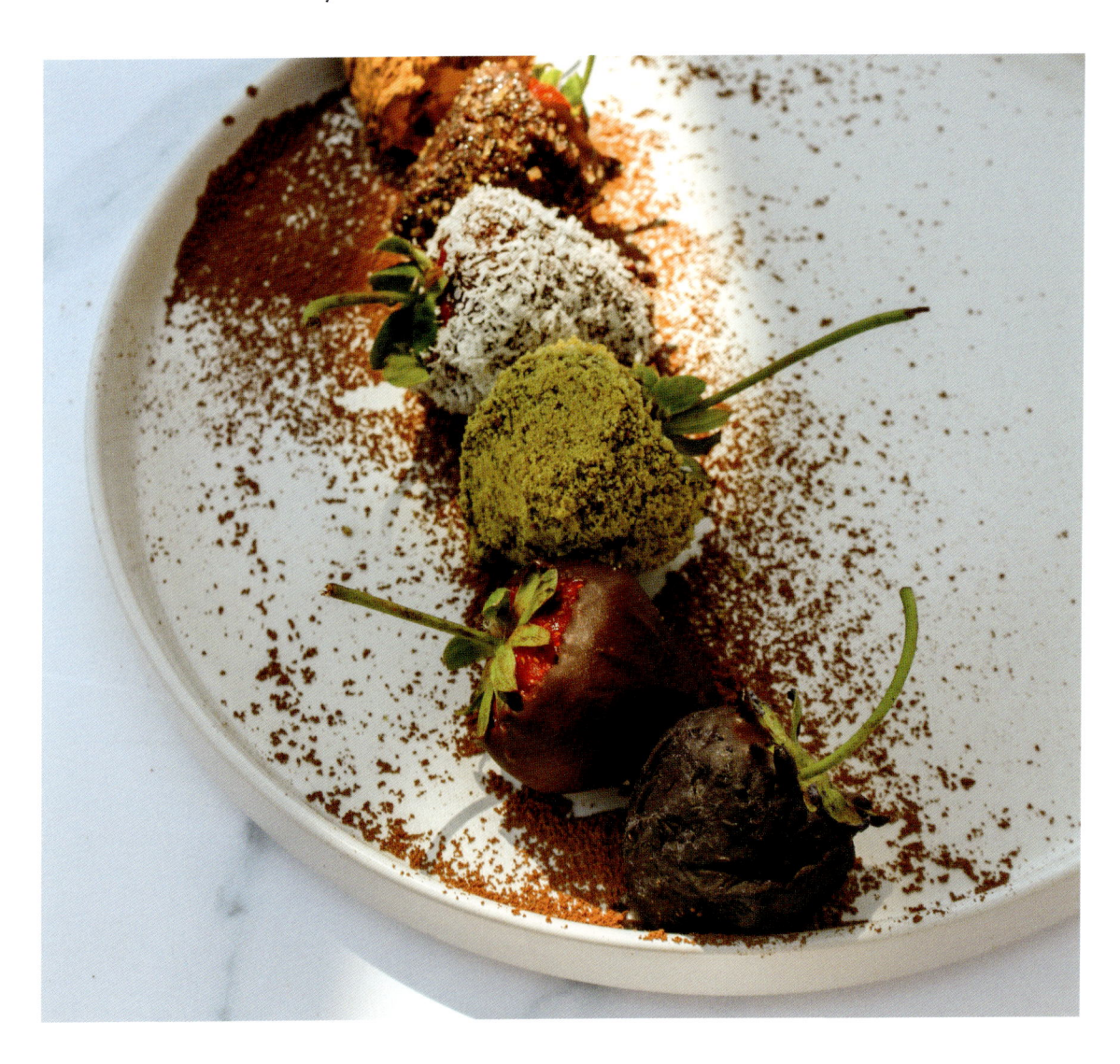

8 large fresh strawberries, with stems if possible
2 tablespoons coconut sugar
2 tablespoons coconut flakes
2 tablespoons goji berry powder
2 tablespoons ground pistachios
2 teaspoons lava salt
¾ cup (130 g) dark chocolate chips or 4½ ounces (130 g) dark chocolate, chopped
1 teaspoon vanilla extract

> **TIPS**
>
> The ideal temperature to melt chocolate for chocolate-covered strawberries is 110° to 115°F (43°–45°C). Avoid overheating, or the chocolate can burn. Maintaining gentle, controlled heat ensures a smooth consistency. And tempering the melted chocolate by adding a small amount of additional solid chocolate to it will ensure a smooth, silky, and dark final result. The tempering process has to happen quickly, so stay focused and be prepared to act immediately once the main batch of chocolate has melted.
>
> You can also make chocolate-covered pineapple chunks, blueberry skewers, or apple slices. They are just as delicious and offer a range of different textures.
>
> It's best not to freeze chocolate-covered strawberries, because the berries will be soggy when thawed and the chocolate coating will be ruined.

1. Remove the strawberries from the refrigerator 15 to 30 minutes before starting this recipe. If they are too cold it may affect the temperature of the chocolate, and they may not be coated as smoothly. Clean the strawberries with a wet cloth and place them on a plate to dry for 1 to 5 minutes. Do not remove the stems from the berries.

2. Prepare the love dusts: Set out the coconut sugar, coconut flakes, goji berry powder, pistachios, and lava salt, each on a separate small plate. Put a baking sheet near the small plates and put a rack on top of the baking sheet.

3. Find a saucepan and a heatproof bowl that fit together so the bowl tightly covers the opening of the pan with open space below the bottom of the bowl sufficient for a few cups of water. Place the saucepan over medium heat and add 3 to 4 cups (approximately 1 L) water. Bring the water to a boil. Reduce the heat to the lowest setting and set the bowl in place on the pan.

4. Pour ½ cup (90 g) of the chocolate chips, or about two-thirds of the chocolate pieces, and the vanilla into the bowl and stir gently until melted and smooth, with no lumps remaining. Remove the bowl from the heat and immediately add the remaining chocolate. Stir until the additional chocolate has melted. Work quickly to avoid allowing the temperature of the melted chocolate to drop too much.

5. Immediately dip each strawberry in the melted chocolate, letting any excess chocolate drip off, and then coat the chocolate-covered strawberry in the love dust of your choice. Allow the coated strawberries to rest on the rack until the chocolate has set. You can store the berries for 1 or 2 days, uncovered, in an open container or on a plate, away from sunlight or heat and ideally in the refrigerator.

Good Sweets ▪ 277

TIPS

I highly recommend using a food processor instead of a blender or mixer for the best texture and flavor with these brownies. When the batter is in the food processor, pause the blending process two or three times and open the lid to stir the mixture. This will make the batter a consistent texture like that of brownie batter made from wheat flour.

Try substituting cooked sweet potato for the black beans in this recipe. Sweet potatoes are also good for bone health because they are an excellent source of vitamin A, which is essential for maintaining healthy bones and cartilage.

Woody, earthy bitter dandelion root powder is a great caffeine-free substitute for coffee or espresso powder. In Traditional Chinese Medicine, dandelions are a liver revitalization remedy, and they are also rich in antioxidants.

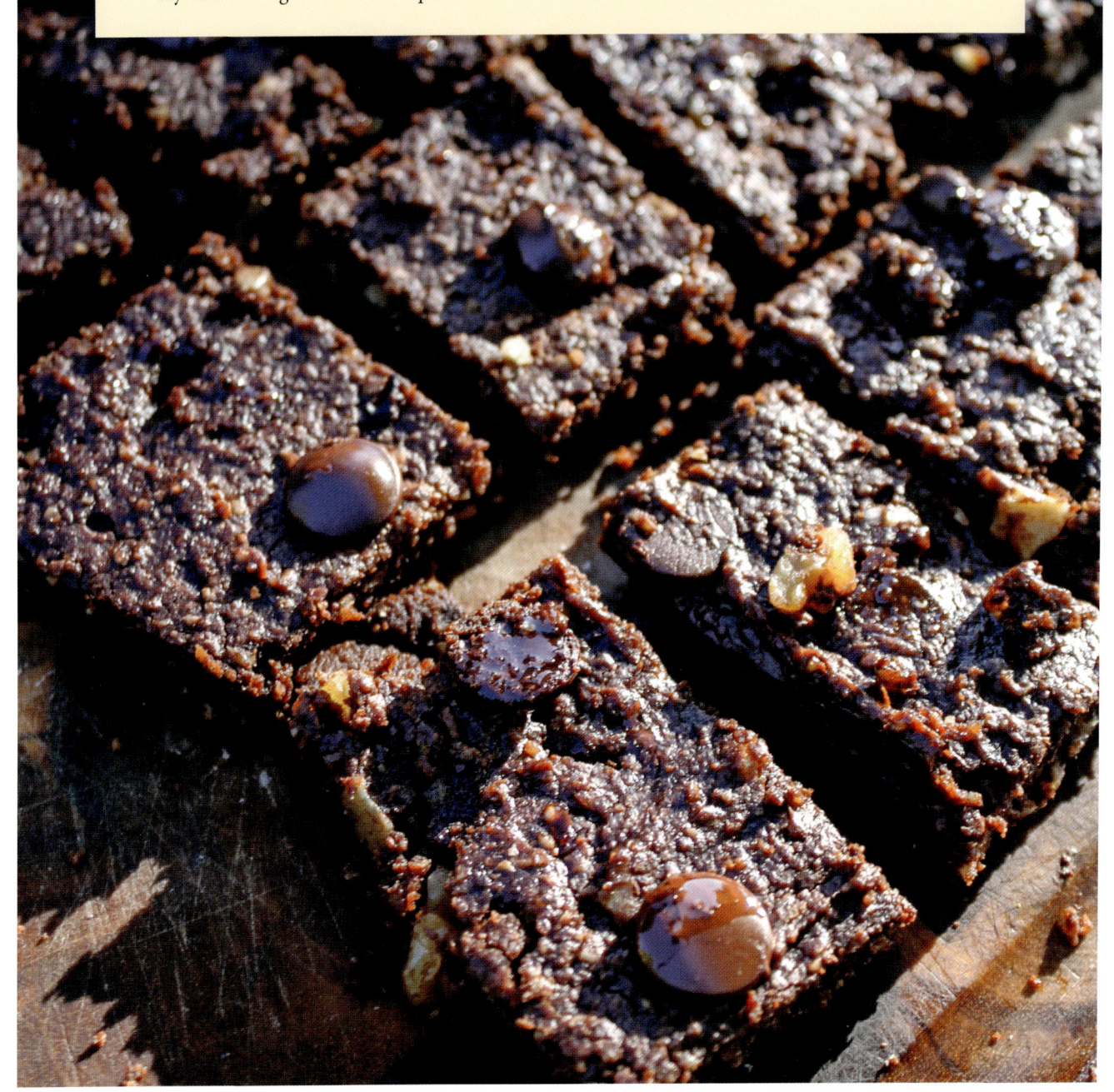

Flourless Black Bean Brownies

MAKES 9 TO 12 BROWNIES

Brownie fans will be flabbergasted when they learn that the main ingredient in these dark, rich brownies is canned black beans. You can't taste any black bean flavor at all! Not only that, but these brownies are grain-free, gluten-free, free of refined sugars, and vegan. They nourish soul and body with a delectable smoky taste from medicinal mushroom powder, an intensified espresso coffee aroma from dandelion root powder, and an extra layer of richness from cacao. For best results, be sure to use a high-quality cacao powder.

1½ cups (250 g) canned black beans
½ cup (50 g) almond flour
⅓ cup (80 ml) maple syrup or date syrup
¼ cup (60 ml) coconut oil or extra-virgin olive oil
1 tablespoon extra-virgin olive oil, plus more for the pan
¼ cup (30 g) chopped walnuts
2 tablespoons cacao powder
2 tablespoons coconut sugar
1½ tablespoons dandelion root powder
1 tablespoon flaxseed meal
2 teaspoons fresh lemon juice
2 teaspoons vanilla extract
1 teaspoon reishi mushroom powder
½ teaspoon baking powder
¼ teaspoon salt
⅛ teaspoon ground cardamom
¾ cup (135 g) vegan sugar-free chocolate chips

1. Preheat the oven to 350°F (180°C). Grease an 8-inch (20 cm) square baking pan. Thoroughly rinse and drain the black beans.
2. In a large bowl, combine the beans, almond flour, maple syrup, coconut oil, olive oil, walnuts, cacao powder, coconut sugar, dandelion root powder, flaxseed meal, lemon juice, vanilla, mushroom powder, baking powder, salt, and cardamom. Mix well by hand, then transfer to a food processor. Blend for 5 to 8 minutes, until the batter has a silky-smooth texture with no lumps.
3. Transfer the brownie batter back into a bowl, add ½ cup (90 g) of the chocolate chips, and gently stir to combine. Spread the dough evenly in the prepared pan. Sprinkle the remaining ¼ cup (45 g) chocolate chips on top. Tap the pan a few times to remove air bubbles and level the surface.
4. Bake for 15 to 18 minutes, then remove from the oven and allow to cool in the pan for at least 10 minutes before cutting. If the brownies seem a bit undercooked, place them in the fridge overnight, and they will firm up magically!

Good Sweets

Oh-Yah Vegan Chocolate Chip Cookies

MAKES TWELVE 2-INCH (5 CM) COOKIES

My chocolate chip cookies have a milky, buttery flavor, but they contain no dairy products, and they support healthy bones, too. The walnuts are a good source of protein, and lion's mane mushroom is a nutrient-rich superfood.

All of the sweetness comes from the coconut sugar, dates, and maple syrup. Note that spelt flour does contain gluten, but oat flour is a fine gluten-free substitute.

Baking these cookies is a great form of mindfulness practice. You mix the dough by hand, watching carefully to judge whether the ingredients are combining evenly. If the dough is too dry, add up to 2 tablespoons of warm milk to make it just the right consistency.

Now you don't have to feel guilty about how many cookies you eat and regret it later. The only side effects of these cookies are increased energy and a sense of satisfaction and well-being.

1 cup (120 g) sprouted spelt flour or (90 g) oat flour
¼ cup (50 g) coconut sugar
½ teaspoon baking soda
¼ teaspoon salt
¼ cup (45 g) vegan chocolate chips
⅓ cup (80 ml) coconut milk or homemade plant-based milk (see page 111), warmed, plus more if needed
3 tablespoons coconut oil
2 tablespoons extra-virgin olive oil, plus more for the pan
¼ teaspoon vanilla extract
3 tablespoons chopped dates
3 tablespoons crushed walnuts
¼ teaspoon lion's mane mushroom powder
¼ teaspoon grated orange zest

1. In a medium-sized bowl, combine the flour, sugar, baking soda, and salt. Add the chocolate chips and stir well. Slowly add the coconut milk, coconut oil, olive oil, and vanilla and continue stirring as the batter forms. Add the dates, walnuts, mushroom powder, and orange zest and mix well. Add 1 or 2 tablespoons extra milk if the dough seems dry.
2. Press the dough into one big ball. Refrigerate for at least 2 hours or overnight, or chill in the freezer for 10 to 20 minutes until the dough is cold.
3. Preheat the oven to 325°F (160°C). Use an ice cream scoop to scoop individual balls of dough, and place the dough balls 2 to 3 inches (5 to 8 cm) apart on a greased cookie sheet.
4. Put the cookies in the oven to bake and begin checking them after about 7 minutes. Total baking time should be 10 to 15 minutes. Remove the pan from the oven when the cookies still look a little underbaked; they will continue to firm up as they cool.
5. Transfer the cookies to a rack and let cool for at least 10 minutes before eating.

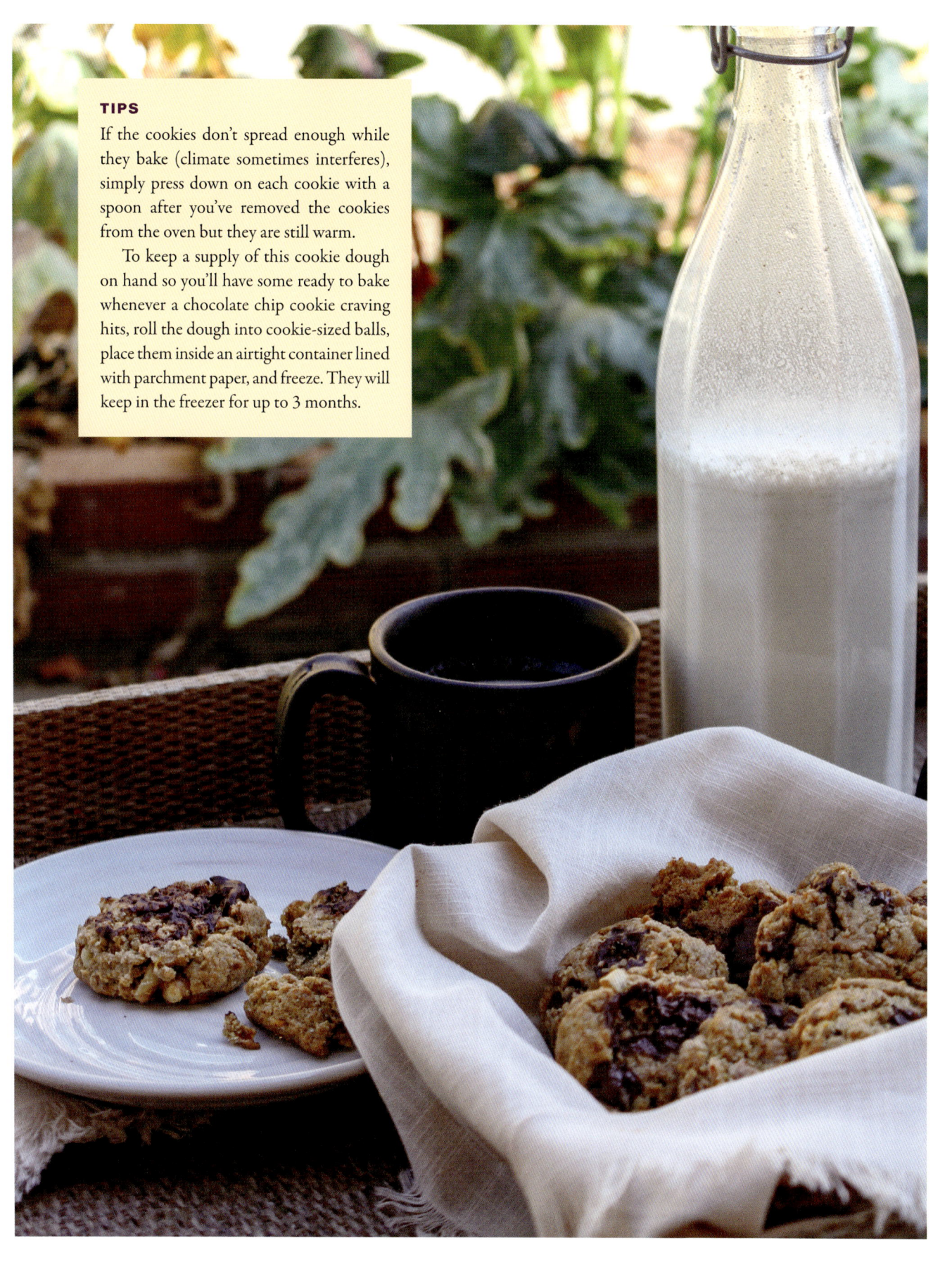

TIPS

If the cookies don't spread enough while they bake (climate sometimes interferes), simply press down on each cookie with a spoon after you've removed the cookies from the oven but they are still warm.

To keep a supply of this cookie dough on hand so you'll have some ready to bake whenever a chocolate chip cookie craving hits, roll the dough into cookie-sized balls, place them inside an airtight container lined with parchment paper, and freeze. They will keep in the freezer for up to 3 months.

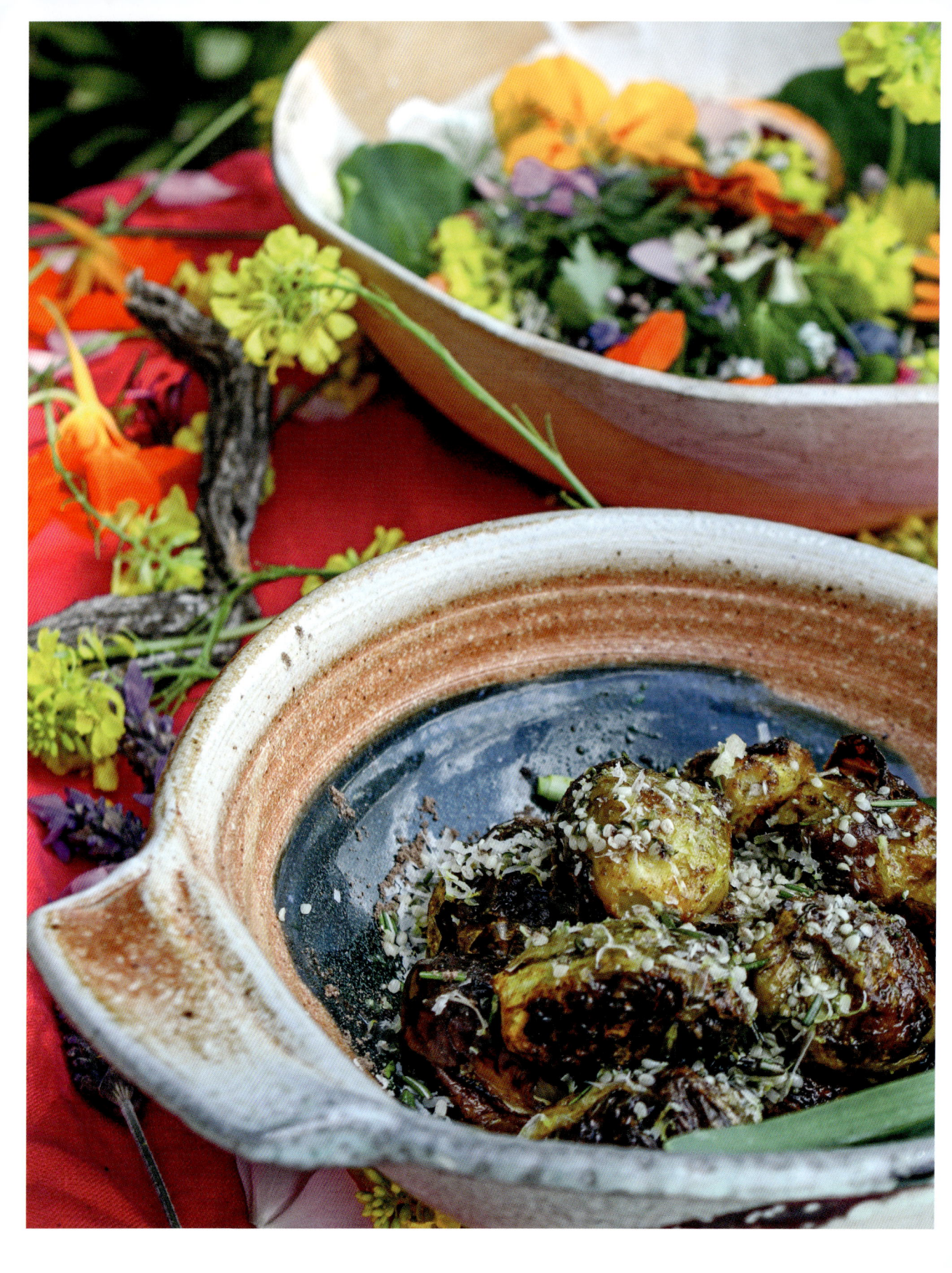

CHAPTER 19

Meal Plans

Down the line you may very well be tailoring dishes and meals to suit your personal needs. However, as you get started on the road to better bone health, you'll have lots of information to absorb. You may do some bone-health testing and arrange conversations with your doctor. While you're considering all of that, relying on meal plans will make it easier to shop, cook, eat with the seasons, and feed your bones. These meal plans also provide models that you can customize over time as you begin to develop your own recipes.

We have organized the meal plans we present here by the four seasons. That's because produce in season—especially produce that you grow or that is locally grown by others—offers the freshest, most nutrient-rich food for body and bones. Most of Jummee's dishes are well balanced according to the Five Elements of Traditional Chinese Medicine and are designed to provide optimal nutrition during the four seasons. You will notice that recommendations for consuming raw food and cooked food change as weather, temperature, and digestion patterns shift.

For example, spring and summer are the choice seasons for raw salads, while hearty soups are best in fall and winter, when your digestion is slower and raw foods will be more challenging to digest. This is because when it is cold outside, our bodies use more energy to keep our body temperature around a toasty 98°F (37°C), with less energy for other functions.

We hope you enjoy these meal plans—designed to help you jump-start your bone-healthy seasonal meal planning.

Spring

The suggested balance of cooked versus raw foods for springtime meals is 40 percent cooked and 60 percent raw.

If you aim to reset your system and activate autophagy to clear out senescent cells (see page 51), then spring is the time to do so. Most ritual fasting is done in spring, as fasting has a profound impact on blood sugar, gut health, immune system health, and much more.

Once your fast is done, then you can enjoy the pleasures of spring foods. Avoid heavy, greasy foods; opt for lighter seasonal fare; and focus on fresh green foods like leafy vegetables, sprouts, and herbs. These foods support liver health and detoxification.

Summer

During those endless summer days, adjust your balance to 80 percent raw foods and 20 percent cooked.

Delicious summer when everything juicy blooms! Take advantage of the cooling, hydrating fruits of the season, like watermelon and cucumbers, to balance the body's internal heat, as well as the leafy green vegetable bounty. Avoid excessively spicy or greasy foods, as they can exacerbate heat-related issues.

Fall

In the fall, you'll shift back to cooking more of what you eat. Aim for 60 percent cooked and 40 percent raw.

As the natural world begins to slow, so does our digestion. This is a good time to transition to more nutrient-dense foods to help our bodies rest.

Now is the time to be more measured in energy expenditure and reflect on what you have learned from the exuberant summer in preparation for new growth next year.

Focus on foods such as pears, apples, white mushrooms, and white beans. Incorporate pungent and spicy flavors to stimulate energy circulation and balance the body for the season.

Table 19.1. Spring Weekly Meal Plan

	Breakfast	Lunch	Snack	Dinner
Monday	Morning March Matcha Latte	Saffron Cauliflower Rice Immortal Root Kimchi	Triple Kale Chips	Vegan Delight Matcha Curry with pickled red onion
Tuesday	Green Shield Smoothie	Snap Peas with Tempeh Dust Green and Red Everyday Sauerkraut	Savory Mung Bean Flatbread with almond butter	California Sushi Roll Licorice Sweet Brown Rice with ginger pickles
Wednesday	Sunny Carrot Juice	California Rainbow Spring Rolls with pickled ginger	Chia Berry Cup	Golden Dal Moringa Khichuri
Thursday	Awakening Golden Smoothie	Ageless Macrobiotic Salad with natto and sautéed shiitake mushrooms	Celery and carrot sticks Silky Tofu–Spinach Dip	Buckwheat Linguine with Kale-Macadamia Pesto
Friday	Morning Ritual Green Juice	Mouthful Quinoa-Carrot Burger Pineapple-Turmeric Kimchi	C-Packed Pink Latte	Broccoli Rabe Restaurant-Style Miso Soup with Dashi Broth
Saturday	C-Packed Pink Latte	Mung Bean Pizza with Hemp Seed Pesto	Crazy Nutty Nut Bark	Wok Express Crunchy Green Beans
Sunday	Basic Green Juice	Herb and Wildflower Garden Salad with hemp seeds and soaked pistachios	Feel-Good Banana Bread with ghee or honey	Edamame Spread Avocado Toast with Mushroom Cashew Pâté radish sprouts with Basil-Walnut Pesto Pineapple-Turmeric Kimchi

Winter

In the winter, shift the balance to 80 percent cooked foods and just 20 percent raw.

Now it is time to conserve energy: to rest, slow down, and sleep well. As things slow in winter, it is best to try to flow like water around obstacles.

Consume warming, nourishing foods like root vegetables, hearty grains, and slow-cooked stews. Include black beans, dark leafy greens, and salty flavors. Stay hydrated with warming teas like ginger to support the kidneys and mushrooms to maintain immunity during the cold season.

Table 19.2. Summer Weekly Meal Plan

	Breakfast	Lunch	Snack	Dinner
Monday	Follow Your Gut Juice	Fennel-Radicchio Salad Sweet Potato–Scallion Pancakes	Feel-Good Banana Bread with nut spread	Sweet and Savory Grilled Peaches and Zucchini
Tuesday	Berry Paradise Smoothie	Chickpea-Cucumber Salad with a Hint of Mint	seasonal fresh berries with coconut yogurt	Steamed Eggplant with Apple-Tahini Sauce and mixed sprouts salad
Wednesday	Golden Milk Latte	Broccoli and Mushroom Buffalo "Wings" shaved fennel salad Kale-Cashew Pesto	Green Shield Smoothie	Happy-Go-Lucky Caesar Salad Meaty Meatless Meatballs with Marinara Sauce
Thursday	Immortal Acai Bowl	Endive Canoes with Guacamole Boiled eggs	Oh-Yah Vegan Chocolate Chip Cookies Pistachio-Mint Milk	Vegan Delight Matcha Curry Almond-Orange-Cacao Cake
Friday	Hearty Cacao Latte	Beefy Tomato Salad with Cherry Vinaigrette	Cherry Velvet Muffin Cashew-Goji-Vanilla Milk	Watermelon-Mint Gazpacho
Saturday	Go Bananas Flourless Pancakes	Maple Syrup BBQ Tempeh New Classic Rainbow Coleslaw	Avocado-Date Chocolate Mousse	California Creamy Corn Chowder
Sunday	Rainbow Veggie Frittata with Feta	Golden Triangle Indian Mash Seaweed Flower Cucumber Salad	Hearty Cacao Latte with cacao nibs	Wok Express Crunchy Green Beans Sweet and Salty Chocolate Strawberries

Meal Plans

Table 19.3. Fall Weekly Meal Plan

	Breakfast	**Lunch**	**Snack**	**Dinner**
Monday	Sea Greens and Shiitake Soup	BBQ Jackfruit Tacos with Mango Salsa	Pine Nut–Matcha Latte	Acorn Squash with Forbidden Rice Stuffing Upside-Down Apple Pie with coconut whipped cream
Tuesday	Flourless Mung Bean Olive Loaf with ghee	Crunchy Roasted Brussels Sprouts Flourless Mung Bean Olive Loaf	Oh-Yah Vegan Chocolate Chip Cookies Pistachio-Mint Milk	Cauliflower Steak with Moroccan Spices Sunrise Carrot-Ginger Soup
Wednesday	Golden Milk Latte	Beets with Herbed Goat Cheese Edamame Dip	Triple Kale Chips	Sweet Potato Boats with Creamy Spinach Broccoli-Potato-Leek Soup
Thursday	Pine Nut–Matcha Latte	Arugula and baby kale salad with Hibiscus Passion Vinaigrette	Cashew-Goji-Vanilla Milk Crazy Nutty Nut Bark	Smoky Roasted Rooty Roots Miso Soup with Dashi Broth, alfalfa sprouts, and red radish
Friday	Hemp Seed Chai	Black Bean and Tofu Scramble Wraps on Red Lentil–Saffron Tortilla	chopped apple, celery, and persimmon on Mushroom Cashew Pâté	Borscht with Cashew Cream Sprouted Seeds Bread Edamame Dip
Saturday	Sprouted Seeds Bread with Mushroom Cashew Pâté	Mouthful Quinoa-Carrot Burger Triple Kale Chips	Flourless Black Bean Brownie	California Sushi Roll Licorice Sweet Brown Rice Root and Leaf Magnesium Broth
Sunday	Recover-Restore-Reboot Porridge	Curry Lemon-Pumpkin Kebabs Silky Tofu–Spinach Dip	Oh-Yah Vegan Chocolate Chip Cookies	Tomato Soup with Basil and Capers Savory Mung Bean Flatbread Upside-Down Apple Pie

Creative Cooking for Healthy Bones

Table 19.4. Winter Weekly Meal Plan

	Breakfast	Lunch	Snack	Dinner
Monday	Feel-Good Banana Bread Hemp Seed Chai	Umami Soy-Glazed Portobello Steak Green and Red Everyday Sauerkraut	Triple Kale Chips	Sunrise Carrot-Ginger Soup Sprouted Seeds Bread Mushroom Cashew Pâté
Tuesday	Cashew-Goji-Vanilla Milk Sprouted Seeds Bread	Kale, Cabbage, and White Bean Salad Meaty Meatless Meatballs with Marinara Sauce Immortal Root Kimchi	Oh-Yah Vegan Chocolate Chip Cookies	Golden Dal Moringa Khichuri baby kale with Basil-Walnut Pesto Immortal Root Kimchi
Wednesday	Hearty Cacao Latte	Broccoli and Mushroom Buffalo "Wings" shredded radish and napa cabbage salad with Three Herbs Bone Pesto	Crazy Nutty Nut Bark C-Packed Pink Latte	Hearty Quinoa Minestrone mixed sprouts salad Savory Mung Bean Flatbread with Parsley–Pine Nut Chimichurri Pesto
Thursday	chopped apple on coconut kefir and honey or maple syrup	Sunrise Carrot-Ginger Soup Savory Mung Bean Flatbread Pineapple-Turmeric Kimchi	Flourless Black Bean Brownie	Acorn Squash with Forbidden Rice Stuffing and mung bean sprouts roasted walnuts Root and Leaf Magnesium Broth with chopped scallions
Friday	eggs any style on Flourless Mung Bean Olive Loaf	Deep Purple Hummus Cauliflower Steak with Moroccan Spices	Avocado-Date Chocolate Mousse	Recover-Restore-Reboot Porridge Triple Kale Chips Pineapple-Turmeric Kimchi
Saturday	Morning March Matcha Latte	Red Lentil–Saffron Tortilla with scrambled eggs or tofu scramble Smoky Roasted Rooty Roots	Mushroom Cashew Pâté baby carrots, sliced apples, sliced fennel	Umami Soy-Glazed Portobello Steak Golden Triangle Indian Mash Pineapple-Turmeric Kimchi
Sunday	Go Bananas Flourless Pancakes Hemp Seed Chai	Beets with Herbed Goat Cheese Saffron Cauliflower Rice	Feel-Good Banana Bread with tahini spread	Broccoli-Potato-Leek Soup Crunchy Roasted Brussels Sprouts Acai-Yam "Cheesecake"

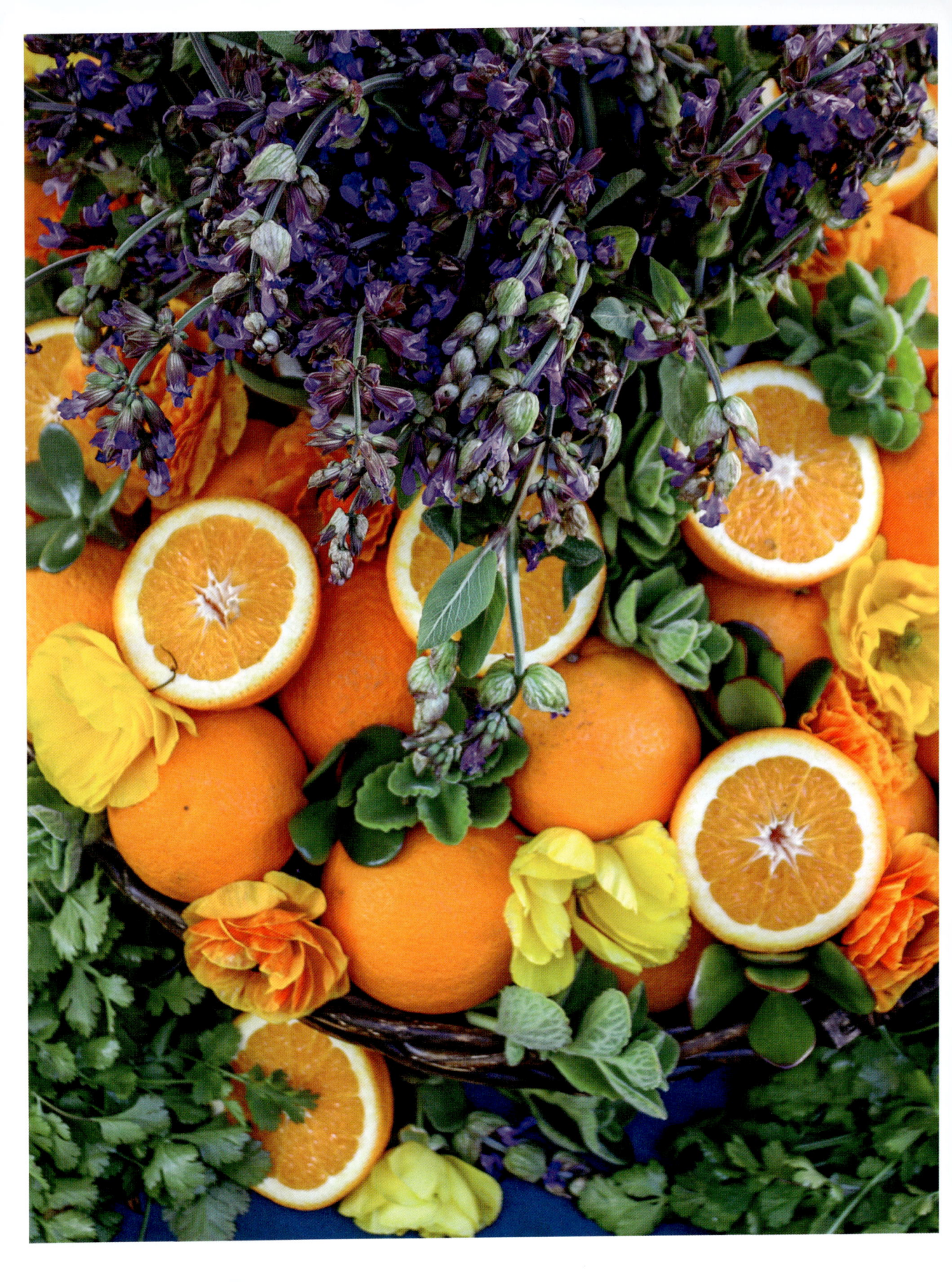

ACKNOWLEDGMENTS

This book would not exist without our editor, Fern Marshall Bradley. We offer our heartfelt thanks for Fern's suggestions, creativity, patience, kindness, and commitment to our success. Many thanks also to Amalia Herren-Lage for editorial support and attention to detail and to publisher Margo Baldwin, whose confidence in this, our second book, we welcome with excitement and deep appreciation.

APPENDIX

Recipes for Paleo and Ketogenic Diets

Nearly every recipe in this book is suitable for vegetarian and vegan diets, and all are made with gluten-free ingredients. This chart indicates which recipes are suitable for those following a paleo or ketogenic diet.

	Page number	Paleo	Ketogenic
Juices, Lattes, Milks, and Smoothies			
Basic Juice Formula	108	■	◆
Basic Green Juice	109	■	◆
Beet to Beat Juice	109	■	◆
Follow Your Gut Juice	109	■	◆
Morning Ritual Green Juice	109	■	◆
Sunny Carrot Juice	110	■	◆
Cashew-Goji-Vanilla Milk	112	■	◆
Hemp Seed Chai	112	■	◆
Pistachio-Mint Milk	112	■	◆
C-Packed Pink Latte	114	■	◆
Golden Milk Latte	114	■	◆
Hearty Cacao Latte	114	■	◆
Morning March Matcha Latte	115	■	◆
Pine Nut–Matcha Latte	115	■	◆

	Page number	Paleo	Ketogenic
Awakening Golden Smoothie	116	■	◆
Berry Paradise Smoothie	117	■	◆
Green Shield Smoothie	117	■	◆
Dressings and Pestos			
Amino-Sesame Vinaigrette	121		◆
Classic Olive Oil–Lemon Vinaigrette	121	■	◆
Hibiscus Passion Vinaigrette	121	■	◆
Mediterranean Herb and Grape Vinaigrette	121	■	◆
Creamy Golden Ranch Dressing	122	■	◆
Yogurt-Orange-Dill Dressing	122	■	◆
Tahini-Apple-Ginger Dressing	122	■	◆
California Vegan Chipotle Sauce	122	■	◆
Basil-Walnut Pesto	125	■	◆
Kale-Cashew Pesto	125	■	◆
Hemp Seed Pesto	125	■	◆
Parsley–Pine Nut Chimichurri Pesto	125		◆
Three Herbs Bone Pesto	125		◆

	Page number	Paleo	Keto-genic
Fermented Slow-Aged Pickles and Bone Vinegar			
Beet-Cauliflower Pickle	128	■	◆
Green and Red Everyday Sauerkraut	130	■	◆
Immortal Root Kimchi	132	■	◆
Jummee's Signature Pineapple-Turmeric Kimchi	134	■	◆
Apple Cider Vinegar	136	■	◆
Dr. Laura's Bone Vinegar	137	■	◆
Molasses-Kale-Herb Vinegar	138	■	◆
Dips and Breads			
Edamame Dip	140		◆
Silky Tofu–Spinach Dip	141	■	◆
Deep Purple Hummus	142	■	◆
Mushroom Cashew Pâté	144	■	◆
Feel-Good Banana Bread	147		◆
Flourless Mung Bean Olive Loaf	148		
Red Lentil–Saffron Tortilla	150		
Savory Mung Bean Flatbread	152		
Sprouted Seeds Bread	154	■	
Small Meals			
Broccoli and Mushroom Buffalo "Wings"	156		
Beets with Herbed Goat Cheese	159	■	◆
California Rainbow Spring Rolls	160		
Golden Triangle Indian Mash	162		
Steamed Eggplant with Apple-Tahini Sauce	163	■	◆
Curry Lemon-Pumpkin Kebabs	165	■	◆

	Page number	Paleo	Keto-genic
Sweet and Savory Grilled Peaches and Zucchini	166		
Sweet Potato–Scallion Pancakes	169	■	
Umami Soy-Glazed Portobello Steak	170		◆
Snap Peas with Tempeh Dust	172	■	◆
Broths, Porridge, and Soups			
Miso Soup with Dashi Broth	174		◆
Root and Leaf Magnesium Broth	177	■	◆
Borscht with Cashew Cream	178	■	◆
Broccoli-Potato-Leek Soup	180		
California Creamy Corn Chowder	182		
Golden Dal Moringa Khichuri	184		
Hearty Quinoa Minestrone	186		
Recover-Restore-Reboot Porridge	188		
Sea Greens and Shiitake Soup	190	■	◆
Tomato Soup with Basil and Capers	192		
Sunrise Carrot-Ginger Soup	194	■	◆
Salad Meals			
Ageless Macrobiotic Salad	197	■	◆
Chickpea-Cucumber Salad with a Hint of Mint	200		
Herb and Wildflower Garden Salad	203	■	◆
Endive Canoes with Guacamole	204	■	◆
Fennel-Radicchio Salad	206	■	◆

Recipes for Paleo and Ketogenic Diets ▪ 291

	Page number	Paleo	Keto-genic
Happy-Go-Lucky Caesar Salad	208	■	◆
Kale, Cabbage, and White Bean Salad	209		
New Classic Rainbow Coleslaw	211	■	◆
Beefy Tomato Salad with Cherry Vinaigrette	212	■	◆
Seaweed Flower Cucumber Salad	214	■	◆
Main Meals			
Acorn Squash with Forbidden Rice Stuffing	216	■	◆
BBQ Jackfruit Tacos with Mango Salsa	218	■	◆
Black Bean and Tofu Scramble Wraps	220		
Buckwheat Linguine with Kale-Macadamia Pesto	222	■	
Cauliflower Steak with Moroccan Spices	224	■	◆
California Sushi Rolls with Licorice Sweet Brown Rice	226	■	
Edamame Spread Avocado Toast	228		
Maple Syrup BBQ Tempeh	230		◆
Meaty Meatless Meatballs with Marinara Sauce	232		◆
Mouthful Quinoa-Carrot Burgers	234		◆
Mung Bean Pizza	236		
Sweet Potato Boats with Creamy Spinach	238	■	
Vegan Delight Matcha Curry	240	■	

	Page number	Paleo	Keto-genic
Super Side Dishes			
Broccoli Rabe Restaurant-Style	244	■	◆
Go Bananas Flourless Pancakes	246	■	
Green Pea and Roasted Red Pepper Mash	248	■	◆
Immortal Acai Bowl	250	■	◆
Crunchy Roasted Brussels Sprouts	251	■	◆
Rainbow Veggie Frittata with Feta	252	■	◆
Saffron Cauliflower Rice	254	■	◆
Smoky Roasted Rooty Roots	256	■	
Triple Kale Chips	258	■	
Watermelon-Mint Gazpacho	261	■	
Wok Express Crunchy Green Beans	262	■	◆
Good Sweets			
Acai-Yam "Cheesecake"	264		
Almond-Orange-Cacao Cake	266		
Upside-Down Apple Pie	268	■	
Avocado-Date Chocolate Mousse	270	■	◆
Chia Berry Cup	272	■	◆
Crazy Nutty Nut Bark	273	■	◆
Cherry Velvet Muffins	275		
Sweet and Salty Chocolate Strawberries	276	■	◆
Flourless Black Bean Brownies	279		
Oh-Yah Vegan Chocolate Chip Cookies	280		

NOTES

Introduction. Plants and Bones: A Dynamic Relationship

1. I. Iguacel, M. L. Miguel-Berges et al., "Veganism, Vegetarianism, Bone Mineral Density, and Fracture Risk: A Systematic Review and Meta-Analysis," *Nutrition Reviews* 77, no. 1 (October 29, 2018): 1–18, https://doi.org/10.1093/nutrit/nuy045.

Chapter 1. Bones Are a Family of Cells

1. C. Palacios, "The Role of Nutrients in Bone Health, from A to Z," *Critical Reviews in Food Science and Nutrition* 45, no. 8 (2006): 621–28, https://doi.org/10.1080/10408390500466174.
2. S. Kim, L. Kelly et al., "Increase in Bone Mineral Density using Precision Data to Drive Targeted Nutrition" (unpublished manuscript, October 2023).
3. A. M. Mohamed, "An Overview of Bone Cells and Their Regulating Factors of Differentiation," *Malaysian Journal of Medical Science* 15, no. 1 (January 2008): 4–12.
4. A. I. Caplan, "Are All Adult Stem Cells the Same?," *Regenerative Engineering and Translational Medicine* 1 (2015): 4–10, https://doi.org/10.1007/s40883-015-0001-4.
5. T. Mizoguchi and N. Ono, "The Diverse Origin of Bone-Forming Osteoblasts," *Journal of Bone and Mineral Research* 36, no. 8 (August 2021): 1432–47, https://doi.org/10.1002/jbmr.4410.
6. E. Balogh et al., "Influence of Iron on Bone Homeostasis," *Pharmaceuticals (Basel)* 11, no. 4 (October 18, 2018): 107, https://doi.org/10.3390/ph11040107.
7. J. O. Hollinger, A. Srinivasan et al., "Bone Tissue Engineering: Growth Factors and Cytokines," in *Comprehensive Biomaterials*, ed. P. Ducheyne (Elsevier, 2011), 281–301, https://doi.org/10.1016/B978-0-08-055294-1.00160-4.
8. M. Fischetti and J. Christiansen, "Our Bodies Replace Billions of Cells Every Day," *Scientific American*, April 1, 2021, https://doi.org/10.1038/scientificamerican0421-76.
9. S. C. Manolagas and A. M. Parfitt, "What Old Means to Bone," *Trends in Endocrinology & Metabolism* 21, no. 6 (June 2010): 369–74, https://doi.org/10.1016/j.tem.2010.01.010.
10. A. Y. Lupatov and K. N. Yarygin, "Telomeres and Telomerase in the Control of Stem Cells," *Biomedicines* 10, no. 10 (2022): 2335, https://doi.org/10.3390/biomedicines10102335.
11. R. K. Rude, H. E. Gruber et al., "Immunolocalization of RANKL Is Increased and OPG Decreased During Dietary Magnesium Deficiency in the Rat," *Nutrition & Metabolism* 2, no. 1 (September 2005), https://doi.org/10.1186/1743-7075-2-24.
12. M. Torrens-Mas and P. Roca, "Phytoestrogens for Cancer Prevention and Treatment," *Biology* 9, no. 12 (2020): 427, https://doi.org/10.3390/biology9120427.

Chapter 2. Feeding Your Bones

1. C. Chaveroux, A. Bruhat et al., "Regulating the Expression of Therapeutic Transgenes by Controlled Intake of Dietary Essential Amino Acids," *Nature Biotechnology* 34, no. 7 (June 2016): 746–51, https://doi.org/10.1038/nbt.3582.
2. A. Negri, V. Naponelli et al., "Molecular Targets of Epigallocatechin—Gallate (EGCG): A Special Focus on Signal Transduction and Cancer," *Nutrients* 10, no. 12 (December 2018): 1936, https://doi.org/10.3390/nu10121936.
3. M. Fenech, "Chapter 4—The Role of Nutrition in DNA Replication, DNA Damage Prevention and DNA Repair," in *Principles of Nutrigenetics and Nutrigenomics* (Academic Press, 2020), 27–32, https://doi.org/10.1016/B978-0-12-804572-5.00004-5.
4. M. Dus, "What You Eat Can Reprogram Your Genes—An Expert Explains the Emerging Science of Nutrigenomics," *The Conversation*, March 1, 2022, https://theconversation.com/what-you-eat-can-reprogram-your-genes-an-expert-explains-the-emerging-science-of-nutrigenomics-165867.

5. V. Locatelli and V. E. Bianchi, "Effect of GH/IGF-1 on Bone Metabolism and Osteoporosis," *International Journal of Endocrinology* (2014): 235060, https://doi.org/10.1155/2014/235060.
6. I. Groenendijk, P. Grootswagers et al., "Protein Intake and Bone Mineral Density: Cross-Sectional Relationship and Longitudinal Effects in Older Adults," *Journal of Cachexia, Sarcopenia, and Muscle* 14, no. 1 (February 2023): 116–25, https://doi.org/10.1002/jcsm.13111.
7. Z. Dai, Y. Zhang et al., "Association between Dietary Fiber Intake and Bone Loss in the Framingham Offspring Study," *Journal of Bone and Mineral Research* 33, no. 2 (February 2018): 241–49, https://doi.org/10.1002/jbmr.3308.
8. Harvard Health, "Precious Metals and Other Important Minerals for Health," February 15, 2021, https://www.health.harvard.edu/staying-healthy/precious-metals-and-other-important-minerals-for-health.
9. Office of Dietary Supplements, "Nutrient Recommendations and Databases," n.d., https://ods.od.nih.gov/HealthInformation/nutrientrecommendations.aspx#dri.
10. G. Guney, B. Sener-Simsek et al., "Assessment of the Relationship between Serum Vitamin D and Osteocalcin Levels with Metabolic Syndrome in Non-Osteoporotic Postmenopausal Women," *Geburtshilfe Frauenheilkd* 79, no. 3 (March 2019): 293–99, https://doi.org/10.1055/a-0767-6572.
11. T. O. Carpenter, S. J. Mackowiak et al., "Osteocalcin and Its Message: Relationship to Bone Histology in Magnesium-Deprived Rats," *American Journal of Physiology-Endocrinology and Metabolism* 263, no. 1 (July 1992): E107–E114, https://doi.org/10.1152/ajpendo.1992.263.1.e107; F. Mammoli, S. Castiglioni et al., "Magnesium Is a Key Regulator of the Balance between Osteoclast and Osteoblast Differentiation in the Presence of Vitamin D_3," *International Journal of Molecular Science* 20, no. 2 (January 2019): 385, https://doi.org/10.3390/ijms20020385.
12. P. Chambers, "Vitamin B6, Magnesium, and Vitamin D: The Triple Play," *Medical & Clinical Research* 8, no. 10 (2023): 1–7.
13. D. A. Bushinsky, D. R. Riordon et al., "Decreased Potassium Stimulates Bone Resorption," *American Journal of Physiology* 272, no. 6 (June 1997): F774–F780, https://doi.org/10.1152/ajprenal.1997.272.6.F774.
14. L. Gambari, B. Grigolo et al., "Dietary Organosulfur Compounds: Emerging Players in the Regulation of Bone Homeostasis," *Frontiers in Endocrinology* 13 (2022), https://doi.org/10.3389/fendo.2022.937956.
15. J. P. O'Connor, D. Kanjilal et al., "Zinc as a Therapeutic Agent in Bone Regeneration," *Materials* 13, no. 10 (May 2020): 2211, https://doi.org/10.3390/ma13102211.
16. M. Rondanelli, M. A. Faliva et al., "Copper as Dietary Supplement for Bone Metabolism: A Review," *Nutrients* 13, no. 2 (June 2021): 2246, https://doi.org/10.3390/nu13072246.
17. M. Rondanelli, M. A. Faliva et al., "An Update on Magnesium and Bone Health," *Biometals* 34, no. 4 (August 2021): 715–36, https://doi.org/10.1007/s10534-021-00305-0.
18. J. S. Walsh, R. M. Jacques et al., "Effect of Selenium Supplementation on Musculoskeletal Health in Older Women: A Randomised, Double-Blind, Placebo-Controlled Trail," *The Lancet Healthy Longevity* 2, no. 4 (2021): e212–e221.
19. C. M. Beukhof, M. Medici et al., "Selenium Status Is Positively Associated with Bone Mineral Density in Healthy Aging European Men," *PLOS One* 11, no. 4 (April 2016): e0152748, https://doi.org/10.1371/journal.pone.0152748.
20. G. C. Chen and Z. X. Wan, "Nut Consumption, Lipid Profile, and Health Outcomes," *American Journal of Clinical Nutrition* 103, no. 4 (April 2016): 1185–86, https://doi.org/10.3945/ajcn.115.128272.
21. M. Rondanelli, M. A. Faliva et al., "Essentiality of Manganese for Bone Health: An Overview and Update," *Natural Product Communications* 16, no. 5 (2021), https://doi.org/10.1177/1934578X211016649.
22. M. M. F. Yee, K. Y. Chin et al., "Vitamin A and Bone Health: A Review on Current Evidence," *Molecules* 26, no. 6 (March 2021): 1757, https://doi.org/10.3390/molecules26061757.
23. D. D. Bikle, "Vitamin D Metabolism, Mechanism of Action, and Clinical Applications," *Chemical Biology* 21, no. 3 (March 2014): 319–29, https://doi.org/10.1016/j.chembiol.2013.12.016.
24. Y. Yamamoto, T. Yoshizawa et al., "Vitamin D Receptor in Osteoblasts Is a Negative Regulator of Bone Mass Control," *Endocrinology* 154, no. 3 (March 2013): 1008–20, https://doi.org/10.1210/en.2012-1542.
25. S. Akbari and A. A. Rasouli-Ghahroudi, "Vitamin K and Bone Metabolism: A Review of the Latest Evidence in Preclinical Studies." *BioMed Research International* 2018: 4629383, http://doi.org/10.1155/2018/4629383.

26. J. M. Geleijnse, C. Vermeer et al., "Dietary Intake of Menaquinone Is Associated with a Reduced Risk of Coronary Heart Disease: The Rotterdam Study," *Journal of Nutrition* 134, no. 11 (2004).

27. C. Lampropoulos, I. Papaioannou, et.al., "Osteoporosis—A Risk Factor for Cardiovascular Disease?," *Nature Reviews Rheumatology* 8 (2012): 587–98, https://doi.org/10.1038/nrrheum.2012.120.

28. A. N. Panche, A. D. Diwan et al., "Flavonoids: An Overview," *Journal of Nutritional Science* 5 (December 2016): e47, https://doi.org/10.1017/jns.2016.41.

29. N. Yoshimi, H. Kohzaki et al., "Anti-Osteoporotic Mechanisms of Polyphenols Elucidated Based on In Vivo Studies Using Ovariectomized Animals," *Antioxidants* 11, no. 2 (2022): 217, https://doi.org/10.3390/antiox11020217.

30. T. Sato, N. Inaba et al., "MK-7 and Its Effects on Bone Quality and Strength," *Nutrients* 12, no. 4 (March 2020): 965, https://doi.org/10.3390/nu12040965.

31. F. Zhang, N. Hu et al., "The Correlation of Urinary Strontium with the Risk of Chronic Kidney Disease among the General United States Population," *Frontiers in Public Health* 11 (September 2023): 1251232, https://doi.org/10.3389/fpubh.2023.

32. U. Schött, C. Solomon et al., "The Endothelial Glycocalyx and Its Disruption, Protection and Regeneration: A Narrative Review," *Scandinavian Journal of Trauma, Resuscitation and Emergency Medicine* 24 (April 2016): 48, https://doi.org/10.1186/s13049-016-0239-y.

33. Schött, "The Endothelial Glycocalyx."

34. J. Øyen, C. G. Gjesdal et al., "Dietary Choline Intake Is Directly Associated with Bone Mineral Density in the Hordaland Health Study," *Journal of Nutrition* 147, no. 4 (April 2017): 572–78, https://doi.org/10.3945/jn.116.243006.

35. P. Uribe, A. Johansson et al., "Soluble Silica Stimulates Osteogenic Differentiation and Gap Junction Communication in Human Dental Follicle Cells," *Scientific Reports* 10, no. 1 (June 2020): 9923, https://doi.org/10.1038/s41598-020-66939-1.

36. R. Jugdaohsingh, "Silicon and Bone Health," *Journal of Nutrition, Health, and Aging* 11, no. 2 (March–April 2007): 99–110.

37. Jugdaohsingh, "Silicon and Bone Health."

38. M. Rondanelli, M. A. Faliva et al., "Pivotal Role of Boron Supplementation on Bone Health: A Narrative Review," *Journal of Trace Elements in Medical Biology* 62 (December 2020): 126577, https://doi.org/10.1016/j.jtemb.2020.126577.

39. L. Pizzorno, "Nothing Boring about Boron," *Integrative Medicine (Encinitas)* 14, no. 4 (August 2015): 35–48.

Chapter 3. Managing Antinutrients and Acrylamide

1. W. Petroski and D. M. Minich, "Is There Such a Thing as 'Anti-Nutrients'? A Narrative Review of Perceived Problematic Plant Compounds," *Nutrients* 12, no. 10 (September 2020): 2929, https://doi.org/10.3390/nu12102929.

2. M. Alhujaily, W. Dhifi et al., "An Overview of the Potential of Medicinal Plants Used in the Development of Nutraceuticals for the Management of Diabetes Mellitus: Proposed Biological Mechanisms," *Processes* 10, no. 10 (2022): 2044, https://doi.org/10.3390/pr10102044.

3. M. Afifi, "A Review on the New Trends of Acrylamide Toxicity," *Biomedical Journal of Scientific and Technical Research*, Biomedical Research Network, April 27, 2020, https://doi.org/10.26717/bjstr.2020.27.004480.

4. N. Veronese, F. Bolzetta et al., "Dietary Acrylamide and Incident Osteoporotic Fractures: An 8-year Prospective Cohort Study," *Aging Clinical and Experimental Research* 34, no. 10 (October 2022): 2441–48, https://doi.org/10.1007/s40520-022-02214-9.

5. D. Benford, M. Bignami et al., "Assessment of the Genotoxicity of Acrylamide," *European Food Safety Authority Journal* 20, no. 5 (May 2022): e07293, https://doi.org/10.2903/j.efsa.2022.7293.

6. F. Xu, M. J. Oruna-Concha et al., "The Use of Asparaginase to Reduce Acrylamide Levels in Cooked Food," *Food Chemistry* 210 (November 2016): 163–71, https://doi.org/10.1016/j.foodchem.2016.04.105.

7. ScienceDaily, "A Little Rosemary Can Go a Long Way in Reducing Acrylamide in Food," February 8, 2008.

8. J. Kubala, "What Are Cacao Nibs? Nutrition, Benefits, and Culinary Uses," *Healthline*, March 28, 2019, https://www.healthline.com/nutrition/cacao-nibs#nutrition.

9. K. S. George and J. Munoz, "The Short-Term Effect of Prunes in Improving Bone in Men," *Nutrients* 14, no. 2 (January 2022): 276, https://doi.org/10.3390/nu14020276; A. Becalski and B. Brady, "Formation of Acrylamide at Temperatures Lower than 100°C: The Case of Prunes and a Model Study," *Food Additives and Contaminants. Part A, Chemistry, Analysis, Control, Exposure, and Risk Assessment* 28, no. 6 (June 2011): 726–30, https://doi.org/10.1080/19440049.2010.535217.

Chapter 4. Healthy Body, Healthy Bones

1. Penn State Extension, "Cool Season vs Warm Season Vegetables," https://extension.psu.edu/cool-season-vs-warm-season-vegetables.
2. M. Ogrodnik, S. A. Evans et al., "Whole-Body Senescent Cell Clearance Alleviates Age-Related Brain Inflammation and Cognitive Impairment in Mice," *Aging Cell* 20 (2021): e13296, https://doi.org/10.1111/acel.13296.
3. A. E. Hoban and R. M. Stilling, "The Microbiome Regulates Amygdala-Dependent Fear Recall," *Molecular Psychiatry* 23, no. 5 (May 2018): 1134–44, https://doi.org/10.1038/mp.2017.100.
4. M. N. Weitzmann, "Bone and the Immune System," *Toxicologic Pathology* 45, no. 7 (October 2017): 911–24, https://doi.org/10.1177/0192623317735316.
5. D. D. Weisenburger, "A Review and Update with Perspective of Evidence that the Herbicide Glyphosate (Roundup) Is a Cause of Non-Hodgkin's Lymphoma," *Clinical Lymphoma, Myeloma, and Leukemia* 21, no. 9 (2021): 621–30, https://doi.org/10.1016/j.clml.2021.04.009.
6. Y. M. Naguib, "Antioxidant Activities of Astaxanthin and Related Carotenoids," *Journal of Agricultural and Food Chemistry* 48, no. 4 (2000): 1150–54, https://doi.org/10.1021/jf991106k.
7. R. S. Hardy, H. Zhou et al., "Glucocorticoids and Bone: Consequences of Endogenous and Exogenous Excess and Replacement Therapy," *Endocrine Reviews* 39, no. 5 (October 2018): 519–48.
8. K. J. O'Riordan, M. Collins, G. M. Moloney et al., "Short Chain Fatty Acids: Microbial Metabolites for Gut-Brain Axis Signalling," *Molecular and Cellular Endocrinology* 546 (April 2022): 111572, https://doi.org/10.1016/j.mce.2022.111572.
9. S. L. Gray, A. Z. LaCroix, J. Larson, et al, "Proton Pump Inhibitor Use, Hip Fracture, and Change in Bone Mineral Density in Postmenopausal Women: Results from the Women's Health Initiative," *JAMA Internal Medicine* 170, no. 9 (2010): 765–71, http://doi.org/10.1001/archinternmed.2010.94.
10. A. B. Berenson, M. Rahman, C. R. Breitkopf, et al., "Effects of Depot Medroxyprogesterone Acetate and 20-Microgram Oral Contraceptives on Bone Mineral Density," *Obstetrics & Gynecology* 112, no. 4 (2008):788–99, http://doi.org/10.1097/AOG.0b013e3181875b78.
11. D. Gulayan, "8 Foods Containing the Highest Quantity of Glutathione," *Longevity.Technology*, October 27, 2022, https://longevity.technology/lifestyle/8-foods-containing-the-highest-quantity-of-glutathione.
12. J. Gao and T. Hou, "Cardiovascular Disease Treatment Using Traditional Chinese Medicine: Mitochondria as the Achilles' Heel," *Biomedicine & Pharmacotherapy* 164 (2023): 114999, https://doi.org/10.1016/j.biopha.2023.114999.
13. A. Dave, E. J. Park et al., "Consumption of Grapes Modulates Gene Expression, Reduces Non-Alcoholic Fatty Liver Disease, and Extends Longevity in Female C57BL/6J Mice Provided with a High-Fat Western-Pattern Diet," *Foods* 11, no. 3 (July 2022): 1984, https://doi.org/10.3390/foods11131984.
14. Mount Sinai Health System, "Dandelion," n.d., https://www.mountsinai.org/health-library/herb/dandelion.
15. Mount Sinai Health System, "Milk Thistle," n.d., https://www.mountsinai.org/health-library/herb/milk-thistle.
16. X. Chen, S. Wang et al., "Adverse Health Effects of Emerging Contaminants on Inflammatory Bowel Disease," *Frontiers in Public Health* 11 (February 2023): 1140786, https://doi.org/10.3389/fpubh.2023.1140786.
17. M. Boland, "Developmental PFAS Exposures Affect Bone Health," National Institute of Environmental Health, February 2023, https://www.niehs.nih.gov/research/programs/geh/geh_newsletter/2023/2/spotlight/developmental_pfas_exposures_affect_bone_health_study_suggests.cfm.
18. H. S. Kim, Y. J. Kim et al., "An Overview of Carcinogenic Heavy Metal: Molecular Toxicity Mechanism and Prevention," *Journal of Cancer Prevention* 20, no. 4 (December 2015): 232–40, https://doi.org/10.15430/JCP.2015.20.4.232.
19. M. Shahid, B. Pourrut et al., "Heavy-Metal-Induced Reactive Oxygen Species: Phytotoxicity and Physicochemical Changes in Plants," *Reviews of Environmental Contamination and Toxicology* 232 (2014): 1–44, https://doi.org/10.1007/978-3-319-06746-9_1.
20. J. Rodríguez, P. M. Mandalunis et al., "A Review of Metal Exposure and Its Effects on Bone Health," *Journal of Toxicology* 2018 (December 2018): 4854152, https://doi.org/10.1155/2018/4854152.
21. H. Zhou, W. T. Yang et al., "Accumulation of Heavy Metals in Vegetable Species Planted in Contaminated Soils and the Health Risk Assessment," *International Journal of Environmental Research and Public Health* 13, no. 3 (March 2016): 289, https://doi.org/10.3390/ijerph13030289.

22. A. Sattar, M. Wahid et al., "Concentration of Selected Heavy Metals in Spices, Dry Fruits and Plant Nuts," *Plant Foods and Human Nutrition* 39, no. 3 (September 1989): 279–86, https://doi.org/10.1007/BF01091938.
23. A. Andersen and H. N. Hansen, "High Cadmium and Nickel Contents in Sunflower Kernels," *Zeitschrift für Lebensmittel Untersuchung und Forschung* 179, no. 5 (November 1984): 399–400, https://doi.org/10.1007/BF01043439.
24. Cleveland Clinic Medical, "Heavy Metal Test," Cleveland Clinic, n.d., https://my.clevelandclinic.org/health/diagnostics/22797-heavy-metal-test.
25. CK-12 Foundation, "Fruits and Flowering Plants," n.d., https://www.ck12.org/book/ck-12-biology-advanced-concepts/section/13.47; H. Zhou, W. T. Yang et al., "Accumulation of Heavy Metals in Vegetable Species Planted in Contaminated Soils and the Health Risk Assessment," *International Journal of Environmental Research and Public Health* 13, no. 3 (March 2016): 289, https://doi.org/10.3390/ijerph13030289.
26. W. Kalt, A. Cassidy et al., "Recent Research on the Health Benefits of Blueberries and Their Anthocyanins," *Advances in Nutrition* 11, no. 2 (March 2020): 224–36, https://doi.org/10.1093/advances/nmz065.

Chapter 5. Healthy Bones on a Vegan Diet

1. I. Sela, M. A. Yaskolka et al., "*Wolffia globosa*–Mankai Plant-Based Protein Contains Bioactive Vitamin B12 and Is Well Absorbed in Humans," *Nutrients* 12, no. 10 (October 2020): 3067, https://doi.org/10.3390/nu12103067.
2. N. Li, G. Zhao et al., "The Efficacy and Safety of Vitamin C for Iron Supplementation in Adult Patients with Iron Deficiency Anemia: A Randomized Clinical Trial," *JAMA Network Open* 3, no. 11 (2020): e2023644, https://doi.org/10.1001/jamanetworkopen.2020.23644.
3. L. Grinder-Pedersen, K. Bukhave et al., "Calcium from Milk or Calcium-Fortified Foods Does Not Inhibit Nonheme-Iron Absorption from a Whole Diet Consumed over a 4-D Period," *American Journal of Clinical Nutrition* 80, no. 2 (August 2004): 404–9, https://doi.org/10.1093/ajcn/80.2.404.

Chapter 6. Creating a Bone-Health Nutrition Plan

1. "CTX—Overview: Beta-CrossLaps, Serum," n.d., https://www.mayocliniclabs.com/test-catalog/overview/83175#Clinical-and-Interpretive.
2. "PINP—Overview: Procollagen I Intact N-Terminal, Serum," n.d., https://www.mayocliniclabs.com/test-catalog/overview/61695#Clinical-and-Interpretive.

Chapter 7. Ancient Medicine for Bone Health

1. Food and Agriculture of the United Nations, "Fermented Foods: A Global Perspective," n.d., https://www.fao.org/3/x0560e/x0560e05.htm.
2. A kingdom is the penultimate taxonomic group. The taxonomy from smallest to largest is species, genus, family, order, class, phylum, kingdom, and domain.
3. People eat mushrooms rather than all fungi because so many fungi are toxic, and while edible mushrooms may contain trace amounts of toxins, an edible mushroom's trace toxins are extinguished by heat. Mushrooms in powder or extract form are many times more powerful than the culinary fruiting body and in the presence of chronic illness or condition requiring a daily pharmaceutical medicine, should be taken with the advice of a health care provider.
4. People can be allergic to mushrooms just as some people can be allergic to just about any chemical in any plant food or otherwise. In fact, unless one is tested by a pharmacogeneticist, reactions to chemistry are so unpredictable, people can be allergic to other people.
5. C. A. Janeway Jr., P. Travers et al., *Immunobiology: The Immune System in Health and Disease*, 5th ed. (New York: Garland Science, 2001), https://www.ncbi.nlm.nih.gov/books/NBK27092/.
6. C. Lull, H. J. Wichers et al., "Anti-inflammatory and Immunomodulating Properties of Fungal Metabolites," *Mediators of Inflammation* 2005, no. 2 (June 2005): 63–80, https://doi.org/10.1155/MI.2005.63.
7. G. Törős, H. El-Ramady et al., "Modulation of the Gut Microbiota with Prebiotics and Antimicrobial Agents from *Pleurotus ostreatus* Mushroom," *Foods* 12, no. 10 (May 2023): 2010, https://doi.org/10.3390/foods12102010.
8. X. Dai, J. M. Stanilka et al., "Consuming *Lentinula edodes* (Shiitake) Mushrooms Daily Improves Human Immunity: A Randomized Dietary Intervention in Healthy Young Adults," *Journal of the American College of Nutrition* 34, no. 6 (2015): 478–87, https://doi.org/10.1080/07315724.2014.950391.
9. Memorial Sloan Kettering Cancer Center, "Shiitake Mushroom," February 14, 2023, https://www.mskcc.org/cancer-care/integrative-medicine/herbs/shiitake-mushroom.

10. H. S. Tuli, S. S. Sandhu et al., "Pharmacological and Therapeutic Potential of Cordyceps with Special Reference to Cordycepin," *3 Biotech* 4 (February 2014): 1–12, https://doi.org/10.1007/s13205-013-0121-9.

11. P. L. Lai, M. Naidu et al., "Neurotrophic Properties of the Lion's Mane Medicinal Mushroom, *Hericium erinaceus* (Higher Basidiomycetes) from Malaysia," *International Journal of Medicinal Mushrooms* 15, no. 6 (2013): 539–54. https://doi.org/10.1615/intjmedmushr.v15.i6.30.

12. A. Panossian and G. Wikman, "Effects of Adaptogens on the Central Nervous System and the Molecular Mechanisms Associated with Their Stress-Protective Activity," *Pharmaceuticals* 3, no. 1 (January 2010): 188–224, https://doi.org/10.3390/ph3010188.

13. S. J. Jung, M. R. Oh et al., "Effect of Ginseng Extracts on the Improvement of Osteopathic and Arthritis Symptoms in Women with Osteopenia: A Randomized, Double-Blind, Placebo-Controlled Clinical Trial," *Nutrients* 13, no. 10 (2021): 3352, https://doi.org/10.3390/nu13103352.

14. P. R. Nagareddy and M. Lakshmana, "*Withania somnifera* Improves Bone Calcification in Calcium-Deficient Ovariectomized Rats," *Journal of Pharmacy and Pharmacology* 58, no. 4 (April 2006): 513–19, https://doi.org/10.1211/jpp.58.4.0011.

INDEX

Note: Page references in *italics* indicate recipe photographs.

A

Acai
    Bowl, Immortal, 250
    -Lemon Vinaigrette, 159
    -Yam "Cheesecake," 264–65, *265*
Acetyl groups, 19–20
Acrylamide, 45–47, 48
Adaptogens, 97–98
Advanced-glycation end products (AGEs), 45
Alcohol, 46
Almond(s)
    -Orange-Cacao Cake, *266*, 266–67
    sprouted, health benefits, 35
Alpha-linolenic acid (ALA), 79
Amino acid calculator, 69
Amino acids, 71
Amino-Sesame Vinaigrette, 121
AMPK, 50, 51
Ancient medicine for bone health, 91–98
Antinutrients, 41–45, 47–48
Antioxidants, 42, 63–66
Antiseizure drugs, 62
Apple(s)
    Apple Cider Vinegar, 136
    Green Shield Smoothie, 117, *117*
    Pie, Upside-Down, *268*, 268–69
    reducing tannins in, 47
    -Tahini-Ginger Dressing, 122
    -Tahini Sauce, Steamed Eggplant with, 163
Appliances, small, 104–5
Arsenic, 68
Ashwagandha, 97
Asparaginase, 46

Asparagine, 46
Asparagus
    Vegan Delight Matcha Curry, *240*, 240–41
Astaxanthin, 56
Autophagy, 51
Avocado(s)
    California Rainbow Spring Rolls, 160–61, *161*
    California Sushi Rolls with Licorice Sweet Brown Rice, *226*, 226–27
    -Date Chocolate Mousse, 270, *271*
    Edamame Spread Toast, *228*, 228–29
    Green Shield Smoothie, 117, *117*
    Guacamole, *204*, 204–5

B

Bacterial infections, 62
Banana(s)
    Bread, Feel-Good, *146*, 147
    Go Bananas Flourless Pancakes, *242*, 246–47
Bark, Crazy Nutty Nut, 273, *273*
Basil-Walnut Pesto, 125
BBQ Jackfruit Tacos with Mango Salsa, *218*, 218–19
BBQ Tempeh, Maple Syrup, *230*, 230–31
BCM01 gene, 78
Bean(s). *See also* Edamame; Mung Bean
    antinutrients in, 73
    Black, and Tofu Scramble Wraps, *220*, 220–21

    Black, Flourless Brownies, *278*, 279
    Chickpea-Cucumber Salad with a Hint of Mint, 200, *201*
    easy Mexican-style dishes with, 73
    Golden Triangle Indian Mash, 162, *162*
    Green, Wok Express Crunchy, *262*, 262
    pairing with rice, 25
    soaking, 102–3
    White, Kale, and Cabbage Salad, 209
Beet(s)
    Beet to Beat Juice, 109, *110*
    Borscht with Cashew Cream, *178*, 178–79
    -Cauliflower Pickle, 128–29
    C-Packed Pink Latte, 114
    Deep Purple Hummus, *142*, 142–43
    with Herbed Goat Cheese, *158*, 159
    reducing oxalates in, 47
Berry(ies)
    Cup, Chia, 272
    health benefits of blueberries, 68
    Herb and Wildflower Garden Salad, *202*, 203
    Immortal Acai Bowl, 250
    Paradise Smoothie, 117, *117*
    Sweet and Salty Chocolate Strawberries, *276*, 276–77
Beta-carotene, 78
Black pepper, 25, 103
Blood pH, 74

Blueberries, 68
Bok choy, 48, 76
Bone anatomy, 13
Bone cells, 13–15
Bone density genetics, 84
Bone density loss
   assessing severity of, 86–88
   from chronic inflammation, 52–53
   considering actions for, 86–88
   natural medicine plan, 88–89
   osteoporosis, 12, 17, 86, 89–90
   reasons behind, 16–17
   scoring, worksheet for, 87
   sex-based patterns, 11–12
   treating with herbal principles, 93
Bone disorders, 62–63
Bone flexibility, 86
Bone health
   ancient medicine for, 91–98
   and commonly-used medicines, 62
   creating nutrition plan for, 81–90
   favorite foods for, 22–25
   hormonal influences, 56–59
   and inflammation, 52–55
   and the microbiome, 59–61
   nutrients for, 25–39
   and pH balance, 61
   RDA values, 25–26
   testing, 84–86
Bone-lining cells, 15
Bone mineralization, 26
Bone turnover (remodeling), 13–14, 15–16
Boron, 28, 38
Borscht with Cashew Cream, *178*, 178–79
Bovine leukemia virus (BLV), 60
Brain health, 60
Brazil nuts, 34, 35
Bread(s)
   Banana, Feel-Good, *146*, 147
   Edamame Spread Avocado Toast, *228*, 228–29
   Flourless Mung Bean Olive Loaf, 148, *149*

   making croutons with, 193
   Red Lentil–Saffron Tortillas, 150–51, *151*
   Savory Mung Bean Flatbread, 152–53
   Sprouted Seeds, 154
   toasted, note about, 45
Broccoli
   and Mushroom Buffalo "Wings," *155*, 156–57
   -Potato-Leek Soup, 180–81, *181*
Broccoli Rabe Restaurant-Style, 244–45, *245*
Broth
   Dashi, 174–75, *175*
   Root and Leaf Magnesium, 177
Brownies, Flourless Black Bean, *278*, 279
Brussels Sprouts, Crunchy Roasted, 251, *251*
Buckwheat Linguine with Kale-Macadamia Pesto, *222*, 222–23
Burdock root
   Follow Your Gut Juice, 109
   Immortal Root Kimchi, *132*, 132–33
   Root and Leaf Magnesium Broth, 177
Burgers, Mouthful Quinoa-Carrot, 234–35
B vitamins, 26, 28

C

Cabbage
   Green and Red Everyday Sauerkraut, 130–31
   Jummee's Signature Pineapple-Turmeric Kimchi, 134–35
   Kale, and White Bean Salad, 209
   New Classic Rainbow Coleslaw, *210*, 211
   Recover-Restore-Reboot Porridge, *188*, 188–89
Cacao
   -Almond-Orange Cake, *266*, 266–67

   Avocado-Date Chocolate Mousse, 270, *271*
   Flourless Black Bean Brownies, *278*, 279
   Latte, Hearty, 114, *114*
Cacao nibs, 48
Cadmium, 67
Cake, Almond-Orange-Cacao, *266*, 266–67
Calcitonin, 56
Calcitriol, 35
Calcium, 26–32
   effect on iron absorption, 76
   pairing with Vitamin D, 24
   -regulating hormones, 56
   sources and bone RDA, 28
   supplements, 27, 32
California Rainbow Spring Rolls, 160–61, *161*
Cancer, 54, 61
Carbohydrates, 21
Carnosine, 79
Carotene, 21
Carotenoids, 34, 56, 78
Carrot(s)
   California Rainbow Spring Rolls, 160–61, *161*
   California Sushi Rolls with Licorice Sweet Brown Rice, *226*, 226–27
   -Ginger Soup, Sunrise, 194
   Juice, Sunny, 110, *110*
   Maple Syrup BBQ Tempeh, *230*, 230–31
   -Quinoa Burgers, Mouthful, 234–35
   Smoky Roasted Rooty Roots, *256*, 256–57
Cashew(s)
   Acai-Yam "Cheesecake," 264–65, *265*
   commercially available, note about, 48
   Cream, Borscht with, *178*, 178–79
   -Goji-Vanilla Milk, 112
   -Kale Pesto, 125
   Mushroom Pâté, 144–45, *145*

-Parsley Pesto, 231
-Pineapple Dressing, 211
roasted unsalted, choosing, 35
selenium in, 34
Three Herb Bone Pesto, 125
urushiol in, 35, 48
Cast-iron cookware, 104
Cauliflower
   -Beet Pickle, 128–29
   Golden Triangle Indian Mash, 162, *162*
   Mung Bean Pizza, *236,* 236–37
   Rice, Saffron, 254–55, *255*
   Steak with Moroccan Spices, 224–25, *225*
Celiac disease, 53
Cell danger response, 52
Chaga, 95
Chai, Hemp Seed, 112
Cheese
   Blue, Dressing, *155,* 156–57
   Bone Health Classic Pesto, 124
   California Rainbow Spring Rolls, 160–61, *161*
   California Sushi Rolls with Licorice Sweet Brown Rice, *226,* 226–27
   Crunchy Roasted Brussels Sprouts, 251, *251*
   Herbed Goat, Beets with, *158,* 159
   Mung Bean Pizza, *236,* 236–37
   Rainbow Veggie Frittata with Feta, *252,* 252–53
   Snap Peas with Tempeh Dust, 172, *172*
"Cheesecake," Acai-Yam, 264–65, *265*
Chelating foods, 68
Cherry
   Velvet Muffins, *274,* 275
   Vinaigrette, 212, *213*
Chia Berry Cup, 272
Chickpea(s)
   -Cucumber Salad with a Hint of Mint, 200, *201*
   Golden Triangle Indian Mash, 162, *162*
   Chimichurri Sauce, 170, *171*

Chipotle Sauce, California Vegan, 122
Chocolate
   Almond-Orange-Cacao Cake, *266,* 266–67
   Chip Cookies, Oh-Yah Vegan, 280–81, *281*
   commercially available, heavy metals in, 48, 67
   Crazy Nutty Nut Bark, 273, *273*
   dark, acrylamide in, 48
   dark, health benefits, 48
   dark, magnesium in, 35
   Flourless Black Bean Brownies, *278,* 279
   Mousse, Avocado-Date, 270, *271*
   Strawberries, Sweet and Salty, *276,* 276–77
Cholesterol, 22
Choline, 28, 37, 78, 83–84
Chowder, California Creamy Corn, *182,* 182–83
Chromium, 28, 38–39
Chutney, Sweet and Tangy Mint, *184,* 185
Clotting genetics, 85
Coconut
   -Lemon-Caesar Dressing, 208
   -Orange Ranch Dressing, *216,* 217
   Whipped Cream, *242,* 247
Coffeeless Lattes
   Cacao, Hearty, 114, *114*
   C-Packed Pink, 114
   Golden Milk, 114, *114*
   Morning March Matcha, 115, *115*
   Pine Nut–Matcha, 115, *115*
   preparing, 113
Coleslaw, New Classic Rainbow, *210,* 211
Collagen, 13, 23, 36
Community-supported agriculture (CSA), 50
Companion eating, 24–25
Cookies, Oh-Yah Vegan Chocolate Chip, 280–81, *281*
Cooking basics and tips, 101–3
Copper, 28, 33

Corn Chowder, California Creamy, *182,* 182–83
Cortisol, 58
Creatine, 79
CTx, 84–85, 88
Cucumber(s)
   California Rainbow Spring Rolls, 160–61, *161*
   -Chickpea Salad with a Hint of Mint, 200, *201*
   Seaweed Flower Salad, 214
   Watermelon-Mint Gazpacho, *260,* 261
Curry, Vegan Delight Matcha, *240,* 240–41
Curry Lemon-Pumpkin Kebabs, *164,* 165
Cybernetic system, 52
Cytokines, 94

D

Dairy milk, 60
Dan Shen, 64
Dashi Broth, Miso Soup with, 174–75, *175*
Date-Avocado Chocolate Mousse, 270, *271*
Denaturing, 72
Depo-Provera, 62
Desserts and sweets
   Acai-Yam "Cheesecake," 264–65, *265*
   Almond-Orange-Cacao Cake, *266,* 266–67
   Avocado-Date Chocolate Mousse, 270, *271*
   Cherry Velvet Muffins, *274,* 275
   Chia Berry Cup, 272
   Crazy Nutty Nut Bark, 273, *273*
   Flourless Black Bean Brownies, *278,* 279
   Oh-Yah Vegan Chocolate Chip Cookies, 280–81, *281*
   Sweet and Salty Chocolate Strawberries, *276,* 276–77
   Upside-Down Apple Pie, *268,* 268–69
DEXA scan, 84, 86

DHA, 79
Diabetes, 57–58
Diet, early human, 74
Dips
    Deep Purple Hummus, *142,* 142–43
    Edamame, *139,* 140
    Silky Tofu–Spinach, 141, *141*
DNA, 19, 20
DNA methylation, 19
Dressings
    Blue Cheese, *155,* 156–57
    California Vegan Chipotle Sauce, 122
    Coconut-Lemon-Caesar, 208
    Pineapple-Cashew, 211
    preparing, 122
    Ranch, Creamy Golden, 122
    Ranch, Orange-Coconut, *216,* 217
    Ranch, Papaya–Hemp Seed, *164,* 165
    Tahini-Apple-Ginger, 122
    Tahini-Ginger, 209
    Yogurt-Orange-Dill, 122
Drinks. *See* Coffeeless Lattes; Juices; Smoothies

E

Early human diet, 74
Edamame
    Dip, *139,* 140
    Meaty Meatless Meatballs with Marinara Sauce, *232,* 232–33
    Spread Avocado Toast, *228,* 228–29
Edestin, 71
EGCG, 20
Eggplant, Steamed, with Apple-Tahini Sauce, 163
Eggs
    flaxseed, preparing, 146
    Rainbow Veggie Frittata with Feta, *252,* 252–53
    on toast ("soldiers"), 45
Eggshell calcium, 32
Endive Canoes with Guacamole, *204,* 204–5

Essential amino acids, 71
Estrogen, 16, 58
Estrogen detoxification test, 85
Estrogen therapy, 85
Eternal Bone-Healing Formula, 92
Exercise, 17, 51, 64

F

Fasting, 49, 51, 64
Fat, 21–22
Fennel
    health benefits, 77
    -Radicchio Salad, 206–7, *207*
Fermentation, 44–45, 78, 127
Fiber, 21
Fibrils, 13
Flavonoids, 36
Flaxseed meal egg substitute, 146
Fluoride, 29, 37
Folate, 21, 83–84
Food allergies, 53
Food intolerances, 53
Food pairings, 24–25
Foraging, 48
Fractures, treating, 92–93
Free radicals, 63–64
Frittata, Rainbow Veggie, with Feta, *252,* 252–53
Fruit. *See also specific fruits*
    dried, health benefits, 48
    dried, soaking, 103
    fresh, how to clean, 102
    phytochemicals in, 55
Fulvic acid, 38

G

Garlic, 68
Gazpacho, Watermelon-Mint, *260,* 261
Gene expression, 2, 19–21
Ginger
    -Carrot Soup, Sunrise, 194
    -Miso Vinaigrette, 197
    -Tahini Dressing, 209
Ginseng, 97
Glucocorticoids, 58–59
Glucose, 21
Glucosinolates, 42

Glutathione, 64–66
Gluten-free flours, 54
Gluten intolerance, 53–54
Glycidamide, 45
Glyphosate, 54, 61
GMO foods, 61
Goitrogens, 42, 43
Grains. *See also specific grains*
    Plant-Based Milks, *111,* 111–12
    soaking, 102–3
Grapefruit, 76
Grape(s)
    Green, Vinaigrette, 200
    health benefits, 65
    and Herb Vinaigrette, Mediterranean, 121
Green Beans, Wok Express Crunchy, *262,* 262
Greens. *See also specific greens*
    Basic Green Juice, 109, *110*
    Bone Health Classic Pesto, 124
    Root and Leaf Magnesium Broth, 177
Green tea, 48
Growth hormone, 58
Guacamole, *204,* 204–5
Gum inflammation, 62
Gut
    -brain axis, 60
    health, testing for, 86
    microbiome, 59–61

H

HbA1c levels, 85
The Healthy Bones Nutrition Plan and Cookbook (Kelly and Kelly), 3
Heavy metals, 66–68
Hemp Seed
    Chai, 112
    health benefits, 71
    –Papaya Ranch Dressing, *164,* 165
    Pesto, 125
Herbicides, 54, 61, 66–68
Herb(s). *See also specific herbs*
    Bone Health Classic Pesto, 124
    Chimichurri Sauce, 170, *171*
    Dr. Laura's Bone Vinegar, 137
    fresh, storing, 102

and Grape Vinaigrette,
Mediterranean, 121
-Molasses-Kale Vinegar, 138
Three, Bone Pesto, 125
and Wildflower Garden Salad, *202,* 203
Hibiscus Passion Vinaigrette, 121
High-density lipoprotein (HDL), 22
Highly processed foods, 61
Honeybees, 20
Hormone replacement therapy, 85
Hormones, and bone health, 56–59
HPA axis, 97
Humic acid, 38
Hummus, Deep Purple, *142,* 142–43
Hyperparathyrodism, 57
Hypothyroidism, 56

I
IBS, 61
Immune system, 59, 94
Inflammation
    chronic, 52–53
    controlling, strategies for, 53–55
    from food allergies, 53
    in the gut, 59
    managing, with ashwagandha, 97
    from physical injury, 93
    reducing, with shiitakes, 96
Insecticides, 61
Insulin, 57–58
Insulin-like growth factor-1 (IGF-1), 58
Intermittent fasting, 49, 52, 64
Iodine, 29, 42, 56
Iron
    enhancing absorption of, 70, 75–77
    meeting daily goal for, 83
    non-heme, 29, 76–77
    pairing with Vitamin C, 24
    sources and bone RDA, 29

J
Jackfruit, BBQ, Tacos with Mango Salsa, *218,* 218–19
Juices
    basic formula, 108–9

Beet to Beat, 109, *110*
Carrot, Sunny, 110, *110*
Follow Your Gut, 109
Green, Basic, 109, *110*
Green, Morning Ritual, 109
pH levels in, 120

K
Kale
    Cabbage, and White Bean Salad, 209
    -Cashew Pesto, 125
    -Macadamia Pesto, 222–23
    -Molasses-Herb Vinegar, 138
    Morning Ritual Green Juice, 109
    Triple, Chips, 258, *259*
Kefir
    Immortal Acai Bowl, 250
Khichuri, Golden Dal Moringa, *184,* 184–85
Kimchi
    Immortal Root, *132,* 132–33
    Pineapple-Turmeric, Jummee's Signature, 134–35
Kitchen tools, 103–4
Knives, 105

L
Lactose intolerance, 60
Lattes. *See* Coffeeless Lattes
Lead, 67, 68
Leaky gut, 43, 54, 59
Lectins, 42, 43
Leek-Broccoli-Potato Soup, 180–81, *181*
Lemon
    -Coconut-Caesar Dressing, 208
    –Olive Oil Vinaigrette, Classic, 121
Lentil(s)
    bioavailable protein in, 73
    Red, –Saffron Tortillas, 150–51, *151*
Lettuce
    Happy-Go-Lucky Caesar Salad, *123,* 208
Linguine, Buckwheat, with Kale-Macadamia Pesto, *222,* 222–23

Lovastatin, 95
Low-density lipoprotein (LDL), 22

M
Macadamia(s)
    Crunchy Roasted Brussels Sprouts, 251, *251*
    -Kale Pesto, 222–23
Macrominerals, 25
Macronutrients, 21–22
Magnesium
    bone RDA, 29
    Broth, Root and Leaf, 177
    deficiency in, effects of, 16–17, 32, 34, 57
    favorite foods for, 32
    plant-food sources, 29
Maillard reaction, 45
Manganese, 29, 33–34
Mango
    Awakening Golden Smoothie, 116, *116*
    Salsa, *218,* 218–19
Mankai duckweed, 72
Maple Syrup BBQ Tempeh, *230,* 230–31
Marinara Sauce, *232,* 232–33
Marrow, 13
Matcha
    Curry, Vegan Delight, *240,* 240–41
    Latte, Morning March, 115, *115*
    –Pine Nut Latte, 115, *115*
Meal plans, 283–87
Meatballs, Meaty Meatless, with Marinara Sauce, *232,* 232–33
Medications, 12, 62
Men, and bone loss, 11–12, 17
Mercury, 67–68
Metabolic acidosis, 61
Metabolism, 50
Metabolomix micronutrient test, 85
Methylfolate, 21
Methyl groups, 19–20
Microbiome, 59–61
Micronutrients, 21–22
Milk, 60. *See also* Plant-based milks

Index ▪ 303

Minerals, 25, 26, 38
Mint Chutney, Sweet and Tangy, *184*, 185
Miso
   -Ginger Vinaigrette, 197
   Soup with Dashi Broth, 174–75, *175*
   Umami Soy-Glazed Portobello Steak, 170, *171*
Mitochondria, 52, 64
Molasses-Kale-Herb Vinegar, 138
Molybdenum, 29
Moringa Khichuri, Golden Dal, *184*, 184–85
Mousse, Avocado-Date Chocolate, 270, *271*
MTHFR, 21
mTor, 50–52
Muffins, Cherry Velvet, *274*, 275
Mulberries, 48
Mung Bean
   Flatbread, Savory, 152–53
   Golden Dal Moringa Khichuri, *184*, 184–85
   Olive Loaf, Flourless, 148, *149*
   Pizza, *236*, 236–37
Mushroom(s)
   agaricus blazei, 96
   amino acids in, 72
   antiviral and antifungal, 94
   beneficial effects of, 94–97
   and Broccoli Buffalo "Wings," *155*, 156–57
   California Creamy Corn Chowder, *182*, 182–83
   Cashew Pâté, 144–45, *145*
   cautionary note, 93
   cordyceps, 96
   Edamame Spread Avocado Toast, *228*, 228–29
   iron in, 76
   lion's mane, 96
   maitake, 94–95, 96
   medicinal, 93–97
   Miso Soup with Dashi Broth, 174–75, *175*

Mung Bean Pizza, *236*, 236–37
   oyster, 95
   pairing with bok choy, 48
   Recover-Restore-Reboot Porridge, *188*, 188–89
   regulating immune system with, 54
   reishi, 95
   Root and Leaf Magnesium Broth, 177
   Sea Greens and Shiitake Soup, 190–91, *191*
   shiitake, 95–96
   turkey tail, 97
   Umami Soy-Glazed Portobello Steak, 170, *171*
MyFoodData, 39, 81–82

N

Non-Hodgkin's lymphoma (NHL), 54
Nori, 70
Nutrients. *See also specific nutrients*
   for bone health, 25–39
   online nutrient calculators, 69, 81
   testing for nutritional deficiencies, 25, 82
Nutrigenetics, 2–3, 20–21
Nutrigenomics, 2–3
Nutrition plan for bone health, 81–90
Nut(s). *See also* Cashew(s); Pine Nut(s); Walnut(s)
   Almond-Orange-Cacao Cake, *266*, 266–67
   Bark, Crazy Nutty, *273*, 273
   Bone Health Classic Pesto, 124
   Brazil, notes about, 34, 35
   Crunchy Roasted Brussels Sprouts, 251, *251*
   health benefits of sprouted almonds, 35
   Kale-Macadamia Pesto, 222–23
   Pistachio-Mint Milk, 112
   Plant-Based Milks, *111*, 111–12
   sprouting, 44, 47–48
   weakening antinutrients in, 74

O

Oats
   eating with mixed seeds, 72–73
   Go Bananas Flourless Pancakes, *242*, 246–47
   Upside-Down Apple Pie, *268*, 268–69
Olive Mung Bean Loaf, Flourless, 148, *149*
Olive oil, 24
Omega-3 fatty acids, 30, 79
Onions, 77
Opal Health, 82, 85
Orange(s)
   -Almond-Cacao Cake, *266*, 266–67
   Awakening Golden Smoothie, 116, *116*
   Blood, –Hazelnut Oil Vinaigrette, 203
   -Coconut Ranch Dressing, *216*, 217
   Herb and Wildflower Garden Salad, *202*, 203
   -Yogurt-Dill Dressing, 122
Organically grown produce, 55
Osteoblasts, 14, 16
Osteocalcin, 26–27
Osteoclastogenesis, 14
Osteoclasts, 14
Osteocytes, 14–15
Osteogenesis imperfecta, 63
Osteomyelitis, 62–63
Osteopetrosis, 63
Osteoporosis
   diagnosis of, 86
   family history of, 86
   in men, 12, 17
   quick-start suggestions for, 89–90
Osteoporotic fractures, 46
Osteoprogenitor cells, 14
Osteoprotegerin (OPG), 16, 17
Oxalates, 42, 43, 76

P

P1NP, 85, 88
Paget's disease, 63

Pancakes
    Go Bananas Flourless, *242,* 246–47
    Sweet Potato–Scallion, *168,* 169
Pancreas, 57
Pantry list, 105–6
Papaya–Hemp Seed Ranch Dressing, *164,* 165
Parathyroid hormone (PTH), 32, 56–57
Parsley
    -Cashew Pesto, 231
    –Pine Nut Chimichurri Pesto, 125
Pâté, Mushroom Cashew, 144–45, *145*
Peaches and Zucchini, Sweet and Savory Grilled, 166, *167*
Pears, reducing tannins in, 47
Pea(s)
    Green, and Roasted Red Pepper Mash, *248,* 248–49
    Snap, with Tempeh Dust, 172, *172*
Pepper(s)
    California Rainbow Spring Rolls, 160–61, *161*
    Roasted Red, and Green Pea Mash, *248,* 248–49
    Vegan Delight Matcha Curry, *240,* 240–41
Periodontal disease, 62
Periosteum, 13
Personalized nutrition plan, 82
Pesto
    Basil-Walnut, 125
    Bone Health Classic, 124
    Cashew-Parsley, 231
    Hemp Seed, 125
    Kale-Cashew, 125
    Kale-Macadamia, 222–23
    Parsley–Pine Nut Chimichurri, 125
    Three Herbs Bone, 125
PFAS, 66–68
pH balance, 61, 74–75
Phosphorus, 30, 32
Phytates, 42, 43, 44

Phytochemicals, 55
Phytoestrogens, 17, 42, 43
Pickle, Beet-Cauliflower, 128–29
Pie, Upside-Down Apple, *268,* 268–69
Pineapple
    Awakening Golden Smoothie, 116, *116*
    bromelain in, 72
    -Cashew Dressing, 211
    -Turmeric Kimchi, Jummee's Signature, 134–35
Pine Nut(s)
    Green Pea and Roasted Red Pepper Mash, *248,* 248–49
    –Matcha Latte, 115, *115*
    –Parsley Chimichurri Pesto, 125
Pistachio-Mint Milk, 112
Pizza, Mung Bean, *236,* 236–37
Plant-based milks, 60, *111*
    basic formula, 111
    Cashew-Goji-Vanilla, 112
    Hemp Seed Chai, 112
    Pistachio-Mint, 112
Plant foods. *See also specific plant foods*
    with complete protein, 71
    high in protein, 71–72
    locally grown and seasonal, 50
Polyphenols, 36
Porridge, Recover-Restore-Reboot, *188,* 188–89
Potassium, 30, 32–33
Potato(es). *See also* Sweet Potato(es)
    -Broccoli-Leek Soup, 180–81, *181*
    Golden Triangle Indian Mash, 162, *162*
    Smoky Roasted Rooty Roots, *256,* 256–57
Pots and pans, 103–4
Prebiotics, 59
Produce, organic, 55
Protein
    about, 70
    animal, acid residue from, 74–75
    bone health RDA values, 26

    complete, easy vegan recipes for, 72–74
    complete, plant foods with, 71
    daily recommendations, 22–23
    debate over, 22
    denatured, 72
    effect on bone health, 70–71
    meeting daily goal for, 82–83
    nature of, 72
    at night, note about, 51
    role in bone health, 21, 23
    sources and bone RDA, 30
    in vegan diet, 70–75
Proton pump inhibitors, 62
Prunes, 48
Pumpkin-Lemon Kebabs, Curry, *164,* 165

Q

Quercetin, 66
Quinoa
    -Carrot Burgers, Mouthful, 234–35
    Minestrone, Hearty, 186–87, *187*

R

Radicchio-Fennel Salad, 206–7, *207*
Radish(es)
    Beefy Tomato Salad with Cherry Vinaigrette, 212, *213*
    Endive Canoes with Guacamole, *204,* 204–5
    Immortal Root Kimchi, *132,* 132–33
    Miso Soup with Dashi Broth, 174–75, *175*
    Root and Leaf Magnesium Broth, 177
    Sea Greens and Shiitake Soup, 190–91, *191*
RANKL, 16, 17
Reproductive cancer genetic test, 85
Resveratrol, 44, 65
Retinol, 21, 34, 78
Retinol activity equivalent (RAE), 78

Rhodiola, 97–98
Rice
 arsenic in, 68
 brown, 34
 Forbidden, Stuffing, Acorn Squash with, *216,* 216–17
 Golden Dal Moringa Khichuri, *184,* 184–85
 Licorice Sweet Brown, California Sushi Rolls with, *226,* 226–27
 pairing with beans, 25
 Recover-Restore-Reboot Porridge, *188,* 188–89
 Vegan Delight Matcha Curry, *240,* 240–41
 water, how to make, 191
Rosemary, 46–47

S

Saffron
 Cauliflower Rice, 254–55, *255*
 –Red Lentil Tortillas, 150–51, *151*
Salads
 Ageless Macrobiotic, *196,* 197
 Beefy Tomato, with Cherry Vinaigrette, 212, *213*
 Chickpea-Cucumber, with a Hint of Mint, 200, *201*
 Endive Canoes with Guacamole, *204,* 204–5
 Fennel-Radicchio, 206–7, *207*
 Happy-Go-Lucky Caesar, *123,* 208
 Herb and Wildflower Garden, *202,* 203
 Kale, Cabbage, and White Bean, 209
 New Classic Rainbow Coleslaw, *210,* 211
 Persian Shirazi, 224, *225*
 Seaweed Flower Cucumber, 214
Salsa, Mango, *218,* 218–19
Salt, 103
Saponins, 43, 44
Sauces
 Chimichurri, 170, *171*
 Deep Green, 257
 Marinara, *232,* 232–33
Sauerkraut
 Endive Canoes with Guacamole, *204,* 204–5
 Green and Red Everyday, 130–31
 Scallion–Sweet Potato Pancakes, *168,* 169
Sclerostin (SOST), 14
Seasoning with salt, 103
Seaweed
 California Sushi Rolls with Licorice Sweet Brown Rice, *226,* 226–27
 Sea Greens and Shiitake Soup, 190–91, *191*
 Seaweed Flower Cucumber Salad, 214
 for thyroid health, 56
Seeds. *See also specific seeds*
 Bone Health Classic Pesto, 124
 Crazy Nutty Nut Bark, *273,* 273
 pairing with oatmeal, 72–73
 Plant-Based Milks, *111,* 111–12
 soaking, 103
 Sprouted, Bread, 154
 sprouting, best choices for, 198
 sprouting, directions for, 199
 sprouting, effects of, 44, 73
Selenium, 30, 34–35, 64
Serotonin, 60
Sex hormones, 58
Short-chain fatty acids (SCFAs), 21
Silica, 30
Silicon, 37–38
Sleep, 51
Smoothies
 Awakening Golden, 116, *116*
 Berry Paradise, 117, *117*
 Green Shield, 117, *117*
 preparing, 116
Soups
 Borscht with Cashew Cream, *178,* 178–79
 Broccoli-Potato-Leek, 180–81, *181*
 California Creamy Corn Chowder, *182,* 182–83
 Carrot-Ginger, Sunrise, 194
 Hearty Quinoa Minestrone, 186–87, *187*
 Miso, with Dashi Broth, 174–75, *175*
 Sea Greens and Shiitake, 190–91, *191*
 Tomato, with Basil and Capers, *192,* 192–93
 Watermelon-Mint Gazpacho, *260,* 261
Spinach
 Creamy, Sweet Potato Boats with, 238–39, *239*
 Deep Green Sauce, 257
 Green Pea and Roasted Red Pepper Mash, *248,* 248–49
 health benefits, 27
 oxalates in, 34, 47
 pairing with tomatoes, 47
 –Silky Tofu Dip, 141, *141*
Spirulina, 68
Spring Rolls, California Rainbow, 160–61, *161*
Sprouting
 best seeds for, 198
 instructions for, 199
 weakening antinutrients with, 44, 73
Sprouts
 Ageless Macrobiotic Salad, *196,* 197
 Endive Canoes with Guacamole, *204,* 204–5
Squash. *See also Zucchini*
 Acorn, with Forbidden Rice Stuffing, *216,* 216–17
 Curry Lemon-Pumpkin Kebabs, *164,* 165
Strawberries, Sweet and Salty Chocolate, *276,* 276–77
Strontium, 30, 36–37
Sulfur, 30, 33, 68
Sushi Rolls, California, with Licorice Sweet Brown Rice, *226,* 226–27

Sweet Potato(es)
    Boats with Creamy Spinach, 238–39, *239*
    reducing antinutrients in, 47
    –Scallion Pancakes, *168,* 169
    vitamin A in, 78

T

Tacos, BBQ Jackfruit, with Mango Salsa, *218,* 218–19
Tahini
    -Apple-Ginger Dressing, 122
    -Apple Sauce, Steamed Eggplant with, 163
    -Ginger Dressing, 209
Tannins, 42, 43, 44
Taurine, 37, 79
Tea, green, 48
Telomeres, 15
Tempeh
    Dust, Snap Peas with, *172,* 172
    Maple Syrup BBQ, *230,* 230–31
Testosterone, 58
Thyroid hormones, 42, 56
Toast, Edamame Spread Avocado, *228,* 228–29
Tofu
    Happy-Go-Lucky Caesar Salad, *123,* 208
    Meaty Meatless Meatballs with Marinara Sauce, *232,* 232–33
    Miso Soup with Dashi Broth, 174–75, *175*
    Scramble and Black Bean Wraps, *220,* 220–21
    Silky, –Spinach Dip, 141, *141*
Tomato(es)
    Beefy, Salad with Cherry Vinaigrette, 212, *213*
    Marinara Sauce, *232,* 232–33
    Mung Bean Pizza, *236,* 236–37
    pairing with olive oil, 24
    pairing with spinach, 47
    Persian Shirazi Salad, 224, *225*
    Soup with Basil and Capers, *192,* 192–93
    Watermelon-Mint Gazpacho, *260,* 261
Tortillas
    BBQ Jackfruit Tacos with Mango Salsa, *218,* 218–19
    Red Lentil–Saffron, 150–51, *151*
Trabecular bone score (TBS), 86
Trace minerals, 25, 38
Traditional Chinese Medicine (TCM), 92, 98
Triglycerides, 22
T score, 84
Tulsi, 97
Turmeric
    Creamy Golden Ranch Dressing, 122
    Golden Milk Latte, 114, *114*
    Golden Triangle Indian Mash, *162,* 162
    pairing with black pepper, 25
    -Pineapple Kimchi, Jummee's Signature, 134–35

U

Urine pH, 61, 74

V

Vagus nerve, 60
Vegan diet, 69–80
    adjusting to vegan cooking, 79–80
    and choline, 78
    and creatine, carnosine, and taurine, 79
    and DHA, 79
    and iron absorption, 70, 75–77
    nutritional planning for, 82–84
    protein needs, 70–75
    using nutrition calculator for, 69
    and vitamin A, 78
    and vitamin B12, 77–78
Vegetables. *See also specific vegetables*
    fermenting, effect of, 78
    Hearty Quinoa Minestrone, 186–87, *187*
    how to clean, 102
    phytochemicals in, 55
    Rainbow Veggie Frittata with Feta, *252,* 252–53
    Smoky Roasted Rooty Roots, *256,* 256–57
    storing, 102
    Vegan Delight Matcha Curry, *240,* 240–41
Vinaigrettes
    Acai-Lemon, 159
    Amino-Sesame, 121
    Blood Orange–Hazelnut Oil, 203
    Cherry, 212, *213*
    formula for, 120
    Green Grape, 200
    Herb and Grape, Mediterranean, 121
    Hibiscus Passion, 121
    Miso-Ginger, 197
    Olive Oil–Lemon, Classic, 121
Vinegar
    Apple Cider, 136
    Bone, Dr. Laura's, 137
    Molasses-Kale-Herb, 138
Vitamin A
    in animals, 21
    fat-solubility, 26
    meeting daily goal for, 83
    in plants, 21, 34
    sources and bone RDA, 31
    two forms of, 78
Vitamin B12, 70, 77–78, 84
Vitamin C, 24, 26, 31, 76
Vitamin D, 24, 26, 31, 34–35, 85
Vitamin D3, 27
Vitamin E, 26, 31
Vitamin K1, 35, 36
Vitamin K2, 26–27, 31, 35–36
Vitamins, 25–26. *See also specific vitamins*

W

Walnut(s)
    -Basil Pesto, 125
    Chimichurri Sauce, 170, *171*
    Flourless Black Bean Brownies, *278,* 279

Walnut(s) (*continued*)
    Upside-Down Apple Pie, *268*, 268–69
Water, 21, 101–2
Watermelon-Mint Gazpacho, *260*, 261
Wheat products, 54, 61
Whipped Cream, Coconut, *242*, 247
Wildflower and Herb Garden Salad, *202*, 203
Wraps, Black Bean and Tofu Scramble, *220*, 220–21

Y

Yam(s)
    -Acai "Cheesecake," 264–65, *265*
    Vegan Delight Matcha Curry, *240*, 240–41
Yin and yang, 98
Yogurt
    California Vegan Chipotle Sauce, 122
    -Orange-Dill Dressing, 122

Z

Zinc, 31, 33
Zonulin, 54
Zoopharmacognosy, 91
Zucchini
    Mung Bean Pizza, *236*, 236–37
    and Peaches, Sweet and Savory Grilled, 166, *167*
    Vegan Delight Matcha Curry, *240*, 240–41

ABOUT THE AUTHORS

Dr. Laura Kelly is a Traditional Chinese Medicine physician-scientist, CEO, activist educator, and the coauthor of *The Healthy Bones Nutrition Plan and Cookbook*. She draws on principles and practices of precision medicine, integrative medicine, and Chinese medicine to investigate and treat malfunctioning mechanisms in the body. In her private practice, Dr. Kelly has worked with hundreds of people, from age 30 to 93, tailoring nutrition to prevent, mitigate, or reverse bone loss. To make her approach more widely available, in 2019 Dr. Kelly developed Opal, a protocol that offers the public access to testing and specifies treatment in the form of a personalized nutrition plan.

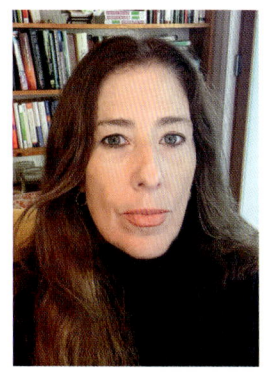

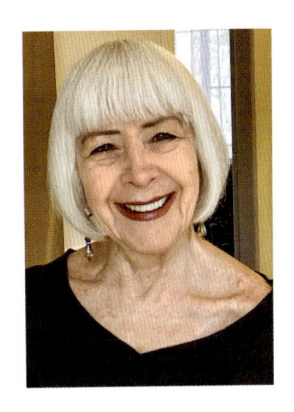

Nick Brooks

Helen Bryman Kelly is the coauthor of *The Healthy Bones Nutrition Plan and Cookbook*. She writes about health, medicine, and management topics and has worked as an editor for McGraw Hill and as a writer for Yale University's Medical School, Child Study Center, and Joint Program in Medicine and Public Health. Helen also teaches bone health as an adult education instructor. In the 1990s she served as a policy advisor to the UK education minister. She is currently writing *Early Years Learning in the Later Years*, which focuses on the educational methods and materials developed in the course of her work with disadvantaged populations.

Jummee Park, food shaman and wellness consultant, is the founder of Jummee's Bliss Kitchen, where she has developed authentic Korean food remedies that cater to Western palates, including a line of kimchi. Jummee shares her insights as a speaker in cooking classes and lectures, emphasizing the benefits and significance of food as a remedy, promoting longevity, health, and spiritual practices. She was born in An Dong, South Korea, but eventually departed Korea for the United States, where she became an executive at a Fortune 500 multimedia company. Later, listening to her inner calling, she left her corporate position to pursue culinary training, Eastern medicine, and the healing arts.

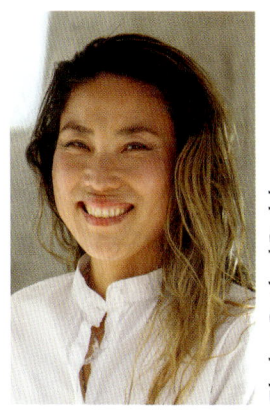

Elyabou Raphael Bialobos

the politics and practice of sustainable living

CHELSEA GREEN PUBLISHING

Chelsea Green Publishing sees books as tools for effecting cultural change and seeks to empower citizens to participate in reclaiming our global commons and become its impassioned stewards. If you enjoyed reading *The Healthy Bones Plant-Based Nutrition Plan and Cookbook*, please consider these other great books related to cooking and wellness.

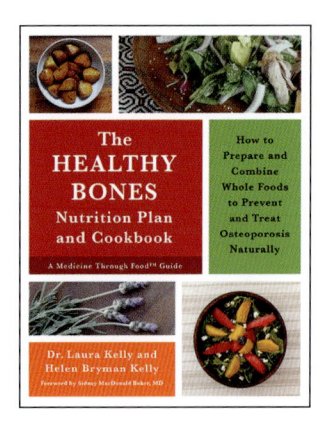

**THE HEALTHY BONES
NUTRITION PLAN AND COOKBOOK**
*How to Prepare and Combine Whole Foods
to Prevent and Treat Osteoporosis Naturally*
DR. LAURA KELLY and HELEN BRYMAN KELLY
9781603586245
Paperback

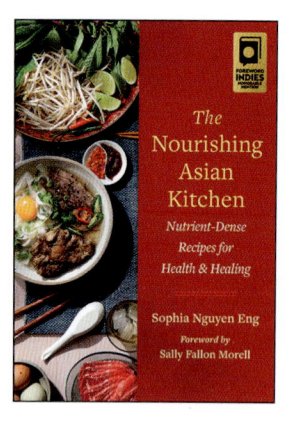

THE NOURISHING ASIAN KITCHEN
*Nutrient-Dense Recipes for
Health and Healing*
SOPHIA NGUYEN ENG
9781645022169
Paperback

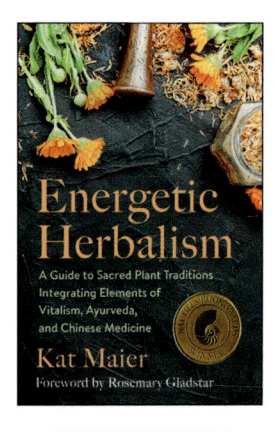

ENERGETIC HERBALISM
*A Guide to Sacred Plant Traditions Integrating Elements
of Vitalism, Ayurveda, and Chinese Medicine*
KAT MAIER
9781645020820
Paperback

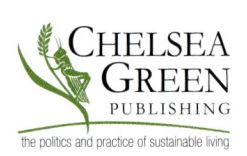

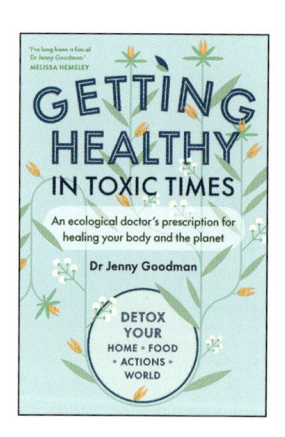

GETTING HEALTHY IN TOXIC TIMES
*An Ecological Doctor's Prescription for
Healing Your Body and the Planet*
DR. JENNY GOODMAN
9781915294333
Paperback

CHELSEA GREEN PUBLISHING
the politics and practice of sustainable living

For more information,
visit **www.chelseagreen.com**.